Oxford Handbook of
Orthopaedics and Trauma

Edited by

Gavin Bowden

Consultant Orthopaedic and Spinal Surgeon
Nuffield Orthopaedic Centre and John Radcliffe Hospital
Honorary Senior Lecturer
Nuffield Department of Orthopaedics, Rheumatology and
Musculoskeletal Sciences
Oxford, UK

Martin A. McNally

Consultant in Limb Reconstruction
Nuffield Orthopaedic Centre
Honorary Senior Lecturer in Orthopaedic Surgery
University of Oxford
Oxford, UK

Simon R.Y.W. Thomas

Consultant in Children's Orthopaedics
Bristol Royal Hospital for Children
University Hospitals Bristol
Bristol, UK

Alexander Gibson

Consultant Surgeon
Royal National Orthopaedic Hospital
Stanmore, UK

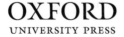

OXFORD
UNIVERSITY PRESS

OXFORD
UNIVERSITY PRESS

Great Clarendon Street, Oxford OX2 6DP

Oxford University Press is a department of the University of Oxford.
It furthers the University's objective of excellence in research, scholarship,
and education by publishing worldwide in

Oxford New York

Auckland Cape Town Dar es Salaam Hong Kong Karachi
Kuala Lumpur Madrid Melbourne Mexico City Nairobi
New Delhi Shanghai Taipei Toronto

With offices in

Argentina Austria Brazil Chile Czech Republic France Greece
Guatemala Hungary Italy Japan Poland Portugal Singapore
South Korea Switzerland Thailand Turkey Ukraine Vietnam

Oxford is a registered trade mark of Oxford University Press
in the UK and in certain other countries

Published in the United States
by Oxford University Press Inc., New York

British Library Cataloguing in Publication Data
Data available

Library of Congress Cataloging-in-Publication Data
Data available

Typeset by Glyph International, Bangalore, India
Printed in China
on acid-free paper through
C&C Offset Printing Co., Ltd.

ISBN 978-0-19-856958-9

10 9 8

Preface

'The scientist is a builder. Collecting scientific data can be compared
to gathering stones for a house; a stack is no more 'science' than a
heap of stones is a house. Unstudied scientific results are just a
dead heap of stones.'
Kristian Birkeland, Norwegian Physicist, 1867–1917.

In recent decades, orthopaedic surgeons, rheumatologists, and musculoskeletal scientists have amassed an enormous collection of clinical and
scientific data relating to the skeleton, to joints and muscles and to the
wide variety of conditions and injuries which affect all of us. This book is
intended for those who are beginning to learn about these common conditions and who may be daunted by the size of the 'heap of stones'.

It is tempting, as an experienced specialist, to present detail and complexity in order to illustrate why we find musculoskeletal medicine and
surgery fascinating. This may be inspirational, but it often fails to provide
a good structure for learning, for those struggling to understand the basics
of our subject. We have tried to avoid this temptation.

This book provides many 'stones' which can be studied with the patients,
in the operating room, in tutorials and together with more detailed
descriptions of conditions in larger textbooks. The sections have been
edited to ensure that the salient features of each condition are presented
clearly (often as lists), to give the student a knowledge base which allows
further consideration and discussion of the condition in a clinical setting.
The established Handbook format, with blank pages adjacent to each
topic, encourages annotation and addition of detail at a level which the
student should find helpful and comfortable. This detail can be found in
many excellent, larger orthopaedic textbooks and we would particularly
recommend the *Oxford Textbook of Orthopaedics and Trauma* and *Apley's
System of Orthopaedics and Fractures*.

The locomotor system and its diseases require a hands-on and practical
approach to learning. We hope that this book gives the student the con-
fidence to take the knowledge within (in a pocket) and apply it in clinical
activities. It is the interaction of acquired factual knowledge with clinical
experience which will give the student the beginnings of a 'house' rather
than a 'heap of stones'.

The nature of the topics and the speed of change in our specialty mean
that there will undoubtedly be errors, omissions and areas which could be
improved within the text. We would welcome feedback from readers, so
that these may be corrected and addressed in future editions.

Martin A. McNally
2010

Acknowledgements

We would like to thank Caitlin Bowden for encouraging us to undertake the project and for reviewing completed chapters. Louise Hailey assisted in completing the book by reviewing material, searching for new material and re-writing chapters and we would like to thank her for her contribution.

We thank Patrick McNally and Maria Dudareva for giving a fresh view on learning orthopaedics as medical students.

We would like to thank the Editorial staff at OUP, especially Liz Reeve, Sara Chare, Beth Womack, and Jamie Hartmann-Boyce. Without their encouragement and support the book would never have been completed.

Contents

Detailed contents

Section 4 **Paediatrics**

11 Paediatric trauma   **549**

Contributors

James R. Barnes
Bristol Royal Infirmary
Bristol, UK

Meg Birks
Northern General Hospital
Sheffield, UK

Petros J. Boscainos
University of Dundee and NHS
Tayside
Perth, UK

Iona Collins
Queen's Medical Centre
Nottingham, UK

Tim Coltman
Queen Alexandra Hospital
Portsmouth, UK

Joel David
Nuffield Orthopaedic Centre
Oxford, UK

Kate David
Birmingham Medical School
Birmingham, UK

Charles Docker
Worcester Acute Hospitals
NHS Trust
Worcester, UK

Matt D.A. Fletcher
NE Department of Surgical
Services
Dawson Creek & District Hospital
Dawson Creek, BC, Canada

Robert Freeman
Oxford, UK

Campbell Hand
Southampton University Hospital
Southampton, UK

David Hollinghurst
Great Western Hospital
Swindon, UK

Catherine F. Kellett
NHS Tayside
Perth Royal Infirmary & Dundee
Ninewells Hospital, UK

Ravi Kirubanandan
Bristol Royal Hospital
for Children
Bristol, UK

Rohit Kotnis
Nuffield Orthopaedic Centre
Oxford, UK

Christopher Little
Nuffield Orthopaedic Centre
Oxford, UK

Jeremy Loveridge
Bristol, UK

Saadia Afzal Mir
North Central School of
Anaesthesia
London, UK

Shobhana Nagraj
General Practice and Primary Care
Research Unit
University of Cambridge
Cambridge, UK

Lorraine Michelle Olley
Nuffield Orthopaedic Centre
Oxford, UK

Neil M. Orpen
Great Western Hospital
Swindon, UK

Tom Palser
Nottingham, UK

Chandra Pasapula
King's Lynn NHS Trust
King's Lynn, UK

Thomas C.B. Pollard
Nuffield Orthopaedic Centre
NHS Trust
Headington
Oxford, UK

David Stubbs
Nuffield Orthopaedic Centre
Oxford, UK

Andrew Wood
Department of Surgery
University of Auckland
Auckland
New Zealand

Symbols and abbreviations

📖	cross reference
<	less than
>	greater than
~	approximately
↑	increased
→	leading to
↓	fewer
AARS	atlantoaxial rotatory subluxation
ABPI	ankle–brachial pressure index
ACE	angiotensin-converting enzyme
ACJ	acromioclavicular joint
ACL	anterior cruciate ligament
ACTH	adrenocorticotrophic hormone
AD	autosomal dominant
ADL	activities of daily living
A&E	accident and emergency
AF	annulus fibrosus
AFO	ankle–foot orthosis
AIIS	anterior inferior iliac spine
ALL	acute lymphoblastic leukaemia
AML	acute myelogenous leukaemia
ANA	antinuclear antibody
ANCA	antinuclear cytoplasmic antibody
AP	antero-posterior
APL	abductor pollicis longus
APTT	activated partial thromboplastin time
AR	autosomal recessive
ARDS	adult respiratory distress syndrome
AS	ankylosing spondylitis
ASIS	anterior superior iliac spine
ATLS	Advanced Trauma Life Support
AVN	avascular necrosis
BMD	bone mineral density
BMI	body mass index

BP	blood pressure
CABG	coronary artery bypass graft
CC	coracoclavicular
CIA	carpal instability adaptive
CIC	carpal instability combined
CID	carpal instability dissociative
CIND	carpal instability non-dissociative
CLL	chronic lymphocytic leukaemia
CMCJ	carpometacarpal joint
CMT	congenital muscular torticollis
CNS	central nervous system
COPD	chronic obstructive pulmonary disease
CP	cerebral palsy
CPAP	continuous positive airway pressure
CPK	creatine phosphokinase
CREST	**C**alcinosis of subcutaneous tissues, **R**aynaud's phenomenon, disordered o**E**sophageal motility, **S**clerodactyly and **T**elangiectasia
CRP	C-reactive protein
CSF	cerebrospinal fluid
CT	computed tomography
CVA	cerebrovascular accident
CVP	central venous pressure
CXR	chest X-ray
DDH	developmental dysplasia of hip
DIPJ	distal interphalangeal joint
DMAA	distal metatarsal articular angle
DMARDs	disease-modifying antirheumatic drugs
DVT	deep vein thrombosis
ECRB	extensor carpi radialis brevis
ECRL	extensor carpi radialis longus
ECU	extensor carpi ulnaris
ED	extensor digitorum
EDC	extensor digitorum communis
EDL	extensor digitorum longus
EDM	extensor digiti minimi
EEG	electroencephalogram
EHL	extensor hallucis longus
EI	extensor indicis
EIP	extensor indicis proprius
EMG	electromyography

EPB	extensor pollicis brevis
EPL	extensor pollicis longus
ESR	erythrocyte sedimentation rate
EUA	examination under anaesthesia
FBC	full blood count
FCR	flexor carpi radialis
FCU	flexor carpi ulnaris
FDG	fluorodeoxyglucose
FDP	flexor digitorum profundus
FDS	flexor digitorum superficialis
FFD	fixed flexion deformity
FFP	fresh frozen plasma
FHL	flexor hallucis longus
FPL	flexor pollicis longus
GCS	Glasgow Coma Scale
GCTTS	giant cell tumour of tendon sheath
GHJ	glenohumeral joint
HAGL	humeral avulsion of inferior glenohumeral ligament
HbS	haemoglobin S
HDU	high dependency unit
HEPA	high efficiency particulate air
HIV	human inmmunodeficiency virus
HLA	human leukocyte antigen
HME	hereditary multiple exostoses
HMSN	hereditary motor and sensory neuropathy
HVA	hallux valgus angle
IBD	inflammatory bowel disease
ICP	intracranial pressure
ICU	intensive care unit
IFS	interferential stimulation
IM	intramedullary
INR	international normalized ratio
IPA	interphalangeal angle
IPJ	interphalangeal joint
IMTA	intermetatarsal angle
ITU	intensive therapy unit
JVP	jugular venous pressure
LCH	Langerhans cell histiocytosis
LCL	lateral collateral ligament
LFT	liver function test

LMN	lower motor neuron
LMWH	low molecular weight heparin
MCL	medial collateral ligament
MCPJ	metacarpophalangeal joint
MCV	mean cell volume
MI	myocardial infarction
MRA	MR angiography
MRI	magnetic resonance imaging
MRSA	meticillin-resistant *S. aureus*
MTPJ	metatarsophalangeal joint
NAI	non-accidental injury
NCS	nerve conduction studies
NEMS	neuromuscular electrical stimulation
NF	neurofibromatosis
NIBP	non-invasive blood pressure monitoring
NICE	National Institute for Health and Clinical Excellence
NP	nucleus pulposus
NSAIDs	non-steroidal anti-inflammatory drugs
OA	osteoarthritis
OCD	osteochondritis dissecans
OI	osteogenesis imperfecta
OP	osteoporosis
ORIF	open reduction internal fixation
OS	Osgood–Schlatter disease
PCL	posterior cruciate ligament
PE	pulmonary embolism
PET	positron emission tomography
PFFD	proximal femoral focal deficiency
PG	proteoglycan
PIN	posterior interosseous nerve
PIPJ	proximal interphalangeal joint
PL	palmaris longus
PLL	posterior longitudinal ligament
PPV	pes planovalgus
PQ	pronator quadratus
PRUJ	proximal radioulnar joint
PSA	prostate-specific antigen
PT	prothrombin time
PTH	parathyroid hormone
RA	rheumatoid arthritis

RCJ	radiocapitellar joint
RCT	randomized controlled trial
RF	radiofrequency
RhF	rheumatoid factor
RICE	rest, ice, compression bandage, elevation
ROM	range of movement
RTA	road traffic accident
RVAD	rib vertebral angle difference
SAD	subacromial decompression
SCD	sickle cell disease
SCFE	slipped capital femoral epiphysis
SCIWORA	spinal cord injury without radiographic abnormality
SCJ	sternoclavicular joint
SIJ	sacroiliac joint
SIRS	systemic inflammatory response syndrome
SLE	systemic lupus erythematosus
SLJ	Sinding–Larsen–Johanssen disease
SLR	straight leg raise
SMN	survival motor neuron
TAR	thrombocytopenia–absent radius
TCL	transverse carpal ligament
TED	thromboembolic disease
TFL	tensor fasciae latae
TFT	thyroid function test
THR	total hip replacement
TKR	total knee replacement
U&E	urea & electrolytes
UMN	upper motor neuron
USS	ultrasound scan
UTI	urinary tract infection
VACTERL	Vertebral, Anorectal, Cardiac, Tracheo-oesophageal, Renal and Limb abnormalities
VCL	volar carpal ligament
VMO	vastus medialis oblique
vWD	von Willebrand's disease
vWF	von Willebrand factor
WCC	white cell count
WTD	Wall–tragus distance
ZPA	zone of polarizing activity

Principles of orthopaedics and trauma

Orthopaedic history and examination

General principles

The key to the diagnosis of musculoskeletal disorders is a thorough history and examination. A comprehensive clinical approach will help to establish an accurate differential diagnosis if a specific diagnosis is not immediately evident and help focus further investigations.

History

- Presenting complaint: traumatic or non-traumatic, acute or chronic, congenital or acquired, night pain (associated with severity and malignancy), relieving and exacerbating factors (e.g. movement, positions)
- Social history and functional status
- Activities of daily living (ADL)—shopping, cooking, washing, dressing. Ask if they find difficulty in performing an activity. Ask about their normal mobility. Use of any walking aids. Have any adaptations been made to their home because of disability?
- Social history: who do they live with, where do they live (flat with working lift) and can they manage stairs? Do they smoke or drink?
- Past medical history: co-morbidities, previous trauma, surgery or hospital admissions, medication. With children ask their mother about problems during pregnancy, delivery and about developmental milestones
- Family history is important
- Treatment history and drug allergies
- Review of systems: important to look for co-morbidities and associated disorders to assist with the differential diagnosis.

Examination

- Look, feel, move
- Compare with other side where possible
- Assess function—ability to dress and undress, grip objects comfortably. Can they hold a pen, can they do buttons with arthritic fingers?
- Perform specific tests—assess movements, stability (e.g. anterior draw for anterior cruciate ligament (ACL) injury of the knee), functional status, pain (provocative tests)
- Systemic examination—look for co-morbidities.

Look. Scars, skin changes (erythema, ulcers, pressure areas), swelling, deformity, gait, balance, posture, muscle wasting.

Feel. Temperature, pain on palpation, joint effusion (patellar tap test), abnormal movement, measure (limb length discrepancy).

Move. Assess both active and passive range of movement. Assess power; a full neurological examination is indicated in musculoskeletal disorder.

Presentation of patients with musculoskeletal disorders

Musculoskeletal disorders may present to the general practitioner (GP), specialist or accident and emergency (A&E) department as an isolated joint problem (e.g. septic arthritis) or systemic disease (e.g. systemic lupus erythematosus (SLE), rheumatoid arthritis (RA)).

They affect all age groups, races, genders, socioeconomic groups and present in a broad range of circumstances. These may be categorized as below.

Trauma
- Blunt—blast, road traffic accident (RTA), sports related
- Penetrating—shotgun, stab wound
- Burns
- Isolated injury or multiple injuries
- Trauma may affect bone, muscle, soft tissues (haematoma, compartment syndrome, infection), nerves, and vessels
- Sequelae of previous trauma—non-union, malunion, arthritis
- Systemic complications of trauma (fat embolus, pulmonary embolism (PE) or deep vein thrombosis (DVT)).

Orthopaedic disorders
- Congenital: developmental dysplasia of the hip, spina bifida
- Acquired: degenerative disease
- Oncology: sarcoma.

Rheumatological disorders
- RA
- Seronegative arthropathies
- Osteoarthritis
- Gout
- Reactive arthritis
- Fibromyalgia
- Metabolic bone disease.

Patients with these conditions present to both rheumatologists and orthopaedic surgeons.

Typical presenting features of musculoskeletal disorders
- Pain
- Deformity
- Loss of function
- Stiffness
- Developmental delay
- Trauma
- Infection
- Neurological disturbance
- Iatrogenic problems or complications of trauma.

Systematic history and examination

History taking
Is the most critical part of the assessment. A good, clear history will often suggest a specific pathology and the examination is then used to confirm that provisional diagnosis.

Presenting complaint
- pain—site (although may not correlate to site of pathology); radiation; sudden/gradual onset; severity; aggravating/relieving factors
- stiffness—localized/generalized. Often not distinguished from pain
- swelling—acute/chronic, variable/constant, painful
- sensory disturbance—from compression neuropathy, local ischaemia, peripheral neuropathy
- weakness or loss of function
- ask about any treatment for a current complaint, its effectiveness, possible side effects, and assess compliance.

Past history
- previous operations, illnesses or injuries, and also general health
- define pre-morbid function.

Occupational/social history
- occupation/current work status
- understand the patient's expectation—do they want reassurance, advice or treatment?
- home circumstances for rehabilitation after surgery.

Other
- drug, alcohol, and smoking history
- allergies
- family history.

Examination
Orthopaedic examination follows the 'look, feel, move, X-ray' approach of *Apley*[1]. It begins the moment you lay eyes on the patient—posture, gait, and ease of movement can all be observed as the patient walks in from the waiting room.
- always examine in room or cubicle with adequate light and privacy
- ask patient to undress and provide them with hospital gown
- always have a chaperone available. Male doctors should always use one when examining females
- examine the relevant part of the body gently, systematically and thoroughly
- start with the good limb first then the symptomatic one
- always examine joints above and below the site of pathology.

Look
- the skin for scars, swelling, sinuses, bruising, erythema
- measure limb lengths and girth (for muscle wasting), size of any masses
- the resting posture of the limb and look for any disturbance in the normal contours of the part (suggests fracture or dislocation).

Feel

- the affected part for temperature, joint effusion, masses, tenderness, abnormal anatomy (e.g. tendon defect), crepitus on movement
- the regional lymph nodes
- the distal pulses.

Move

- passive range of movement possible at joints
- active movement (range that patient can achieve by muscular contraction—if less than the passive range = a lag sign)
- abnormal movement (e.g. in a fracture or non-union)
- joint stability
- functional assessment, e.g. gait, simple tasks with hands
- relevant neurological findings—power, sensation, tone, reflexes.

Special tests

There are many more specialized examination tests which are specific to particular areas or joints (e.g. Thomas' test in the hip, impingement tests in the shoulder). Some of these are explained in the examination subsections later in this chapter, but most can be categorized as:

- Tests of a particular muscle or musculo-tendinous unit (which may require a specific position or action to assess power/integrity)
- Tests to assess range of movement in a joint
- Provocation tests which are designed to be painful in specific conditions
- Local anaesthetic tests to remove pain as a cause of dysfunction of a joint or muscle
- Ligament tests to assess stability.

Reference

1 Warwick DJ, Solomon L, Nayagam S. *Apley's System of Orthopaedics and Fractures*, 8th rev. edn. London: Hodder Arnold, 2001.

Spine examination

Ask patient to undress down to underwear and put on hospital gown untied at the back. Observe walking, standing from sitting, ease of movement.

Look

- skin—scars (remember chest and abdomen), sinuses/erythema, midline hair tuft/dimpling, café au lait spots or nodules
- soft tissue—masses, paravertebral and limb musculature
- bone—plumb line from occiput should drop to natal cleft, shoulders and pelvis should be level (correct any limb length discrepancy with blocks). Look from side at lumbar lordosis/thoracic kyphosis. If any scoliosis suspected, bend forward to assess if of structural origin.

Feel

- further define any abnormalities, e.g. masses/asymmetry/steps in between spinous processes
- tenderness—may be midline or paravertebral.

Move

- Gait—ask patient to walk normally, then on tip-toes, then on heels
- Assess movement of cervical and thoracolumbar spine separately. When assessing the neck ensure shoulders are immobilized. When assessing movements of trunk ensure that pelvis is immobilized. All movements should be symmetrical.

Normal cervical spine movements
- flexion such that chin touches chest, extension to 30°
- lateral rotation should be to 70–90° on either side
- lateral flexion ('put ear on shoulder') should be to at least 40°.

Normal thoracolumbar movements
- flexion/extension occurs mainly in the lumbar spine. Simple assessment made by asking patient to touch toes, but much of this movement may come from the hips. Better to mark two points 15cm apart on the lumbar spine when erect—should increase to 20cm on forward flexion (Schober's test)
- rotation mainly in thoracic spine—normal ~60°
- lateral flexion measured as how far hands can reach down either thigh (ensure that movement is truly lateral not forward)
- chest expansion (limited in ankylosing spondylitis (AS))—normal expansion ≥5cm on full inspiration.

Neurological examination
- Sensation—all dermatomes, light touch and pin-prick
- Motor power—all myotomes, graded 0–5 on MRC scale
- Tone—and clonus if present
- Reflexes—biceps, triceps, supinator (brachioradialis) in upper limbs, knee and ankle jerks, and plantar response in lower limbs

- Perform perianal pin-prick and rectal examination (sensation, sphincter tone and sphincter grip strength) in cases of suspected cord or cauda equina compression.

Special tests

- straight leg raise (SLR) test[1]—limitation because of sciatic (leg) pain suggests radiculopathy. If SLR of pain-free leg causes pain down the opposite leg (crossed SLR) this is more specific for disc herniation
- femoral stretch test—with patient prone, hip extension with knee flexed produces pain
- Spurling's test—in cervical nerve root compression—exacerbation of pain on axial compression of the head with the neck extended and rotated to the side of the radicular pain
- Waddell's signs[2]—three or more suggestive of non-organic low back pain:
  - superficial or non-anatomic tenderness
  - low back pain on axial head compression or simulated rotation
  - discrepancy of SLR in supine and seated position
  - regional weakness (cogwheel giving way) or non-dermatomal sensory disturbance
  - patient over-reaction.

References

1 Devillé WL, van der Windt DA, Dzaferagić A, *et al.* The test of Lasègue: systematic review of the accuracy in diagnosing herniated discs. *Spine* 2000;**25**:1140–7.
2 Waddell G, McCulloch JA, Kummel E, *et al.* Nonorganic physical signs in low-back pain. *Spine* 1980;**5**:117–25.

Shoulder examination

Examine both from in front and behind (include axilla—joint effusions are best seen here).

Look
- skin: scars/sinuses/erythema
- soft tissues: wasting of deltoids, hands, pectorals, rotator cuff muscles
- bones: resting position—anteromedial mass (?anterior glenohumeral dislocation), internally rotated (?posterior dislocation). Sternoclavicular joint (SCJ) and acromioclavicular joint (ACJ) deformity, winging of scapula.

Feel
- skin: warmth, tenderness
- soft tissue: rotator cuff defects, supraspinatus tendon, tendon to long head of biceps, subacromial bursa
- bone: SCJ, clavicle, ACJ, acromion, greater and lesser tuberosities, glenohumeral joint (GHJ): anterior and posterior aspects, spine of scapula and coracoid process.

Move
Examine strength and range of movements. Normals: abduction 0–180°, flexion 0–180°, extension 0–40°, external rotation to 0–60° (arm by side, elbow flexed at 90°), internal rotation 0–55° (at 90° shoulder abduction). Observe abduction in front and behind through full range—note difficulty initiating or painful arc. Assess relative movements of scapulothoracic joint and GHJ.

Special tests

There are a multitude of tests of shoulder function. Some of the more common tests are described below (Fig. 1.1).

Rotator cuff tests
- Supraspinatus—shoulder flexed 30° and abducted 30°, thumb down. Resisted abduction to assess strength—also palpate muscle belly (may also be weak because of impingement)
- Subscapularis—Gerber's lift off test—dorsum of hand against buttock and lift off against resistance
- Infraspinatus and teres minor—arm by side of body, elbow at 90°, external rotation against resistance.

Other muscles
- Biceps—elbow flexion against resistance
- Serratus anterior—push against wall ?winged scapula
- Deltoid—resisted shoulder abduction.

Instability tests
- Anterior apprehension test—with patient supine, abduct, externally rotate and extend shoulder then push on head of humerus (from behind) with opposite hand. Subluxation and protective muscle contraction with discomfort indicate anterior instability. Abolished by anterior pressure over humeral head when arm in same position.

Impingement tests

- Painful arc of abduction (60–120°) worse with thumb pointing down (empty can), better with thumb up (full can)
- Hawkin's test—90° flexion, elbow flexed to 90°, support elbow and internally rotate arm—gives pain
- Neer's sign—pain with passive elevation beyond 90°
- Jobe's test—supraspinatus muscle test produces pain
- As an adjunct to the above impingement tests, abolition of pain after injection of 10ml of 1% lidocaine into the subacromial space and repeat testing is further evidence of subacromial bursitis.

Acromioclavicular joint

- High painful arc—compare arc of impingement
- Scarf test—take arm across opposite shoulder with a bent elbow and pull gently—pain indicates pathology of ACJ.

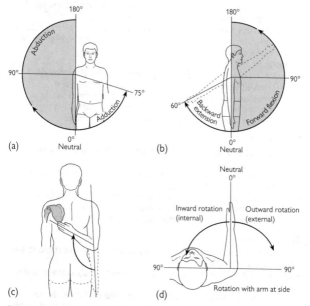

Fig. 1.1 Range of movement. (a) Abduction; (b) flexion; (c) internal rotation; (d) external rotation.

Reproduced from Bulstrode et al., Oxford Textbook of Orthopaedics and Trauma, with permission from Oxford University Press.

Elbow examination

Look

From the front with both arms fully extended and supinated, then with elbows fully flexed. Next inspect from medial and lateral sides and then from behind

- resting posture and any deformity or asymmetry
- skin for scars, sinuses, erythema
- soft tissues for swellings/muscle bulk
- bone for malalignment or bony swelling
- carrying angle.

Feel

- warmth or swelling/masses, e.g. enlarged olecranon bursa, rheumatoid nodules, gouty tophi, effusion
- three bony prominences—medial and lateral epicondyles and tip of olecranon—palpate from posteriorly with elbow flexed to 90°— should form a triangle—compare with other side. Altered by posterior dislocation or fractures of olecranon, epicondyles or condyles but not by a supracondylar fracture
- olecranon and radial head
- medial and lateral epicondyles for point tenderness (?epicondylitis)
- ulnar nerve behind the medial epicondyle for thickening and tenderness. Assess for subluxation in flexion and extension
- between the lateral epicondyle, olecranon and radial head is region where more subtle effusions/synovial thickening palpable.

Move—active

- fully extend both elbows and then touch shoulders with finger tips. Normal range: 0–150° of flexion
- elbows flexed 90° and arms at side to assess pronation and supination. Normal range: 180° of rotation
- pain on resisted wrist flexion in supination implies golfer's elbow
- pain on resisted wrist extension in pronation or resisted extension of middle finger (extensor carpi radialis brevis) implies tennis elbow.

Special tests

- medial collateral ligament (MCL) laxity assessed by valgus stress to the fully supinated elbow
- lateral collateral ligament (LCL) laxity assessed by valgus stress to the fully pronated elbow
- posterolateral rotatory instability best assessed by pivot-shift test, similar to the knee, with patient supine and arm above the head. Apply valgus and supinating force whilst flexing[1].

Reference

1 O'Driscoll SW, Bell DF, Morrey BF. Posterolateral rotatory instability of the elbow. *J Boint Join Surg Am* 1991;**73**:440–6.

Wrist and hand examination

Look
- general—posture, wasting, deformity
- skin and nails—colour, scars, wounds, clubbing, ridges and pitting
- soft tissue—swelling, muscle atrophy, contractures, lumps, nodules
- bones/joints—deformity, osteoarthritis (OA) (Heberden's nodes), RA (ulnar deviation, rheumatoid nodules, Boutonniere/swan neck/Z deformities), mallet finger, rotational deformity (in extension look at the nail beds end on, in flexion look for scissoring of the fingers).

Feel
- for swellings/deformity of or near tendons or joints
- identify and define any tender areas; scaphoid tenderness is elicited in the anatomical snuff box or on axial compression of the thumb
- for crepitus on movement
- palpate palmar fascia for nodules or cords of Dupuytren's disease
- vascular examination—capillary refill time, radial pulse at the wrist. Allen's test (occlude both radial and ulnar arteries by direct pressure whilst making tight fist, open fingers and release pressure over one artery, repeat with the other artery to assess each one's contribution to palmar arch), can also be adapted to test digital arteries of a finger
- sensation—especially in context of penetrating trauma (2-point discrimination is most sensitive).

Move
Requires careful examination as subtle abnormalities can produce significant functional impairment:
- assess flexion, extension, abduction and adduction of all fingers, and circumduction and opposition of thumb. Extension of index and small fingers whilst keeping middle and ring fingers flexed tests extensor indicis proprius (EIP) and extensor digiti minimi (EDM)
- assess flexion (0–80°), extension (0–70°), radial (0–20°) and ulnar (0–30°) deviation, pronation (0–90°) and supination (0–90°) of wrist joint (note supination and pronation also limited by elbow pathology)
- identify separate action of flexor digitorum superficialis (FDS) and flexor digitorum profundus (FDP) on fingers: splint middle phalanx to assess flexor action of FDP at distal interphalangeal joint (DIPJ); hold other fingers in full extension to assess flexion of FDS at proximal interphalangeal joint (PIPJ) of each isolated finger
- assess power in main nerve territories
  - Radial nerve: wrist and metacarpophalangeal joint (MCPJ) extension
  - Ulnar nerve: 1st dorsal interosseus and small finger abduction
  - Median nerve: with palm upward abduct (antepose) the thumb
- functional assessment—ask patient to write their name, hold a key, drink from a glass, do up a button, pick up a small object.

Special tests

- Tinel's test over course of median or ulnar nerve
- Phalen's test: fully flex wrist for 30s—suggests carpal tunnel syndrome if pain and paraesthesia develop
- Watson's test (scaphoid shift test)—examiner grasps forearm with one hand, scaphoid with the other, thumb pressing on scaphoid tubercle and resisting its movement on radial and ulnar deviation of the wrist. Painful click in scaphoid instability. Also painful in scaphoid fracture
- Froment's test—grab paper between thumb and radial border of index—if weakness in ulnar innervated adductor pollicis, then patient will grip by flexing the thumb IPJ
- Finkelstein's test—flex thumb into palm and clasp with fingers, ulnar deviation of the wrist produces great pain in De Quervain's disease.

Hip examination

Watch walking (do they use a stick?), ease of movement, sitting and standing posture. Undress down to underwear. Examine standing and lying.

Standing

Look

- skin of pelvis, hips and legs: ischaemic or trophic changes, scars, sinuses
- swelling/mass, e.g. lipoma, trauma, tumour, infection, hernia
- muscle atrophy (especially buttocks) or hypertrophy
- deformity (leg length inequality, pes cavus, scoliosis). Position and degree of rotation of the leg.

Feel

Trendelenberg's test—identify the anterior superior iliac spine (ASIS) on both sides with patient standing. Ask to stand on one leg—normally both ASIS will stay at the same level because of the contraction of the abductors on the standing side. If the abductors fail to hold the pelvis level (because of pain, neurological impairment or detachment from the greater trochanter) the tilt of the pelvis will be detected by the examiner (ASIS of the opposite side will drop) and the patient will compensate by moving their trunk (i.e. centre of gravity) over the standing leg and/or seek support by taking weight via their arms.

Move

Ask the patient to walk and assess their gait (see Gait analysis, 🕮 p. 25).

Lying

Look

Leg lengths—an apparent leg length discrepancy disregards the contribution of any pelvic tilt. Thus the skeletal length of the lower limbs may actually be equal, but one leg be *apparently* longer than the other. A true discrepancy exists where the bones of the lower limbs are of different lengths, and is measured clinically by holding the pelvis level and legs symmetrical—ideally straight and in neutral position but if there is a resting deformity in one leg, match it in the contralateral limb.

Feel

Palpation over the joint is of limited value: assess tenderness over the greater trochanter as this may imply trochanteric bursitis or a fracture.

Move

- flexion of each hip. Normal 0–120°. Assess for any rotation occurring during the course of the flexion arc
- Thomas's test—flex contralateral hip such that lumbar lordosis is eliminated; hip under examination should be able to extend fully (leg flat on bed) otherwise fixed flexion deformity (FFD) is present

- extension (0–10°) assess with patient prone—best left until end of examination
- rotation of each hip—normal 0–45° internal/0–60° external. Commonly performed with hip and knee both flexed to 90° but can also be done in extension or at 45° mid-flexion where capsule is most lax
- abduction (normal 0–40°)/adduction (normal 0–25°). Assess with hip and knee extended, pelvis neutral and immobilized.

Knee examination

Inspect whilst standing: include front, back and sides, and assess gait.

Look
- Skin: wounds, scars, erythema, sinuses
- Supra-/infra-/prepatellar swelling—?bursitis
- popliteal fossa: Baker's cyst, aneurysm, lymphadenopathy
- calf swelling: ruptured Baker's cyst, DVT, cellulitis
- knee joint: effusion, synovial thickening or meniscal cyst
- muscle bulk: quadriceps and calf muscles
- Alignment of the leg: varus/valgus deformity (measure intermalleolar distance if valgus).

Feel
Whilst lying down, assess:
- Temperature using dorsum of hand
- Tenderness with knee extended: suprapatellar pouch, patella, patellar tendon, tibial tuberosity, condyles of femur and tibia including attachments of collateral ligaments
- Tenderness with knee flexed to 90°: medial and lateral joint lines and popliteal fossa
- Effusion—3 methods to assess this
  - Stroke test—squeeze suprapatellar pouch then move any fluid by stroking it from medial to lateral side of the knee (and back again)—look for it bulging—for a small effusion
  - Patellar tap—squeeze suprapatellar pouch then push on patella and try to ballotte it against the femur—medium sized effusion
  - Cross fluctuance—large amount of fluid (effusion or blood).

Move
- active range of movement: normal 0–130°
- active extension: tests integrity of extensor mechanism—inability to extend knee fully implies FFD or quadriceps lag
- passively flex and extend knee and assess for crepitus
- collateral ligaments—varus and valgus stress testing in extension and in 30° of flexion: painful minimal joint opening = partial tear, gross opening with less pain = full tear
- cruciate ligament tests
  - anterior and posterior draw tests: flex knee to 90°. Look from the side to see if any posterior sag (posterior cruciate ligament (PCL) injury), then pull proximal tibia forward whilst stabilizing the foot—assess amount of displacement and quality of 'end-point' (for ACL injury)
  - Lachman test—variant of anterior draw performed at 15° of flexion
  - pivot-shift—with valgus force and internal rotation of the tibia, moving from flexion to extension produces visible jump of tibia on femur

- menisci—there are many tests, none has 100% accuracy. Most well known is probably McMurray's test[1]—medial meniscus: flex hip and knee, externally rotate tibia, then extend. (+)ve if painful click over medial joint line. Lateral meniscus: start with knee flexed and internally rotated, then extend
- patella glide test: knee flexed to 30° move medially and laterally. Apprehension on lateral movement suggests recurrent dislocation.

Reference

1 McMurray TP. The semilunar cartilages. *Br J Surg* 1942;**29**:407–14.

Ankle and foot examination

Expose the whole leg and foot; inspect front/back/sides/sole of foot; standing (normally and then on tip-toes) and then sitting—patient sat on examination couch with legs over the side—examiner sat on a chair at a lower level than the couch.

Look

- examine soles of shoes for signs of asymmetrical wear
- assess gait—look specifically for high stepping gait (e.g. foot drop), antalgic gait and short propulsive phase (forefoot pain)
- skin for scars, swelling, bruising, vascular disease, ulcers, gangrene, callosities
- nails for colour, deformity, infection (paronychia), pitting (psoriasis)
- soft tissue—masses/swelling/muscle atrophy or hypertrophy
- foot size—unilaterally small ?clubfoot, bilaterally large ?marfanoid
- limb alignment (especially genu valgus with flat feet)
- look at the foot shape and position. Common foot shapes:
  - neutral ('rectus') foot
  - skew foot: hindfoot valgus with forefoot adduction
  - cavus foot: high arch with hindfoot varus and pronated forefoot
  - flat foot (pes planus): low medial longitudinal arch with hindfoot valgus and abducted forefoot
- common toe deformities:
  - clawing: hyperextended metatarsophalangeal joint (MTPJ), flexed IPJs
  - mallet: flexion deformity at DIPJ only
  - hammer: flexion at PIPJ, extension at DIPJ
  - hallux valgus.

Feel

- palpate the foot and ankle to define areas of tenderness
- feel pedal pulses
- assess sensation.

Move

- ankle dorsiflexion: normal 0–25°
- ankle plantarflexion: normal 0–45°
- inversion/eversion at subtalar joint—hold ankle joint dorsiflexed and grasp calcaneus with examining hand. Passively invert and evert
- mid-tarsal joint. Heel is held with one hand—passively flex/extend and move side-to-side with other hand holding forefoot
- flexion/extension of toes—MTPJ and IPJs.

Special tests

- Simmonds test—calf squeeze test for assessing integrity of tendo-achilles
- Coleman block test—in cavovarus deformity a block placed laterally under the foot accommodates a plantarflexed first ray—hindfoot varus will correct if flexible
- Ankle stability tests—medial and lateral stress testing and anterior draw (tests anterior talofibular ligament).

Neurological history and examination 1

History

A neurological history is important in completing a full assessment of patients with musculoskeletal conditions. The history should be directed by presenting symptoms, location of symptoms and their severity. It is essential to have a sound knowledge of disorders that cause or are associated with musculoskeletal problems. On completion of the neurological assessment one must have established:

- site of the lesion
- likely pathology
- available treatment options
- prognosis.

Common presentations

Pain: site, onset, characteristics, radiation, aggravating factors, relieving factors, associated factors, course.

Upper motor neuron (UMN) signs: increased tone, brisk tendon reflexes, Babinski sign (hallux extends with stimulation of the sole of the foot), Hoffman's sign (flicking DIPJ induces thumb flexion).

Lower motor neuron (LMN) signs: decreased tone, areflexia or hyporeflexia, fasciculations, fibrillations, paresis or paralysis.

Neurological symptoms

- Higher functions—cognition
- Sensory symptoms—altered sensation can be described in a similar way to pain. Distinguish between acute and chronic symptoms. They may be due to central or peripheral nervous system disorders or the disorder may affect both systems. Symptoms may develop as a neurological manifestation or systemic disease
- Motor symptoms—attempt to establish if there is a myotomal or nerve root distribution. Acute or chronic, fluctuating, static or progressive, exacerbating or remitting? Results of prior treatment and the therapeutic response important.

Examination

Level of consciousness

Glasgow Coma Scale (GCS; scoring maximum of 15):

- Eyes: opens spontaneously = 4, verbal command = 3, pain = 2, no response = 1
- Motor: obeys = 6, localizes = 5, flexion withdrawal = 4, flexion (decorticate) = 3, extension (decerebrate) = 2, no response = 1
- Voice: orientated = 5, disorientated = 4, inappropriate = 3, incomprehensible = 2, no response = 1.

Higher functions and speech

Mental status

Abbreviated mental test score (<6 suggestive of dementia). Easy to use at end of consultation. Each question carries 1 point: age, time to nearest hour, an address (repeated at the end of the test), year, hospital name, recognition of two, date of birth, First World War started, name of Queen, counting backwards from 20 to 1.

Speech

- Dysphasias—distinguish by command, repeat statement and naming object
- Conductive—repeat statements and names poorly, follows commands
- Expressive—often hesitant and non-grammatical but comprehension usually preserved (Broca's lesion)
- Receptive—fluent, nonsensical, with poor comprehension (Wernicke's lesion)
- Nominal—specifically cannot name objects
- Dysarthria—difficulty of articulation only (alcohol, cerebellar, bulbar or pseudobulbar palsy, extrapyramidal).

Cerebellar signs

- Ataxia
- Intention tremor
- Dysdiadochokinesis
- Dysarthria
- Dysmetria
- Poor heel–toe coordination (dysdiabkinesia).

Cranial nerves must be examined

- I Olfactory—assess smell
- II Optic—visual accuracy, visual fields, pupillary reaction to light (in conjunction with assessment of other cranial nerves) and fundoscopy
- III, IV, VI Oculomotor, trochlea, abducens—assess movements of eyes and eyelids
- V Trigeminal—assess muscle of mastication and facial sensation
- VII Facial—assess facial muscles
- VIII Auditory—assess hearing (differentiate between conduction and sensineural hearing loss with Rinne and Weber's tests) and vestibular function
- IX Glossopharyngeal—assess swallowing
- X Vagus nerve—assess for palatal deviation
- XI Accessory—assess shoulder shrug
- Hypoglossal—assess tongue movement and wasting.

Neurological history and examination 2

Limbs

Examine upper and lower limbs.

Motor system: power, tone, reflexes.

Inspection: Look for muscle wasting, attitude of the limb, trophic changes. Look for fibrillation, fasciculation, asterexis, choreiform movement.

MRC grading power
- 0 No voluntary contraction
- 1 Flicker of contraction
- 2 Movement with gravity eliminated
- 3 Movement against gravity
- 4 Movement against partial resistance
- 5 Full strength.

NB: this must be through the full range of joint movement.

Myotomes
- C3–5 Supply the diaphragm
- C5 Deltoid and biceps
- C6 Extension of the wrist
- C7 Extension of the elbow
- C8 Flexion of the fingers
- T1 Abduction of the fingers
- T2—T12 Supply the chest wall and abdominal muscles
- L2 Flexion of the hip
- L3 Extension of the knee
- L4 Dorsiflexion of the foot
- L5 Extension of the hallux
- S1 Plantarflexion of the foot
- S3, 4, 5 Important in the bladder and bowel control and sexual function.

Tone: grasp under elbow and at wrist and rotate the two joints to assess resistance. Parkinson's disease have lead pipe rigidity. Clonus occurs with UMN lesions.

Sensory (Fig. 1.2)

The test for light touch (cotton wool), pin-prick (pin or 'millinery' wheel) sensation and vibration sense (tuning fork).

Assess proprioception. Always looking for sensory distribution, dermatomal, peripheral nerve, or glove and stocking distribution.

Reflexes

Deep tendon reflexes
- Biceps (musculocutaneous nerve) C5, 6.
- Supinator (radial nerve) C5, 6 root.
- Triceps (radial nerve) C7.
- Knee L3, 4 (femoral nerve).
- Ankle (tibial nerve) S1, 2.

Superficial reflexes
- Abdominal, upper T8, 9 and lower T10, 11
- Cremasteric L1, 2 and anal S4, 5.

Meningeal irritation
- Babinski sign
- Kernig's sign
- (+)ve SLR (pain aggravated). (+)ve stretch test
- Bowstring sign.

Gait
- Hemiparetic gait: shoulder or leg flexed, internally rotated, forearm pronated, knee flexed and equinus foot
- Ataxic gait: legs spread, wide base and staggering gait
- Shuffling gait: very short steps. Occurs in cerebral or long tract disease
- High stepping gait: takes high steps, increased knee flexion in swing
- Antalgic gait: pain aggravated by weight bearing.

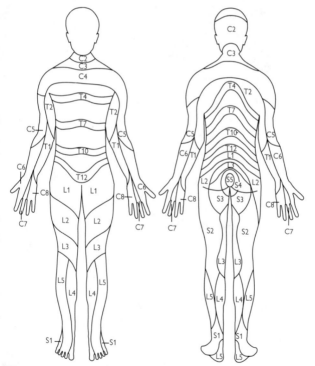

Fig. 1.2 Dermatome chart.

Reproduced from Bulstrode et al., *Oxford Textbook of Orthopaedics and Trauma*, with permission from Oxford University Press.

Orthopaedic investigations

Haematological and biochemical tests

Principles
The clinical assessment should direct what investigations are used. Routine preoperative investigation in healthy patients is usually not useful; however some commonly performed tests are frequently necessary in major surgeries, those with known or suspected co-morbidities and in emergency situations. For elective surgery, local protocols should be available, based on the NICE guidelines[1].

Interpretation of results
All laboratory measurements vary, and reference levels must be known when interpreting results.

Haematological tests

Full blood count
Useful if:
- Surgery is likely to lead to sizeable blood loss
- History of significant blood loss or cardiorespiratory disease
- Infection suspected.

Erythrocyte sedimentation rate (ESR)
Non-specific marker of inflammation—useful when normal; less useful when abnormal.

Sickle cell test
Although most affected patients are of Afro-Carribbean or African ethnic origin, those of Middle Eastern, Asian and some Mediterranean groups are also affected and should be screened.

Clotting profile
- Prothrombin time (PT): measures the extrinsic pathway components. Increased when on warfarin, in liver disease and disseminated intravascular coagulation (DIC)
- Activated partial thromboplastin time (APTT): measures the intrinsic pathway components. Increased in haemophilia, DIC, and in patients on heparin.

Biochemistry

Urea and electrolytes
- In all patients over 65
- Those with known cardiopulmonary, renal or hepatic disease
- Those taking diuretics, steroids, or cardiac drugs.

C-reactive protein (CRP)
Acute phase protein and general marker of inflammation/infection.

Bone profile
Liver and renal function tests may be necessary, but in metabolic disorders affecting bone it is always important to measure levels of Ca^{2+}, PO_4 and alkaline phosphatase (ALP) in the serum. Serum vitamin D levels and urinary calcium levels are sometimes indicated.

Reference

1 http://www.nice.org.uk/guidance/CG3.

Principles of diagnostic imaging: X-ray

X-rays are produced by the sharp deceleration of high-speed electrons, which are emitted when a high voltage is placed between a heated cathode and a tungsten anode, both placed in a vacuum. The X-ray beam is part of the electromagnetic spectrum and is absorbed preferentially by calcium-containing materials, including bone; gas and water absorb virtually no X-rays. X-rays are, therefore, ideal for assessing bone structure.

When passing through tissue, the X-ray beams produce free radicals, which damage cellular DNA. There is a low risk that the altered cellular DNA can lead to neoplasia—the risk is proportional to the concentration of X-rays absorbed by the body and is cumulative over a lifetime. X-rays are also teratogenic.

Radiation protection

As X-rays are not risk free, guidelines on their use are routinely applied and are based on the following principles:
- Necessity—Will the radiograph influence the patient's treatment?
- Minimize irradiated area—What's the smallest irradiated area which will give the necessary information?—i.e. localize the body area to be X-rayed
- Minimize repeat irradiation—limit repeat X-rays to minimize the cumulative X-ray dose. Make sure that the request form clearly conveys to the radiographer what you are looking for on the X-ray, so that an adequate X-ray is obtained with one exposure alone.

The X-ray request

- The X-ray film is a 2-D representation of a 3-D structure. The depth of the structure is assessed by taking a second X-ray at right angles to the first X-ray. The most common X-ray requests are an antero-posterior (AP) film and lateral projection
- When assessing a suspected fractured bone, include the joint above and below the fracture for a complete appreciation of the injury. This practice avoids missing joint dislocations associated with displaced fractures, e.g. distal ulna dislocation with a radial shaft fracture (Galeazzi fracture)
- State whether the body part to be imaged contains metalware, as this influences the X-ray penetration setting used by the radiographer to acheive the best quality film
- When requesting emergency X-rays of a seriously unwell patient consider a request for 'mobile X-rays', where the radiographer takes a mobile X-ray machine to the patient who remains in a controlled environment.

Principles of diagnostic imaging: CT scanning

Introduced to clinical practice in the 1970s, the CT (computed tomography) scan is a set of images produced by multiple X-rays. The patient is passed through a large ring, which contains a rotating X-ray tube and a gas or crystal X-ray detector. The CT X-ray detectors create a higher definition picture than the photographic film used with standard X-rays and a larger range of shades is therefore achieved. This gives greater definition of various tissue densities in the body part scanned. An axial section of the scanned body part is taken with slice thickness of between 1mm and 1cm. The thicker 1cm sliced CT produces a lower quality image, but involves less radiation exposure. The thinner sectioned CTs are used to detect subtle pathology, e.g. undisplaced cervical spine fractures, whereas thicker slices are used to screen for large lesions, e.g. to rule out an intracranial haematoma.

CT reconstructions

The horizontal, or axial, images are converted into coronal or sagittal images, which facilitate visual interpretation of the body part under investigation. Sophisticated computer manipulation can also construct a 3-D image to further facilitate interpretation of, for example, displaced fracture fragments in complex trauma; however, the image resolution is reduced.

Applications of CT

- Spine—plain X-rays tend to under-represent the extent of bony injury compared with CT, so high-energy spine fractures are usually investigated by CT as well as initial X-rays. Certain areas are difficult to visualize on X-ray and CT is therefore employed, such as the cervicothoracic junction and high thoracic spine which is commonly overlapped by the shoulders on lateral views
- Intra-articular fractures—CT is occasionally employed to help decide whether a fracture extending into a joint is displaced and, if so, whether surgery will improve the fracture fragment positions, e.g. os calcis and acetabular fractures
- Tumour surgery—when investigating a bony lesion suspected of being a malignancy, a chest CT is performed to detect any lung metastases which may be undetectable on the conventional chest X-ray (CXR).

Principles of diagnostic imaging: magnetic resonance imaging

Production of a magnetic resonance image

Hydrogen nuclei are spinning protons which rotate in a specific direction. In an MRI scanner, the direction of spin aligns to the direction of the magnetic field. When a short radiofrequency (RF) pulse is directed at tissue, the protons' direction of rotation changes and they then 'relax' as they return to their previous state. The relaxation phase is associated with the emission of a weak radio signal, which can be detected by a detector coil. As water has a high concentration of protons and different tissues have different water saturations, then a highly detailed soft tissue and bony image is constructed by computer interpretation of the differential radio signals detected with each RF pulse.

MRI safety

- No ionizing radiation—no known risk of malignancy
- Contraindications to scanning
  - Cardiac pacemakers
  - Internal hearing devices
  - Intracranial aneurysm clips
  - Metal fragments in eyes—ask and X-ray orbits in, for example, sheet metal workers/grinders
- Joint replacements and spinal implants are generally safe.

Appearances on MRI

By adjusting the frequency and timing of the RF pulses, different tissues are highlighted on the MRI.

T1 weighting
- Dark—water (e.g. cerebrospinal fluid (CSF)), bone, air
- Bright—fat.

T2 weighting
- Dark—cartilage, bone, air
- Bright—water.

Others
- STIR (short T1 inversion recovery)—like T2 but fat appears dark
- Proton density—cartilage appears grey (high signal)
- Gadolinium—intravenous (IV) contrast agent for MRI (with T1 sequence)
- MR angiography (MRA)—uses gadolinium or the flow of blood to highlight vessels.

Applications of MRI

- Spine—prolapsed discs, stenosis, tumours, infection, cord pathology
- Knee—ligament injuries, meniscal tears, cartilage studies
- Hip—labral pathology (with contrast), avascular necrosis (AVN), undisplaced fractures
- Shoulder—rotator cuff anatomy
- Hand and wrist—scaphoid fractures, ligament injuries, AVN
- Others—tumours and infection in all sites.

Principles of diagnostic imaging: bone scintigraphy

Also known as radionuclide imaging, nuclear medicine imaging or 'bone scan'. Technetium 99m (99mTc) radioisotope imaging was developed in 1960.

Production of a bone scan

Radiolabelled elements (radioisotopes) emit gamma radiation, which can be detected by a gamma ray detector. The element chosen is usually preferentially taken up by specific organs, e.g. calcium hydroxyapatite, $Ca_5(PO_4)_3OH$, is the calcified mineral content of bone, so 99mTc-tagged phosphate compounds will be taken up by metabolically active bone. If there is increased bone turnover, more 99mTc accumulates in that particular site.

Bone scan safety

99mTc has a half-life of 6h and emits low doses of gamma radiation, equivalent to ~5yrs of background radiation.

Application of bone scan

- stress fracture detection
- diseases of high bone turnover, e.g. Paget's disease
- detection of most types of bone metastasis
- may fail to detect some lesions, e.g. multiple myeloma.

Positron emission tomography (PET)

Fluorodeoxyglucose (FDG) is a radiolabelled compound containing glucose that and is metabolized in the same manner by the body. Increased metabolism of any kind involves increased glucose metabolism; therefore there is increased FDG uptake in regions of high metabolic activity.

PET is currently thought to be the most sensitive imaging modality for detecting tumour metastases. It also identifies benign tumours when they have little metabolic activity.

Principles of diagnostic imaging: ultrasound

Developed as a medical diagnostic tool in 1940.

Production of an ultrasound scan (USS)

Very high frequency sound waves are produced and received by a transducer and then converted into an electrical signal, producing a 'real-time' moving image.

Fluid allows sound to pass easily through, so very little is reflected back to the transducer. Calcified structures, such as bone, however, reflect most sound waves back to the transducer.

Fluid flow can be detected by the 'Doppler effect' (in vessels or vascularized lesions).

Application of US

- Investigation of a lump, is it solid, cystic or vascular?
- Assessment of tendon integrity e.g. tendo-achilles rupture.
- Delineation of a deep abscess.
- Detection of lower limb venous thromboembolism.
- Evaluation of the cartilaginous neonatal skeletal system.

Paediatric radiology

The immature skeleton differs from that of the skeletally mature adult in that the growing skeleton is undergoing ossification of a cartilage precursor, followed by lengthening via growth plates (endochondral ossification) and widening via the periosteum (appositional, intramembranous growth).

US versus X-ray

The neonatal skeleton is investigated by US rather than X-ray, because cartilage is radiolucent. For example, the suspected developmental dysplastic hip is assessed by US up to the age of ~6 months, because the femoral head does not ossify (and then become identifiable on X-ray) until 4–6 months of age. Neonates with suspected brain abnormalities, such as hydrocephalus, can undergo US of the brain via the anterior fontanelle, which remains open until ~2yrs of age. This may be preferable to irradiating the brain with CT scanning, or anaesthetizing the baby for an MRI scan.

Joints are often incompletely seen on X-ray as they have not fully ossified. This is especially relevant with elbow fractures, where a severely displaced lateral condylar fracture may be missed on X-ray, as the lateral condyle is not fully ossified until the age of ~13yrs old. Arthrogram, US or MRI may be useful.

Ligamentous laxity

Children tend to be ligamentously lax compared with adults. This is relevant when assessing the paediatric cervical spine, where vertebrae appear to be misaligned, or 'pseudosubluxed'. The subluxation is physiological in children, due to ligamentous laxity, but also due to the more horizontal facet joint alignment, compared with adult facet joints. This is especially common at C2–3 and C3–4 levels.

Compliance

A young child will not tolerate a lengthy investigation such as an MRI scan (undereye 5 yrs generally) and may need sedation or a general anaesthetic in order to keep still for the scan.

Neurophysiological tests

The main neurophysiological tests are:
- Nerve conduction studies (NCS)
- Electromyography (EMG)
- Electroencephalogram (EEG)
- Evoked potentials.

Nerve conduction studies

Allow evaluation of peripheral nerves and their sensory and motor response anywhere along their course. Involve stimulation of peripheral nerves and the recording from either the same nerve or the muscle supplied by the nerve.

Terms

- **Latency**—time from the start of stimulation to the start of the response
- **Amplitude**—size of the response
- **Conduction velocity**—speed of the impulse in metres per second.

Measurements can be taken from sensory, motor or mixed nerves. Conduction depends on many factors (age, skin temperature, nerve size).

Technique

Stimulating electrodes are applied to the skin along a nerve, and an electrical stimulus is applied to excite an action potential. Recording electrodes are placed over a muscle for motor nerve studies or over a sensory nerve (e.g. ring electrode for finger digital nerves).

Electromyography

EMG is the study of the electrical characteristics of muscle and is often performed along with NCS. The recording electrode is usually a hollow needle with an insulated wire inside (coaxial needle) that is inserted into the muscle under investigation. The electrical activity of the muscle at rest (normally silent—upon denervation, may show spontaneous activity, e.g. fibrillation), during voluntary contraction and during stimulation can be recorded.

Indications for NCS and EMG

- Localized weakness or altered sensation (e.g. radial nerve palsy after humeral fracture)
- Generalized weakness or altered sensation (peripheral neuropathy vs spinal lesion)
- Weakness alone (motor neuron disease, neuromuscular disease, motor neuropathy or myopathy).

Nerve conduction study results

Condition	Latency	Conduction velocity	Evoked response
Normal	Normal	>40m/s	Biphasic
Axonal neuropathy	Increased	Normal	Prolonged or decreased amplitude
Demyelinating neuropathy	Normal	Decreased	Normal
Anterior horn disease	Normal	Normal	Normal or prolonged
Myopathy	Normal	Normal	Decreased amplitude
Neurapraxia proximal to lesion	Absent	Absent	Absent
Neurapraxia distal to lesion	Normal	Normal	Normal
Axonotmesis proximal to lesion	Absent	Absent	Absent
Axonotmesis distal to lesion	Absent	Absent	Normal
Neurotmesis proximal to lesion	Absent	Absent	Absent
Neurotmesis distal to lesion	Absent	Absent	Absent

Electroencephalogram
- Used in diagnosis of cerebral disease.

Evoked potentials
- Stimulus may be light (visual evoked potentials), sound (brainstem auditory evoked potentials) or electrical stimulation (somatosensory evoked potentials)
- Somatosensory evoked potentials or motor evoked potentials may be used to monitor spinal cord function during spinal surgery.

Outcome assessment in orthopaedics

E. Amory Codman (1869–1940) was a Boston surgeon who pioneered the notion of systematic patient follow-up, to determine whether a given procedure had been successful, at a time when many of his colleagues did not even write any medical notes. Before him only Florence Nightingale had made similar suggestions, and we probably owe the development of the modern 'outcomes movement' to him.

Unfortunately his 'End Result Idea' was not well received during his lifetime; he would later show his colleagues an ostrich with its head in the sand kicking up golden eggs and explain that this typified surgeons and hospital administrators. They had their heads in the sand, never studying their own end results but content as long as they produced the 'golden eggs'. Needless to say, his comments were not well received and he became alienated within his profession despite many great and wide-ranging contributions.

Nowadays, limited healthcare resources are faced with exponential increases in demand and costs. Allied to increasing recognition that a technically and radiographically successful procedure does not automatically confer benefits to overall patient quality of life, as assessed in various domains including pain, function, overall health status and well-being, this has led to the development of increasingly sophisticated measures of outcome.

Scoring systems may be divided into general health status questionnaires and more regionally specific scoring systems[1]. Within these systems, measures may be self-reported (questionnaires) or observed, e.g. range of movement assessment. It is best to use a general health status questionnaire, such as the Short Form 36 (SF-36®), in combination with a specific musculoskeletal scoring system according to type of operation, e.g. hip replacement, or body region, e.g. upper limb.

For a scoring system to be useful it should be designed around the surveyed factors important to the patient group under study and validated to confirm it is:
- Reliable—repeatable without excessive variability
- Valid—the score measures what it is intended to
- Responsive—sensitive to meaningful change
- Quick and easy to perform
- Appropriate for a wide range of patients without significant 'floor' or 'ceiling' effects (whereby large numbers score minimum or maximum scores in any of the domains measured).

Reference

1 Pynsent PB, Fairbank JCT, Carr AJ, eds. *Outcome Measures in Orthopaedics and Orthopaedic Trauma*, 2nd edn. Oxford: Oxford University Press.

Orthopaedic management

Communication in A&E

Communication enables rapid transfer of information between teams to coordinate efforts and optimizes patient care. A&E is often a stressful environment; good communication skills will relieve patient anxiety and reduce the potential for error.

Pre-trauma planning

- Set up and train a trauma team (ideally all ATLS certified)
- Devise and practise a major incident plan.

The ambulance service will generally warn A&E of the impending arrival of any major trauma. A receiving team should be assembled, equipment checked and the team leader should allocate roles to each member of the team.

Typical roles may be

- Team leader who coordinates the whole team
- Airway control; often an anaesthetist
- Circulating doctor who will conduct primary survey
- Runner who may send bloods, set up chest drain, etc.
- Someone to document findings and procedures performed
- Circulating nurse to perform cannulation, remove clothes, etc.
- Radiographer to image as directed by the team leader.

Resuscitation room

When the patient arrives, the team leader needs a succinct but clear handover from the ambulance crew: mechanism and time of injury, basic observations and obvious injuries, procedures performed and fluids/analgesia given.

Communication may be improved by:

- A white board to document handover
- A camera to record open fractures prior to covering them.

Relatives will often accompany the patient. They may have valuable information about the patient's medication and medical co-morbidity. It is important that someone talks to the relatives and keeps them informed of the patient's progress.

Decision making

Once the patient has been resuscitated a decision has to be made on the further management of the patient:

- Transfer to another hospital
- Admission ± transfer to theatre—under the appropriate team
- Observation in A&E followed by discharge
- Discharge with or without follow-up.

Precise communication at this stage saves time and subsequent confusion. Discussion with the relevant team should state the diagnosis accurately and succinctly, and it should be made clear if you are phoning for advice, want the patient to be reviewed or need help now!

If the patient is discharged, careful documentation facilitates future follow-up, and concise legible correspondence should be sent to the patient's GP.

Principles of non-operative management

There is no condition which cannot be made worse by surgery.

Derided by some as 'The Great Rester' in our modern era of operative orthopaedics, Hugh Owen Thomas (1834–91) was a great pioneer in British orthopaedic surgery. Coming to Liverpool from a family of bone-setters on the island of Anglesey off North Wales he strongly advocated the use of rest ('enforced, uninterrupted and prolonged') for treatment of tuberculosis (TB) and fractures. This was against the trend of the time for excision or amputation in chronic bone disorders. He invented several types of splints manufactured in his own workshop by a blacksmith and a saddler. His nephew, Sir Robert Jones, introduced many of his ideas to the surgical community and in the First World War use of the 'Thomas splint' for compound femoral fractures reduced morbidity from 80% to <8%.

While the benefits of rigid, stable fixation and early motion are now undoubted in certain fracture types, for many orthopaedic conditions operation (if indicated) should be considered only after all 'conservative' therapies have been exhausted. These include:

- Rest: reduction in normal activity and avoidance of strain
- Splintage and traction (see 🕮 p. 51)
- Physiotherapy and occupational therapy (see 🕮 Chapter 12, p. 587)
- Medication: analgesics and anti-inflammatory drugs are the mainstays. Also disease-modifying drugs in inflammatory arthropathy, bisphosphonates for fracture prevention in the elderly and to reduce bone pain and fracture risk in osteogenesis imperfecta, botulinum toxin injections for muscle imbalance in cerebral palsy (CP)
- Local injections—usually intra-articular steroid and local anaesthetic, also for tendinopathy, e.g. tennis elbow
- Radiotherapy—treatment of choice for palliation of painful bony metastases. Promotes tumour cell necrosis, collagen proliferation and osteoblastic activity with formation of new woven bone
- Continuous passive motion—invented and expounded by Dr Robert Salter (Hospital for Sick Children, Toronto) based on research findings that joint immobilization is potentially harmful. Motion has a positive effect on cartilage viability and nutrition; machines developed for most joints to move them passively through their physiological range after injury or surgery, or both.

Transport of the injured patient

Pre-hospital to receiving hospital (paramedics) priorities
- Airway maintainance
- Control of external haemorrhage and shock
- Appropriate immobilization
- Rapid, safe transfer to closest appropriate facility.

Inform receiving hospital to enable preparation
- Nature of accident and mechanism of injury
- Number/age/sex of people involved
- Time of accident
- Condition of victims and injuries sustained
- Expected time of arrival.

Transfer to definitive care from receiving hospital
Majority receive all care in receiving hospital; some will need to be transferred for definitive treatment. Timing depends on:
- Distance of transfer
- Available skill levels for transfer
- Circumstances and facilities of local institution
- Intervention required prior to safe transfer.

Aim to treat life-threatening injuries prior to transfer (airway, breathing and circulation (ABCs)) without delaying with unnecessary investigations.

Arrangement of transfer (referring doctor)
- Initiate transfer
- Communicate identity of patient, history and initial assessment
- Stabilize prior to transfer
- Select mode of transportation and level of care for transfer
- Inform transferring personnel of patient's condition and needs
- Ensure medical notes/investigations go with patient.

Receiving doctor
- Ensure receiving facilities appropriate
- Ensure receiving institution willing to accept
- Prepare team for patient arrival.

Transportation
Potentially hazardous; ensure:
- Patient optimally stabilized
- Adequately trained personnel
- Provision made for unexpected crisis.

Adequate monitoring and ongoing management to include:
- Vital signs, pulse oximetry
- Continued cardiorespiratory support
- Continued blood volume replacement if required
- Use of appropriate medications.

Meanwhile communication must be maintained with receiving hospital along with ongoing adequate and contemporaneous documentation. On arrival a complete handover is critical, including details of any problems during transfer.

Injections and aspirations

Local intra-articular injection (usually local anaesthetic ± steroid) may be both therapeutic and diagnostic. Hip joint injection may help differentiate symptoms of radiologically apparent OA from pain of spinal origin. Local (spinal) facet joint injections under X-ray guidance may help relieve pain; nerve root blockade, again with radiological guidance, may identify source of symptoms with multiple level spinal disease.

Aspiration of a joint or collection may also be therapeutic or diagnostic; often the aim is to confirm or exclude infection. Technique must be strictly aseptic[1]; never aspirate a joint through an area of cellulitis. May require X-ray or image intensifier guidance for a joint which is small or deep, e.g. sacroiliac joint (SIJ) or hip joint. US guidance (radiologist) helpful for deep soft tissue collection and joint aspiration in children. CT may be required for deep, inaccessible areas, e.g. paraspinal abscess. Consider likely organism and discuss appropriate culture media with microbiologist if appropriate, e.g. granulomatous disease. Request immediate Gram stain, microscopy and culture.

Indications for synovial fluid aspiration

Diagnostic
- Suspected sepsis
- Gout/pseudogout (send sample for microscopy to identify crystals)
- Inflammatory arthropathy.

Therapeutic aspiration
- Osteoarthritis or inflammatory arthropathy
- Acute haemarthrosis.

Table 3.1 Synovial fluid interpretation

Condition	Opacity	Leukocyte count (per mm³)
Normal	Clear	<200
Osteoarthritis	Clear	1000 (<50% PMNs)
Rheumatoid	Cloudy	1–50 000 PMNs
Crystal arthropathy[1]	Cloudy	5–50 000 PMNs
Sepsis	Cloudy	10–100 000 PMNs
Fracture	Clood + fat	
Bleeding disorders	Blood only	

PMNs, polymorphonuclear leukocytes.

[1] Urate crystals in gout (hyperuricaemia causing recurrent attacks of synovitis) show **negative** birefringence on polarized light microscopy. Calcium pyrophosphate deposition is a condition of the elderly, usually asymptomatic but sometimes causing synovitis mimicking gout, with **positively** birefringent crystals seen on polarized light microscopy.

Site-specific aspiration techniques

- Shoulder—palpate outer inferior edge of the acromion from behind.[1] Thumb-width below and lateral to this is a 'soft spot'; pass needle through this in direction of coracoid (palpate anteriorly with index or middle finger of free hand)
- Elbow—palpate effusion in triangle formed by radial head (felt by rotating forearm with elbow flexed 90°), lateral epicondyle and lateral border of the olecranon. Enter joint at centre of this triangle
- Knee—patient supine, 18 gauge (green) needle is passed into joint between patella and femur medially or laterally. Can infiltrate with 10–20ml of bupivacaine 0.5%, but less effective if infection
- Ankle—plantar flex foot and palpate joint margin between extensor hallucis longus (EHL) and tibialis anterior just above the medial malleolus. Joint is entered between them; neurovascular structures just lateral to EHL.

Drawing appropriate landmarks on the skin with a felt tip marker is often helpful.

Reference

1 Crawley M. Techniques of joint aspiration. *Br Hosp Med* 1974;**11**:747–55.

Slings and casts

Slings

A sling is bandage used to support a part of the body's weight against gravity.

Examples:
- *Broad arm sling*: Traditionally made from a triangular bandage, although more modern designs are available (e.g. Polysling) which are more comfortable. Supports the forearm and elbow; useful in the treatment of shoulder injuries, particularly ACJ disruption and clavicular fractures as it supports the weight of the arm and thus elevates the point of the elbow and shoulder
- *Collar and cuff*: Allows the weight of the arm to act as traction force; useful in non-operative management of humeral shaft and neck fractures.

Casts

A cast is a rigid dressing which immobilizes and protects a body part.

Techniques of cast application are best learnt with the technicians in your local plaster room; they will be amazed and delighted to see you!

Cast materials
- Plaster of Paris rolls, e.g. Cellona™, Gypsona™, consist of fabric weave coated with plaster of Paris (calcium sulphate hemihydrate). They are cheap and readily available but are relatively more opaque to X-rays and susceptible to damage if exposed to moisture
- Synthetics, e.g. Scotchcast™, which consists of knitted fibreglass, or Delta-Cast conformable™ (polyester); both are impregnated with polyurethane resin. They are lighter, more radiolucent and resistant to degradation by moisture. Disadvantages: allow less expansion for swelling after fresh fracture, harder to mould (the material has more 'memory'—will want to return to its original shape).

Note: fresh fractures usually immobilized by a 'plaster slab' (encircling ~70% of the circumference of the limb) to allow for swelling of the injured part. Often this can be 'completed' (wrapping further rolls without removing the slab) after 2–3 days, or exchanged for a new cast using a synthetic casting material. Synthetics are therefore often referred to as intermediate casting materials.

Splintage and traction

Splintage

A splint is a device used either to immobilize a joint or fracture (*static*) or allow movement in a protected way (*dynamic*). A well-moulded above-knee cast for a tibial shaft fracture maintains length and alignment by hydrostatic soft tissue pressure and 3-point moulding against the deformity; including the joint above controls rotation (**static splint**). A **dynamic** finger splint after a flexor tendon repair uses elastic bands to hold the finger passively flexed but permits active extension to preserve joint motion.

Functional bracing is a technique which allows motion and loading in a controlled manner to facilitate healing. Conversion of the above-knee cast described above to a patella–tendon bearing or Sarmiento[1] cast permits weight bearing across the fracture, encouraging axial micromotion[2] which stimulates healing. This is now a functional brace.

Traction

Relies on the phenomenon of creep (Chapter 5, Biomaterials and implants, p. 107); a longitudinal force applies constant load across a fracture and its soft tissue envelope which progressively deforms with time, correcting shortening and angulation together with rotation if correctly applied.

Less popular nowadays because of long associated inpatient stay, but remains an effective temporary means of immobilization and analgesia prior to definitive treatment.

Skin traction—longitudinal tapes (adhesive or non-adhesive) bandaged along the length of the injured limb to which weights are attached. Requires careful and regular skin checks for blistering and breakdown.

Skeletal traction—via a pin (Steinmann-smooth, or Denham-threaded) through bone. Allows more weight and causes fewer soft tissue problems, but beware applying traction across a joint in the zone of injury, e.g. proximal tibial pin for femoral shaft fracture. Also stay extracapsular with pin to prevent risk of seeding the joint with contamination.

Eponymous traction types could be the subject of an entire, if somewhat historical, handbook, but here are two examples you may hear about:
- Thomas splint; fixed traction against a padded ring in the patient's groin. Best avoided because of high risk of pressure sores; better to apply the splint which has a sling for the leg and then attach it directly to weights
- Hamilton Russell traction for femoral shaft fracture; balanced traction with the knee supported by slings.

References

1 Sarmiento A, Latta L. Functional fracture bracing. *J Am Acad Orthop Surg* 1999;**7**:66–75.
2 Kenwright J, Goodship AE. Controlled mechanical stimulation in the treatment of tibial fractures. *Clin Orthop Rel Res* 1989;**241**:36–47.

Organization of a preoperative clinic

The preoperative clinic should provide a suitable environment to counsel and prepare patients for elective orthopaedic surgery. The patient's physical condition and disease process can change between booking and surgery.

A care pathway is a useful means of organizing and documenting the preoperative review, which involves a junior doctor (SHO or FY1/2), a clinic nurse, the operating surgeon, and specialist nurses, physiotherapists and occupational therapists as appropriate.

Medical co-morbidities identified by these health professionals may require assessment by an anaesthetist. This facilitates optimization of the patient's condition, if necessary, with involvement of other specialists, e.g. cardiologist, respiratory physician, in good time prior to surgery.

The likelihood of requiring blood transfusion perioperatively should be assessed. Most hospitals have protocols for guidance as to which patients to group and save and which to cross-match. Potential hazards such as recent transfusion in sickle cell patients must be flagged up at this stage.

Patients should give informed consent to the proposed procedure offered and therefore must gain an adequate understanding of it. The use of skeletal models, radiographs and actual implants or frames in the clinic is very helpful in explaining relevant concepts.

Following orthopaedic surgery a patient's ability to ambulate and self-care may be restricted. Assessment by physiotherapists and occupational therapists allows this to be anticipated so modifications to the home and living environment can be undertaken in advance if necessary. Also, social networks to support the patient can be activated.

The surgeon can plan the operation and ensure any additional instruments, custom implants and bone allograft or substitutes are ordered well in advance of surgery.

Consent

Respect for patient autonomy is a fundamental ethical principle, even if it results in potential harm or death to the patient. Surgeons have an ethical and legal duty to take *informed consent* for any procedure or operation, without which proceeding will constitute an assault. Informed consent requires the provision of sufficient information for the patient to make a balanced decision on their treatment.

Features of informed consent

Patient factors

- The patient must be mentally competent and able to:
  - understand the issues involved
  - retain information to make a rational decision
  - communicate their wishes
- If the patient is mentally competent and above the age for legal consent, nobody else is allowed to make decisions on their behalf; consent by proxy is not provided for in English law
- If a language barrier exists, informed consent must be taken through an interpreter.

Information that should be given

- An explanation of the disease process, its consequences and its prognosis
- What the proposed treatment involves, its intended benefits and practical implications
- Risks of the proposed procedure, both general, e.g. cardiovascular, anaesthetic, and specific, e.g. prosthesis dislocation
- Other treatment options (including no treatment at all) with risks and benefits.

Who can take consent?

- Ideally the doctor performing the actual investigation or operation
- Another doctor who is appropriately trained and qualified in the relevant procedure.

Emergency situations

- When emergency treatment is required and informed consent cannot be obtained, e.g. unconscious trauma patient, the legal duty of the surgeon is to act in the best interests of the patient
- Any valid advance directive should be respected. The relatives should be consulted and information about the patient's premorbid state sought, but the decision on whether to treat or not rests with the surgeon
- Treatment under these circumstances should be restricted to that necessary to save life or limb.

Children
- Any person over the age of 16 is presumed competent to make decisions and can be treated as an adult
- Children under the age of 16 may give consent if competent to understand the issues involved; however if such a child refuses treatment this can be over-ruled by a parent if treatment deemed in the child's best interests. If parents refuse treatment for a child doctors may apply for a court ruling.

Aide mémoire for consent: DIAPER

- **D**iagnosis explained
- **I**ndications for surgery discussed
- **A**lternatives to operation considered
- **P**rocedure explained
- **E**xpected outcome discussed
- **R**isks discussed

Preoperative assessment for anaesthesia

There is more than one way in which anaesthesia for surgery can be performed. These can be broadly categorized under three main headings: local anaesthesia, regional anaesthesia and general anaesthesia.

It is important to remember that there are significant cardiovascular and respiratory changes that occur during general anaesthesia that may increase the risk of morbidity and mortality in susceptible groups such as the elderly. A detailed preoperative assessment is fundamental in assessing and minimizing the anaesthetic risk and planning a safe postoperative course.

Preoperative assessment

History and examination

There are a few anaesthetic considerations that need to be taken into account whilst taking a history from a patient.

- Cardiorespiratory status: essential. Explore symptoms, signs and severity of any ischaemic heart disease, heart failure, hypertension, cerebrovascular disease and respiratory disease. Functional status and exercise tolerance are good measures of physiological reserve
- Aspiration risk: hiatus hernia, reflux disease, obesity, opiates (slow gastrointestinal (GI) motility), diabetes (autonomic neuropathy)
- Neck: at risk during laryngoscopy especially if: RA, AS, fixed deformities
- Teeth: at risk during laryngoscopy, caps, crowns, veneers, bridges, loose teeth, chipped teeth
- Airway: note any obvious features that may make intubation difficult. Facial deformities, receding mandible, small mouth, large tongue, obesity, head and neck surgery/radiotherapy, goitre. Patients with a difficult airway or neck may require an awake fibreoptic intubation
- Drugs: beware of stopping antiplatelet agents such as clopidogrel in patients with a recent stent, or warfarin in patients with valves. Discuss with relevant specialist if in doubt.

Investigations

Investigations should be based on the individual and the surgery involved. In general include:

- Full blood count (FBC) (elderly patients, renal disease, surgery associated with large blood loss)
- Cross-match or order blood
- Urea and electrolytes (U&E) (diabetic patients, renal impairment, patients on medication affecting electrolytes, e.g. antihypertensives)
- Clotting studies (anticoagulants; regional anaesthesia to be performed)
- Electrocardiogram (ECG): on every patient with a cardiac history and in males >40yrs and females >50yrs

- CXR should be performed in patients with an acute deterioration of lung function and considered in patients with longstanding respiratory disease. Lung function tests are more useful in the latter group. Also consider in patients where postoperative admission to the intensive care unit (ICU) is likely. Consult local guidelines if in doubt
- Cervical spine X-ray (flexion/extension views): in patients with RA with persistent neck pain or neurological signs and symptoms
- Specialist investigations such as an echocardiogram, a coronary perfusion scan or a coronary angiogram may be required. Contact a senior anaesthetist or refer patient to the anaesthetic clinic if concerned.

Postoperative course
- Does the patient need a high dependency unit (HDU) or an ICU bed? If so, book in advance. Inform anaesthetist ahead of time if such a patient on an elective list.

Preoperative fasting

- 6h for solid food, infant formula or other milk
- 4h for breast milk
- 2h for clear fluids and non-carbonated fluids

Anaesthesia on the day of surgery

Preoperative management

- Ensure patient is adequately fasted
- Elderly patients are often hypovolaemic. ▶Ensure the patient has an adequate intravascular volume and fluid resuscitate with colloid boluses (250–500ml) if depleted. Signs of intravascular depletion include a prolonged capillary refill time, cold peripheries and a tachycardia. Hypotension and low urine output are late signs
- Continue all regular medication. Angiotensin-converting enzyme (ACE) inhibitors are often omitted on the morning of surgery as they can exacerbate hypotension during general and regional anaesthesia. Consult local guidelines
- Patients on long-term steroids should be administered IV steroid (conversion factor)
- Time thromboprophylaxis appropriately. Regional anaesthesia can only be performed 12h after LMWH. It is therefore often prescribed at 6pm. Aspirin does not need to be stopped for regional anaesthesia.

Intraoperative management

- Positioning: careless positioning with either excessive stretching or direct pressure can lead to iatrogenic peripheral nerve injury. The ulnar nerve, brachial plexus and common peroneal nerve are vulnerable areas. Ensure all pressure areas are padded. Head-up position may cause hypotension
- Antibiotic prophylaxis: must be administered prior to tourniquet inflation
- Cementing/reaming. ▶Communicate to anaesthetist ahead of cementing or reaming as this is associated with hypotension. Thought to be due to fat microembolization during reaming rather than the metabolic effects of methylmethacrylate cement. Also known as cement implantation syndrome (pulmonary hypertension, systemic hypotension and hypoxia). Can be fatal.
- Air embolism: increased risk if venous drainage of the surgical site is above the level of the heart
- Tourniquets: tourniquet time is traditionally considered to be 1h for the arm and 1.5h for the leg, with a maximum time regarded as 2h. Associated with significant systemic (cardiorespiratory, metabolic, haematological) and local (nerve, muscle, vascular, skin injury) effects. If procedure time exceeds this, deflate for at least 10min. Ensure padding beneath the cuff. ☞Not to be used in sickle cell anaemia (avoid use in sickle cell trait). ⚠Remember onset of tourniquet pain after 30–45min in awake patients
- Thromboprophylaxis[1]: graduated compression stockings (unless contraindicated, e.g. peripheral vascular disease, severe neuropathy, massive leg oedema) and intermittent pneumatic device or foot pumps
- Normothermia: hypothermia increases surgical complications. Fluid warmer for >500ml infusion and forced air warming device for all procedures >30min
- Blood loss: may be higher in revision surgery, extracapsular hip fractures, spinal surgery and in patients with Paget's disease (hypervascular bone).

Postoperative management

- Oxygen: hypoxaemia is common in the days following hip fracture surgery. Supplement oxygen for three postoperative nights as this is often when cardiovascular complications occur
- Analgesia. World Health Organization (WHO) analgesic ladder. Avoid non-steroidal anti-inflammatory drugs (NSAIDs) in the elderly, diabetic patients and those with renal impairment. Initially reduce dose of all opioids in the elderly and titrate to pain scores
- Thromboprophylaxis: mechanical and pharmacological. Encourage early mobilization
- Fluids and nutrition. Early oral intake and nutrition has been shown to reduce hospital stay. Supplement with intravenous fluids if poor oral intake or if hypovolaemic
- Epidural. This is normally managed by the anaesthetic and pain team.

A few notes on analgesia

- Paracetamol:
  - Good analgesic to have prescribed regularly
  - Multiple routes available: (IV, PO, PR)
  - 1g 4–6 hourly, max 4g/day
- Codeine:
  - Side effects common (nausea, vomiting, constipation)
  - IV route contraindicated
  - 30–60mg 4–6 hourly, max 240mg/day
- Tramadol:
  - An alternative to codeine with fewer opioid side effects
  - Useful in elderly
  - Caution in patients with a history of epilepsy
  - 50–100mg 4–6 hourly, max 600mg/day. PO, IM and IV routes available
- Morphine:
  - Multiple routes available (PO, SC, IM, IV)
  - Avoid prescribing IV morphine 'as required' on drug chart. If needed for acute severe pain, administer in boluses of 2mg and carefully monitor for drowsiness and respiratory depression
  - Morphine SC or IM: 10mg 2–4 hourly
  - Prescribe appropriate oral dose. Parenteral:oral morphine = 1:2, e.g. morphine 10mg SC/IM = 20mg PO
  - Reduce dose in elderly, e.g. by half
- Oxycodone:
  - Strong opioid
  - Oxycodone 5mg PO = morphine 10mg PO
  - Initial dose PO or SC 5mg 4–6 hourly prn
  - Sustained release oral preparation (oxycotin) has a biphasic action—analgesia within 1h which lasts ~12h
  - Initial prescription: 10mg bd regularly.

Reference

1 National Institute for Health and Clinical Excellence. Venous thromboembolism. Reducing the risk of venous thromboembolism (deep vein thrombosis and pulmonary embolism) in inpatients undergoing surgery. http://www.nice.org.uk/nicemedia/pdf/CG046NICEguideline.pdf.

Regional anaesthesia

Regional anaesthesia can be performed for virtually all orthopaedic procedures. It may occur in conjunction with general anaesthesia as a means of pain relief or as the sole method for anaesthesia.

Indications
- Analgesia
- Patient choice: the patient may prefer to have a regional technique
- Where general anaesthesia may be associated with greater patient risk.

Absolute contraindications
- Patient refusal
- Infection at the site of the block
- Coagulopathy: may increase the risk of haematoma formation at the site of the block. In the case of an epidural, this could be disastrous.

Principle

The peripheral nerve(s) supplying the surgical site is/are blocked by use of a local anaesthetic agent, leading to a combined sensory and motor block. This can be done using a central or peripheral technique.

Central techniques involve blocking spinal nerve roots within the vertebral column (spinal or epidural) and peripheral techniques include blocking nerve plexuses or peripheral nerves. Analgesia to a single joint often requires blocking multiple nerves.

Spinal and epidural anaesthesia

In spinal anaesthesia, the dura is punctured and local anaesthetic solution is injected into the subarachnoid space, which contains the spinal cord, spinal nerve roots and CSF. The local anaesthetic mixes with the CSF and acts on the spinal nerve roots, resulting in a dense and rapid onset block. This typically provides 1.5–2h of surgical time, but may take up to 4h for the effects to start wearing off.

In epidural anaesthesia, the dura is not breached and local anaesthetic solution is injected into the epidural space that also contains spinal nerve roots. A larger volume of solution is required and the block is often less dense but has the advantage of allowing a catheter to remain *in situ* for continuous analgesia. A combined spinal epidural technique is often utilized.

▶There is evidence that regional anaesthesia as the sole technique for hip fracture surgery reduces the risk of DVT, blood loss and acute postoperative confusion in the elderly.

Hypotension and epidurals

A common problem that you may encounter on the ward is hypotension in a patient with an epidural. It is important to understand that both spinal and epidural anaesthesia block sympathetic nerves and that this results in vasodilatation. In a patient who is hypovolaemic this could manifest as hypotension, which in most cases improves with restoration of normovol-aemia. If there is a high block involving T1–T4 spinal nerves (cardioaccel-erator fibres), a bradycardia may be noted and the epidural prescription may need adjusting. ▶In all cases, think of other causes of hypotension such as bleeding. ▶▶If there is severe hypotension, stop the epidural, fluid resuscitate and call for help.

Peripheral nerve blocks: a practical approach

Upper limb
- Shoulder, elbow, wrist, hand: brachial plexus block
- Hand: wrist block (ulnar, median, radial nerves)
- Digit: digital nerve block

Lower limb
- Hip:
  - Anaesthesia: spinal, epidural
  - Analgesia: lumbar plexus block (femoral, genitofemoral, lateral cutaneous, obturator nerves), fascia iliaca block (femoral, obturator and lateral cutaneous nerves)
- Knee:
  - Anaesthesia: spinal, epidural, lumbar plexus and sciatic nerve block
  - Analgesia: combined sciatic and femoral nerve block
- Ankle:
  - Anaesthesia: spinal, epidural, sciatic nerve block (+ saphenous nerve block if medial ankle)
  - Analgesia: ankle block (sural, tibial, superficial peroneal, deep peroneal and saphenous nerves)

Postoperative care

Think of the postoperative period in terms of 3 phases in which specific complications and requirements must be considered:

Immediate—recovery ward (ABCs as per ATLS)

- Oxygenation—patient will be given oxygen in recovery ward and should be breathing normally before transfer to the ward
- Perfusion—if compromised consider blood loss during surgery (overt, i.e. recorded losses, drain output, and covert, e.g. bleeding onto drapes, into soft tissue compartments) to maintain adequate circulating volume with appropriate replacement fluid
- Pain and analgesia—may require patient-controlled or intermittent bolus opiate analgesia in liaison with anaesthetic and pain control team
- Confusion—excess opiates, diabetic control, possible myocardial infarction (MI) or cerebrovascular accident (CVA)
- Urinary retention—if catheterization required after prosthetic joint replacement then follow hospital protocol for antibiotic prophylaxis
- Compartment syndrome—always be alert for this (see 📖 p. 402) and split any dressings or splints to skin as a first measure
- Neurovascular status—if compromised consider damage during time of surgery due to knife, retractor, bleeding or tight dressing, prolonged tourniquet time, also nerve blocks. Discuss with operating and anaesthetic team.

Intermediate—inpatient ward

- Prevention of atelectasis or pneumonia—physiotherapy, sit up and mobilize if possible. Likewise for constipation
- Be vigilant for DVT or PE; embolus classically occurs 10 days postoperatively whilst straining at stool, but not always!
- Mobilization with physiotherapist—*motion is the lotion*; axially load the bone to promote healing and maintain bone density, move the joint to prevent contracture and nourish the cartilage, mobilize the patient to prevent atelectasis, pressure ulceration and promote early discharge
- Wound care—often now devolved to nurses; do not repeatedly remove dressings to satisfy your curiosity as this risks contamination
- Definitive splintage once postoperative swelling receding
- Ongoing and step-down analgesia
- Discharge planning—this process should have started prior to admission, executed now by ward nurses, physiotherapists and occupational therapists.

Long term (home or rehabilitation facility)
- Ongoing occupational and physiotherapy
- Monitor wound healing, in collaboration with GP who should know red flag signs of deep infection requiring referral. Early (within 6 weeks), aggressive washout of infected implants provides the best hope of long-term salvage
- Radiographs—use if clinically indicated to alter management or for surveillance; ensure correct views obtained.

Special circumstances
- Beware of patients at the extremes of age—communication difficulties and confusion, reduced cardiorespiratory reserve
- Co-morbidity, e.g. MI in previous year associated with up to 50% mortality after major surgery (so delay if elective). Patients with metastatic disease are at increased risk of embolism especially after intramedullary instrumentation
- Drug and alcohol misuse—may co-exist with musculoskeletal trauma or osteomyelitis; withdrawal may be disruptive and dangerous in this difficult group of patients.

Cardiac disorders[1]

Cardiac disorders are common in the surgical population. Patients may present with ischaemic heart disease, cardiac failure, hypertension, cardiac dysrhythmias, pacemakers or valvular heart disease.

Preoperative assessment of patients with cardiovascular disease is important to:
- Assess perioperative cardiovascular risk
- Optimize the condition of the patient prior to surgery
- Plan type of operation and anaesthesia given
- Arrange for adequate postoperative monitoring and care.

History

Focus on patient's functional ability. Ask about:
- Previous admissions to hospital for cardiac conditions
- Exercise tolerance on flat ground and 'how many flights of stairs can you climb?'
- 'How many pillows do you sleep with at night?' and symptoms of paroxysmal nocturnal dyspnoea
- 'How often do you use your GTN spray?'
- 'What precipitates your angina?'
- Previous blood pressure (BP) readings
- Any history of palpitations
- Pacemakers: type, when it was last checked, potential problems associated with monopolar or bipolar diathermy, what happens if it stops working?

Examination

- Assess pulse: rate, rhythm, character, and volume
- Check blood pressure ± fundi for hypertensive eye disease
- Look for systemic signs of cardiovascular disease, e.g. cyanosis
- Palpate apex beat—is it displaced? Character?
- Auscultate for murmurs, carotid bruits, third/fourth heart sounds (cardiac failure), also lung fields for crepitations and wheeze (failure)
- Look for evidence of peripheral and sacral oedema
- Palpate the abdomen for hepatomegaly or pulsatile liver.

Investigations

- Blood tests: FBC, U&E, clotting screen, lipid profile
- CXR for evidence of pulmonary oedema or pleural effusion
- Twelve-lead ECG
- Exercise ECG—70% sensitivity and specificity for coronary artery disease
- Echocardiography—cardiac structure, ventricular function, ejection fraction
- Dobutamine echocardiography—dobutamine increases oxygen demand and may induce abnormalities in wall motion which are pathognomic of myocardial ischaemia

- Thallium scan—to assess myocardial blood flow
- Coronary angiography—may be indicated in patients with suspected coronary artery disease.

Management

- All cardiac medication with the possible exception of diuretics should be continued until time of surgery
- Arrange urgent anaesthetic review if:
  - MI <6 months ago
  - Unstable angina
  - Severe exercise limitation
  - Poorly controlled congestive cardiac failure
  - Untreated arrhythmias
  - Murmur (request echocardiogram)
  - Systolic BP >200mmHg or diastolic BP >100mmHg
- Perioperative β-blockers have been shown to decrease cardiac complications in high risk patients[2]
- Control hypertension prior to elective surgery. Acute treatment of hypertension reserved for emergency cases only
- Assess and treat arrhythmias: is it supraventricular or ventricular? Is there evidence of heart block? Is the rate >100 beats/min? Is there evidence of decompensation? (systolic BP <90mmHg)
- Tachycardia + hypotension = emergency medical treatment (Advanced Life Support Protocol)
- If evidence of valvular heart disease:
  - Consider local/field blocks or epidural rather than general anaesthetic in fixed cardiac output states such as severe aortic stenosis
  - Antibiotic prophylaxis for patients with valvular disease or prosthetic valves
  - Patients on anticoagulants for prosthetic heart valves who require surgery may need to be converted to an IV heparin infusion prior to surgery which can be stopped 6h prior to surgery if required. Risk of thrombosis is greater with mitral valve replacement compared with aortic valve replacement.

References

1 Hudson J, Wheeler D, Gupta A. Perioperative management of cardiovascular disease. In: *Core Topics in Perioperative Medicine*. London: Greenwich Medical Media, 2004:2–13.

2 Mangano DT, Layug EL, Wallace A, *et al.* Effect of atenolol on mortality and cardiovascular morbidity after noncardiac surgery. Multicenter Study of Perioperative Ischemia Research Group. *N Engl J Med* 1996;**335**:1713–20.

Respiratory disorders[1,2]

Respiratory disease can be divided into:
- Chronic obstructive pulmonary disease (COPD): emphysema, chronic bronchitis
- Asthma
- Suppurative lung disease: bronchiectasis, pneumonia
- Disorders of reduced lung compliance: pulmonary fibrosis
- Disorders of reduced ventilatory capacity: central nervous system (CNS) depression, neuromuscular disorders.

Preoperative assessment

History
- Current functional ability: 'how far can you walk before getting breathless?'
- 'How often do you use your inhalers?'
- Use of home oxygen and nebulizers?
- Previous admissions to hospital with respiratory problems
- Ever needed intubation or intensive therapy unit (ITU)? Ever had CPAP (continuous positive airway pressure) or BiPAP (biphasic intermittent positive airway pressure)?
- Current treatment—does this include steroids?
- Smoking history
- Previous anaesthetics.

Examination
- Observe for cyanosis, use of accessory muscles of breathing, pursed lip breathing, chest wall deformities
- Inspect, percuss and auscultate chest for crepitations, wheeze, effusions
- Examine for cor pulmonale: right ventricular heave, 3rd heart sound, hepatomegaly, peripheral oedema.

Investigations
- Peak expiratory flow rate: pre- and postbronchodilators
- Spirometry and pulmonary function tests to assess lung capacities
- Pulse oximetry
- 12-lead ECG
- CXR
- FBC for haemoglobin estimation and white cell count in infections
- Arterial blood gas (ABG)—for evidence of respiratory failure.

Preoperative optimization
- Smoking cessation: even 24h will improve oxygen-carrying capability of blood
- Chest physiotherapy to clear secretions both pre- and postoperatively
- Continue regular medications—if on long-term steroids as may need IV hydrocortisone perioperatively to avoid Addisonian crisis
- Medical consultation if inadequate control on current medications
- Treat any current infections, prophylactic antibiotics in bronchiectasis
- Consider booking HDU or ITU bed.

Postoperative management

- Supplemental oxygen; controlled oxygen therapy via a Venturi© mask may be indicated in patients with COPD who retain carbon dioxide
- Restart regular medication promptly
- Analgesia paramount to facilitate coughing and movement
- Monitor patients on opiates postoperatively for respiratory depression
- Chest physiotherapy
- Nutrition instituted as soon as possible—nasogastric feeding may be required
- Monitor for signs of barotrauma postintubation in patients with COPD, e.g. ruptured emphysematous bulla leading to pneumothorax.

References

1 Stanton K, Ghosh S. Perioperative management of respiratory disease. *Surgery* 2005;**23**: 235–8.
2 Hudson J, Wheeler D, Gupta A. Perioperative management of respiratory disease. In: *Core Topics in Perioperative Medicine*. London: Greenwich Medical Media, 2004:14–18.

Gastrointestinal disorders[1]

Perioperative problems in patients with gastrointestinal disorders can be grouped as follows:

Fluid and electrolyte imbalances

- May be due to diarrhoea, vomiting or fluid sequestration secondary to postoperative ileus
- Assess fluid status clinically; ask about symptoms of thirst and oliguria
- Examine for dehydration: decreased skin turgor, sunken eyes, tachycardia, reduced jugular venous pressure (JVP), hypotension, decreased urine output
- Monitor if necessary with:
  - Strict input/output fluid balance charts
  - Hourly urine output—aim for output of >0.5ml/kg/h
  - Central venous pressure (CVP) if indicated (requires central line)
- Investigations include blood tests: FBC for haemoglobin and haematocrit, U&E, plasma osmolality, ABG for acidosis in acute renal failure
- Treatment is by fluid resuscitation and correction of electrolyte imbalances with addition of potassium as required.

Nutritional failure or protein calorie malnutrition

- May be the result of:
  - Catabolic response to trauma
  - Chronic inflammatory bowel disease (IBD)
  - Prolonged ileus
  - Elderly patient with co-morbidities
  - Patient unable to tolerate oral intake
- Effects of malnutrition include:
  - Delayed ambulation postoperatively
  - Respiratory complications
  - Hypoalbuminaemia leading to pulmonary oedema
  - Wound infections
  - Reduced immunity
- Consider perioperative nutritional support in liaison with dieticians
- Enteral feeding is always preferable to parenteral nutrition. If enteral feeding is not possible, ordering of total parenteral nutrition and arrangement for central venous access should be pre-empted.

Respiratory problems

- May occur as a result of diaphragmatic splinting secondary to abdominal distension due to ileus. Also secondary to aspiration of gastric contents, especially in elderly
- Management involves:
  - Resuscitation
  - Decompression of bowel/prevention of aspiration by insertion of nasogastric tube
  - Early treatment of lower respiratory tract infections with antibiotics (remember anaerobic cover if suspected aspiration pneumonia).

Sepsis

May be secondary to gastroenteritis, antibiotic-associated diarrhoea or primary bacterial peritonitis (translocation of bacteria across the intestinal wall) which can lead to a systemic inflammatory response syndrome and multiorgan failure. Principles of management include:

- Resuscitation
- Avoid long-term antibiotics
- Restoration of gut flora by re-instituting oral feeds as soon as patient is able
- Use of probiotics is controversial
- Treat sepsis early[2].

Drug issues

- Enteral route may not be available perioperatively and drug absorption may be altered
- Important medications such as antiepileptics and cardiac medications may be switched to parenteral route.

Other issues to consider include:

- Patients with gastro-oesophageal reflux disease—should be given proton pump inhibitor or a histamine-2 receptor antagonist 2–6h preoperatively.
- Patients with IBD should have adequate hydration, correction of anaemia and may need perioperative steroid cover
- Obesity is a common problem; inform anaesthetist preoperatively.

References

1 Davies DWL, Ziyad A. Perioperative management of gastrointestinal disorders. *Surgery* 2005;**23**:250–6.
2 Rivers E, Nguyen B, Havstad S, *et al.* Early goal directed therapy in the treatment of severe sepsis and septic shock. *N Engl J Med* 2001;**345**:1368–77.

Hepatobiliary disorders

Hepatobiliary disorders can present a number of challenges in the perioperative period.

Chronic liver failure

Surgery should only be undertaken after careful consultation with a gastroenterologist and anaesthetist. These patients may have a number of problems to address prior to surgery:
- Portal hypertension leading to oesophageal varices and risk of gastrointestinal haemorrhage
- Impaired synthesis of clotting factors leading to coagulopathy
- Electrolyte abnormalities including dilutional hyponatraemia
- Risk of hepatic encephalopathy
- Nutritional problems.

History

Ask about:
- Cause of liver failure—alcohol, haemochromatosis, viral hepatitis, autoimmune, drugs
- Previous hospital admissions
- Complete drug history—any hepatotoxic medications?
- Previous history of GI haemorrhage
- Any history suggestive of hepatic encephalopathy?

Examination
- Look for peripheral stigmata of chronic liver disease including: jaundice, spider naevi, encephalopathic tremor, gynaecomastia, leukonychia
- Examine for flapping tremor, anaemia, raised JVP, caput medusae, ascites, hepatomegaly
- Mini-Mental Test score for encephalopathy.

Investigations
- FBC for haemoglobin estimation
- U&E; may show hyponatraemia
- Liver function tests (LFTs) including γ-glutamyltransferase
- Clotting screen: including APTT and PT/international normalized ratio (INR)
- Blood glucose for associated risk of both diabetes mellitus and hypoglycaemia
- Hepatitis serology
- USS abdomen and Doppler studies of portal vein.

Management
- Involve gastroenterologist
- Adequate fluid resuscitation paramount to avoid hepatorenal syndrome and acute renal failure, but give with caution in ascites
- Should be on gastric protection for increased risk of peptic ulceration
- Address nutritional status preoperatively and plan postoperative nutritional care early

- Treat coagulopathies with replacement of clotting factors using fresh frozen plasma (FFP) and IV vitamin K
- Avoid hepatotoxic medications
- Avoid encephalopathy in susceptible individuals by decreasing protein intake. Administration of oral neomycin and lactulose may also be necessary after consultation with medical team.

Obstructive jaundice

Any patient presenting with preoperative jaundice should have their surgery postponed until the cause has been elicited.

Principles of management include:
- Involve gastroenterologist and general surgeon
- Fluid resuscitation
- Antibiotics to prevent ascending cholangitis
- Correct clotting by administering 1mg of IV vitamin K
- FFP for active bleeding
- Investigate underlying cause by performing an ultrasound scan of the liver and biliary tree and proceed to endoscopic retrograde cholangiopancreatography (ERCP) if indicated.

Endocrine disorders[1,2]

Diabetes mellitus

Diabetes may be undiagnosed until a random blood glucose is performed at a preoperative assessment. Alternatively, pre-existing diabetes may be controlled by either diet alone, oral hypoglycaemic agents or insulin therapy.

Preoperative preparation of patients with diabetes mellitus

- Check U&E and glycated haemoglobin (HbA1c)—indicates glycaemic control over previous 8 weeks. Ideally should be <6.5%, although up to 8% is satisfactory
- Assess patient for signs of macrovascular diabetic complications: evidence of peripheral vascular, ischaemic heart and cerebrovascular disease
- Assess for signs of microvascular disease by performing urine dipstick for proteinuria or microalbuminuria, examine fundi for diabetic retinopathy and examine for peripheral neuropathy.

Perioperative management

- Place diabetics first on operating list if possible
- Diet-controlled diabetes:
  - Fast according to usual anaesthetic instructions, should not require insulin sliding scale
- Patients treated with oral hypoglycaemic agents:
  - Morning theatre list: fast from midnight, omit tablets on morning of surgery, start insulin sliding scale (see Table 3.2) at 7am on morning of surgery
  - Afternoon theatre list: fast from 8am, normal tablets before an early breakfast but consult anaesthetist if patient on long-acting sulphonylurea, e.g. glibenclamide (may need to be stopped). Start insulin sliding scale at 11am on day of surgery
- Patients on insulin therapy. Patients on long-acting insulin may need to stop this night before surgery. Ensure good IV access. Otherwise:
  - Morning list: fast from midnight, omit morning insulin, start insulin sliding scale at 7am on morning of surgery
  - Afternoon list: fast from 8am, may have one half of usual insulin dose before an early breakfast. Start insulin sliding scale at 11am
- Monitor blood glucose 2 hourly in the perioperative period
- For minor ops, consult anaesthetist—may not require sliding scales
- Medications can be restarted when patient able to eat and drink again. Generally insulin-dependent patients are given first postoperative dose of subcutaneous insulin before first meal and insulin sliding scale is stopped 30min after meal.

Adrenal failure

- Cortisol is not secreted in response to stress such as surgery, leading to Addisonian crisis
- Causes include 1° Addison's disease, adrenal failure secondary to pituitary pathology or sudden steroid withdrawal

- Patient should be discussed with anaesthetist and arrangements made for perioperative IV hydrocortisone administration. Usually continued 50–100mg 6 hourly for 24–48h postoperatively
- If patient presents as emergency with an Addisonian crisis, ensure adequate fluid rehydration, correction of electrolyte abnormalities and administration of parenteral hydrocortisone.

Thyroid problems

- Ideally, patients should be euthyroid prior to elective surgery
- Hypothyroid patients may be admitted to hospital on levothyroxine therapy. Levothyroxine has a long half-life and may be safely omitted while the patient is nil by mouth prior to surgery
- Hyperthyroidism may be treated prior to surgery with carbimazole or propylthiouracil.

Table 3.2 Example of insulin sliding scale

Blood glucose (mmol/l)	Insulin dose (units/h)	Action
<2.0	None	Give Glucogel® gel or 50% glucose IV. Inform medical team
2–4.0	None	
4.1–6.0	1 unit/h	
6.1–9.0	2 units/h	
9.1–11.0	3 units/h	
11.1–13.0	4 units/h	
13.1–15.0	5 units/h	
>15	6 units/h	Inform endocrine team if persistent problem

50 units of soluble insulin, e.g. Actrapid® in 50ml of 0.9% saline. Given with IV infusion of 5–10% glucose with 20mmol/l of potassium chloride over 8h (refer to local hospital protocol). Aim for blood glucose of 4–7mmol/l (adequate <10mmol/l). Check blood glucose hourly and adjust.

References

1 Ward A, Gatling W. Perioperative management of endocrine disease (including diabetes). *Surgery* 2005;**23**:250–6.
2 Hudson J, Wheeler D, Gupta A. Perioperative management of endocrine disorders and perioperative management of diabetes. In: *Core Topics in Perioperative Medicine* London: Greenwich Medical Media, 2004:74–98.

Neurological disorders[1]

Patients with neurological disorders are at risk of a number of problems in the perioperative period:

- Respiratory complications: ventilatory abnormalities secondary to bulbar weakness, inability to clear secretions, weakness of respiratory muscles, and risk of aspiration leading to lower respiratory tract infections
- Cerebral hypoperfusion: cerebral autoregulation may be impaired due to underlying brain injury, patients also have an increased risk of atherosclerotic blood vessels. Cerebral hypoperfusion may also occur as a result of perioperative hypotension
- Autonomic dysfunction associated with certain neurological disorders: including vasomotor instability in response to sympathetic stimulation, postural change, and arrhythmias
- Increased intracranial pressure
- Deep venous thromboembolism: consider heparin prophylaxis in patients without an intracranial bleed
- Increased risk of prosthetic joint dislocation.

Cerebrovascular accidents

- Patients with a CVA requiring surgery should have their emergency operation delayed for at least 2 weeks following the CVA. Elective surgery should be postponed for at least 2 months
- In the preoperative period, risk factors for CVA including hypertension and atrial fibrillation should be treated and controlled
- In patients with symptomatic cerebrovascular disease, bilateral carotid Dopplers should be performed. If >70% stenosis of the common carotid artery and symptomatic, refer to a vascular surgeon (carotid endarterectomy may be indicated)
- Aspirin may be continued up to surgery—consult surgeon and anaesthetist. Clopidogrel should be stopped 7 days prior to surgery.

Epilepsy

- It is important to ascertain severity of epilepsy from history:
  - When was your last seizure?
  - How often do you get seizures?
  - Seizure type
  - Response to previous anaesthetics
  - Current drug therapy
- Ascertain drug levels prior to surgery to ensure within therapeutic range
- Make anaesthetist aware to avoid drugs which may induce seizures
- Continue anticonvulsants in the perioperative period (even if parenteral route required).

Multiple sclerosis

This demyelinating disorder may be associated with a number of problems in the postoperative period. Take a full history to:

• Determine pattern of relapses and how the disorder affects patient's daily life
• Elicit problems: include spasticity, ocular problems, neuropathic bladder, paraesthesia and limb weakness
• Drug history—current medications including steroids.

Perioperative care should include detail to:

• Respiratory function: can be assessed preoperatively by pulmonary function tests and optimized prior to surgery
• Current medication—if on steroids inform anaesthetist; may need perioperative IV cover
• Sudden withdrawal from baclofen (used for spasticity) may precipitate seizures
• Postoperative urinary retention: may need a urinary catheter in perioperative period (inform patient)
• DVT prophylaxis.

Parkinson's disease

Patients may have associated autonomic dysfunction, rigidity and restrictive lung disease. Important to continue perioperative anti-Parkinsonian drug treatment. Antiemetics such as metoclopramide, which are dopamine antagonists, should be avoided postoperatively as they may exacerbate symptoms.

Dementia

Treat any reversible causes of dementia including alcohol or drug abuse and hypothyroidism.

Important issues include:

• Optimization of medical co-morbidities
• Malnutrition
• Inability to give informed consent
• Increased risk of postoperative confusion.

Reference

1 Fong JJ, Dunsmore J. Perioperative management of neurological and psychiatric conditions. *Surgery* 2005;**23**:258–62.

Haematological disorders

Involve haematologists early in the management of these patients.

Anaemia

Reduction in the haemoglobin concentration (<13.5g/dl for men and <11.5g/dl for women). May be classified according to:

- Mean cell volume (MCV) normal range 76–96fl:
  - Microcytic anaemia, e.g. iron deficiency, thalassaemia
  - Normocytic anaemia, e.g. anaemia of chronic disease
  - Macrocytic anaemia: vitamin B12 and folate deficiency, hypothyroidism, alcohol consumption
- Haemolytic anaemia; red cell membrane defects, enzyme defects or haemoglobinopathies.

Preoperative transfusion of packed red blood cells may be required in patients with a haemoglobin concentration of ≤7g/dl. Threshold may be raised if patient has concomitant systemic disease, e.g. ischaemic heart disease, or is symptomatic of their anaemia, i.e. short of breath, decreased oxygen saturations or hypotension.

Blood transfusion should be completed 2 days preoperatively and an individualized approach should be adopted (especially in renal failure).

Sickle cell anaemia

Individuals carry haemoglobin S (HbS) which is insoluble in the deoxygenated state, leading to vaso-occlusive, visceral sequestration or aplastic crises. A sickle crisis may occur secondary to hypoxia, dehydration or acidosis.

- Identify patients at risk of sickle cell disease (SCD) or trait by a sickle test prior to surgery on all patients of Afro-Caribbean descent
- Consult haematologist and anaesthetist prior to surgery
- Elicit disease severity from the history:
  - Number of admissions to hospital with crisis
  - History of chest crisis or stroke secondary to sickle cell sequestration; if so, inform anaesthetist urgently prior to surgery
  - Current drug treatment
- Patients with SCD may have a resting haemoglobin level of 7–9g/dl; transfusion is rarely indicated
- Important factors in perioperative care include warmth, adequate hydration, analgesia, avoidance of hypoxia and use of antibiotic prophylaxis (as most patients will have autoinfarcted the spleen at a young age). May also have increased analgesic requirements
- Avoid tourniquets during surgery as can precipitate sickling
- Sickle cell trait is usually asymptomatic, but again inform anaesthetist.

Thalassaemia

Patients with thalassaemia often require multiple blood transfusions and therefore are at risk of iron overload. Involve haematologist early in care and inform anaesthetist.

Bleeding tendencies

Haemophilia A

Deficiency of factor VIII leading to coagulopathy. Surgery undertaken only after consultation with haematologist and patient's haemophilia centre.

Issues in care include:
- Administration of factor VIII concentrate prior to and during surgery
- Drugs such as desmopressin (causes rise in endogenous factor VIII)
- Avoidance of aspirin and intramuscular injections.

von Willebrand's disease (vWD)

A family of bleeding disorders caused by abnormality of von Willebrand factor (vWF) gene (Erik Adolf von Willebrand described it in 1926).

vWF carries factor VIII in plasma and mediates platelet adhesion. Deficiency causes prolonged APTT; PT normal.

Management includes:
- Desmopressin for mild bleeding
- Factor VIII concentrate or cryoprecipitate for excessive bleeding
- Fibrinolytic inhibitors, e.g. tranexamic acid may also be helpful.

Thrombocytopenia

Reduction in platelet count ($<140\times10^9$/l). May be idiopathic or secondary to bone marrow failure or increased consumption.
- Platelet transfusion may be required if platelet count $<50\times10^9$/l prior to surgery (aim for count of 100×10^9/l preoperatively)
- Steroids may be useful in idiopathic thrombocytopenic purpura.

Patients on warfarin

- Warfarin is a long-acting oral anticoagulant with a half-life of 30h
- Stop warfarin 3–5 days prior to elective surgery and check INR preoperatively (should be <1.5). Usually restarted postoperatively
- If patient requires perioperative anticoagulation (e.g. mechanical heart valve), commence heparin infusion 24h after last dose of warfarin and stop 6h prior to surgery (monitor PT and APTT ratios).

Emergency surgery for patients on warfarin
- Anticoagulation reversed (after discussion with haematologist) with administration of FFP and IV vitamin K.

Thrombophilia

Surgical patients are at risk of DVT and PE.

Screen for thrombophilia if: positive family history, recurrent thromboses, females with recurrent fetal loss. Most common condition is factor V Leiden deficiency, which affects 5% of population (risk of thrombosis increased 100-fold in homozygotes).
- Ensure adequate thromboprophylaxis—usually subcutaneous injections of LMWHs.

Spinal infections

Pyogenic spinal infection

Can be thought of as a spectrum of disease comprising spondylitis (vertebral inflammation), discitis, spondylodiscitis, pyogenic facet arthropathy and epidural abscess[1]. *Staphylococcus aureus*, the main organism, infection elsewhere the most common predisposing factor. Consider also Gram negatives (*Escherichia coli*, *Pseudomonas* spp, *Proteus*), anaerobes, MRSA (methicillin-resistant *S. aureus*) and fungal infection if immunocompromised. Haematogenous spread may occur via Batson's venous plexus between pelvic and vertebral circulation.

Risk factors

- Age >50yrs
- Immunodeficiency
- Pneumonia, urinary tract infection (UTI) or skin infection
- IV drug addicts (*Pseudomonas*).

Clinical features

Triad of **fever, back pain and tenderness**. Lumbar spine most commonly affected, higher incidence of paralysis if cervical or thoracic. Neurological deficit suggests epidural abscess requiring prompt surgical decompression. Look for associated endocarditis.

Investigation

- Plain X-ray—early disc space narrowing, osteolysis after 6 weeks
- MRI (with gadolinium)—to define involvement, thecal sac compression; aids differentiation from malignancy
- Tissue biopsy—mandatory, especially if blood cultures negative
- Tuberculin skin test.

Management

If possible obtain bacterial diagnosis prior to treatment with IV followed by oral antibiotics for 3 months. Monitor response clinically and with serial ESR and CRP. Surgery indicated for spinal instability, epidural abscess with neurological deficit or failure of medical management.

Epidural abscess

Initial radicular pain with progression to paralysis. Mortality rate is 12%.

Risk factors: immunocompromise, malignancy, diabetes mellitus, alcohol abuse, invasive procedures and vertebral fractures.

Rapid surgical decompression mandatory.

Spinal tuberculosis[2]

50% of all skeletal TB seen in spine. Associated active focus, e.g. pulmonary TB found in <10%. At-risk groups in developed world: recent immigrants, HIV (human immunodeficiency virus) patients, homeless, alcohol and drug abusers, medical professionals.

Clinical features

Presentation usually non-specific and insidious: fever, night sweats, anorexia, and weight loss. Local and then referred pain may follow.

Investigations

- High ESR and possibly white blood cell count
- CXR and tuberculin skin test and quantiferon gold assay
- Biopsy (Ziel–Neelsen stain); cultures visible after 4 weeks
- Plain radiographs; various patterns of involvement
- MRI—delineates extent of involvement, soft tissue mass and extension under anterior and posterior longitudinal ligaments
- Tissue biopsy for histological diagnosis if in doubt.

Clinical course

Vertebral body destruction, progressive deformity ± neurological deficit. Disc destruction occurs early; fusion of bodies above/below may follow. *Cold abscess* is an infected exudate which spreads under the anterior longitudinal ligament (seen in >50%, almost pathognomic). Chemotherapy can arrest changes and expedite consolidation/fusion.

Treatment

Ambulant chemotherapy in 2 phases: intensive (2 months) with 3–4 drugs and continuation (9–12 months) with 2 drugs. Surgery only for progressive deformity, paraplegic complications, or recurrent disease. Most abscesses, however large, clear adequately with chemotherapy, and surgical intervention is rarely required.

References

1 Hadjipavlou AG, Mader JT, Necessary JT, *et al.* Hematogenous pyogenic spinal infections and their surgical management. *Spine* 2000;**25**:1668–79.

2 Rajasekaran R, Shanmugasandarum TK. Spinal tuberculosis. In: Bulstrode C, Buckwater J, Carr A, *et al.*, eds. *Oxford Textbook of Orthopaedics and Trauma.* Oxford: Oxford University Press, 2002:1545–60.

Tetanus

Potentially fatal disease preventable by appropriate immunization.

Exotoxins produced by *Clostridium tetani* (large Gram-positive spore-forming bacillus which is strictly anaerobic) block anterior horn cells of the spinal cord and brainstem causing muscle spasm and hyper-reflexia. Additionally exotoxins are cardiotoxic and cause haemolysis.

Infection via a skin break or mucosal surface. At-risk factors for any wound:
- Deep contamination
- Delay to treatment
- Devitalized, ischaemic tissue
- Co-existent infection with another organism (synergistic infection).

Clinical features
- Pain and stiffness of the jaw
- Generalized facial rigidity
- Rigidity of body musculature causing spinal extension
- Reflex spasms
- Convulsive seizures
- Autonomic dysfunction.

Prophylaxis
Previous immunization

If >10yrs from immunization, give booster of tetanus toxoid for any wound.

Uncertain immunization status

Give human antitoxin (250 units intramuscularly), in addition to toxoid.

Management of tetanus
- Assess ABCs to determine if ventilation and circulatory support are required. Otherwise nurse in quiet environment with careful use of diazepam for spasms (beware respiratory depression)
- 3000–10 000 units IV of human hyperimmune globulin to neutralize circulating toxin. Treat *C. tetani* infection with IV penicillin or tetracycline
- Wound debridement and lavage after obtaining microbiology specimens.

HIV and AIDS in orthopaedics

AIDS is an immune-deficient state associated with HIV

The immune deficiency syndrome may be complicated by *Pneumocystis carinii* pneumonia and Kaposi's sarcoma (nodules or blotches under the skin or in mucous membranes, caused by HHV-8). First recognized in the USA in 1981, causative virus identified in 1983.

May present to orthopaedic surgeons as part of the following[1].

Trauma

Polytrauma: worse outcome from acute lung injury and adult respiratory distress syndrome. Risk of secondary infection is increased, and impaired nutritional status adversely affects the catabolic phase after polytrauma.

Closed fractures: increased risk of infection after internal fixation with late sepsis around implants. *S. aureus* is the most common infecting organism; unusual bacteria/fungi not commonly reported. Delayed or non-union secondary to altered inflammatory response of immunocompromised patients. Whether to remove implants after union to reduce the chance of late sepsis is unclear.

Open fractures: high frequency of wound infections.

Arthroplasty

Unlike trauma implants, joint replacements must be retained once implanted. Due to relative young age of AIDS population, joint replacement is uncommon, with the exception of the haemophiliac population (HIV transmitted via contaminated factor VIII). In this group requiring arthroplasty for haemophilic arthropathy there is a significant rate of late joint sepsis which increases each year postoperatively. The use of antiretroviral therapy is likely to improve outcomes.

Reference

1 Harrison WJ. HIV/AIDS in trauma and orthopaedic surgery. *J Bone Joint Surg Br* 2005;**87**: 1178–81.

Decision making in care of patients with bone and soft tissue tumours

Primary bone and soft tissue tumours are uncommon (<1% of all malignancies). They are best managed in specialist centres by multidisciplinary teams. Varied presentations include: pain, diffuse swelling, discrete mass, neurological or vascular compromise, pathological fracture or as an incidental radiographic finding. In all age groups infection and metabolic bone disease can mimic tumours; in older age groups consider metastatic bone deposits. Investigations aim to obtain a diagnosis, histological grade and stage the spread of the tumour.

History and examination
- Age
- Sex
- Site of lump
- Past history.

Breast, bowel, lung, thyroid, kidney and prostate cancers have a predisposition to metastasize to bone, so these areas should be examined in addition to the liver.

Factors suggesting a malignant lump[1]
- Size >5cm
- Pain at night
- Increase in size
- Deep to deep fascia.

Blood investigations and urinalysis
- FBC and film for leukaemia
- ESR and CRP
- Bone chemistry (calcium, phosphate, liver enzymes and ALP)
- Acid phosphatase
- TFTs (thyroid function tests)
- PSA (prostate-specific antigen)
- Serum protein electrophoresis and urinalysis for Bence-Jones protein (myeloma).

Plain radiographic diagnosis[2]
Age of patient, size and site of lesion within skeleton and then bone (epiphyseal, metaphyseal and diaphyseal, intramedullary, cortical or surface, central or eccentric). Majority of bone tumours are metaphyseal and intramedullary; distal femur, proximal tibia and proximal humerus are common sites.

Describe appearance under the following subheadings:
- Matrix, e.g. cartilage- or bone-forming
- Margin (zone of transition)—well (benign) or poorly defined (malignant)

- Periosteal reaction
- Cortical response
- Soft tissue mass.

Further imaging

- MRI—characterization and staging, e.g. skip lesions, vessel involvement
- CT—further characterization, e.g. osteoid osteoma or to guide biopsy
- USS—to guide biopsy, assess soft tissue mass or look for abdominal secondaries
- CXR or CT chest—for metastases or primary if bone metastasis
- Bone scan—for skeletal metastases
- Abdominal US—visceral metastases
- Angiography or MRA for surgical planning or preoperative embolization.

Biopsy

For histological diagnosis and grade; should be performed in the specialist centre:

- In line of subsequent exposure to facilitate excision of biopsy track at definitive surgery
- Longitudinally through (involved) rather than between muscle compartments to prevent seeding
- Avoiding joint capsule
- Radiological guidance as required
- Adequate size and orientation of sample (consider frozen section to confirm)
- Meticulous haemostasis (tourniquet without exsanguination).

Management

Aim to remove lesion with minimum risk of local recurrence and acceptable risk of complications, e.g. fracture, neurovascular damage. Increasingly, limb salvage procedures preferred to amputation with malignant bone tumours, e.g. osteosarcoma, Ewing's tumour[3] for which neoadjuvant chemotherapy has transformed survival. Large bone defects created by radical resection can be reconstructed with endoprostheses or allograft/allograft–cement composites. Soft tissue reconstruction may require local or distant soft tissue transfer by a plastic surgeon.

References

1 Damron TA, Beauchamp CP, Rougraff BT, *et al.* Soft tissue lumps and bumps. *Instr Course Lect* 2004;**53**:625–37.
2 Helms CA. *Fundamentals of Skeletal Radiology*, 2nd edn. Phildelphia, PA: Saunders.
3 Simon MA, Aschliman MA, Thomas N, *et al.* Limb-salvage treatment versus amputation for osteosarcoma of the distal end of the femur. *J Bone Joint Surg Am* 1986;**68**:1331–7.

Oncological emergencies

Cord compression

Clinical signs of spinal cord compression (disturbance of bladder or bowel function, altered lower limb neurology, perianal anaesthesia) with known or presumed malignancy is a surgical emergency requiring urgent MRI of the whole spine. Causes include: enlarging extradural mass, angular deformity secondary to vertebral collapse, vertebral dislocation from pathological fracture.

IV high dose steroids (dexamethasone) can reduce vasogenic oedema, giving temporary benefit.

Most metastatic disease can be treated with external beam irradiation.

Indications for surgery are:
• Disease progression despite radiotherapy
• Anterior and posterior column disease with spinal instability
• Anterior disease with cord compression
• Tissue biopsy required for histological diagnosis.

Contraindications as follows:
• More than one area of epidural compression
• Inadequate bone stock
• Life expectancy less than 3 months.

Hypercalcaemia

Seen in the following malignancies:
• Solid tumours with bone metastases
• Humoral hypercalcaemia of malignancy
• Haematological malignancy, e.g. myeloma.

>3.5mmol/l is a medical emergency; symptoms and signs
• Nocturia, polyuria, thirst
• Nausea, anorexia, constipation
• Depression, confusion, psychosis
• Dehydration.

Treatment
• Early recognition
• Copious fluid rehydration (beware if renal failure in myeloma) ± CVP and urinary catheter
• Consider furosemide (increased renal calcium excretion), monitor electrolytes (potassium and magnesium)
• Need to block excessive bone resorption with appropriate bisphosphonate, e.g. pamidronate, clodronate
• Judicious use of steroids in myeloma, sarcoidosis.

Pathological fracture

Impending fracture around a metastatic deposit in a long bone requires prompt prophylactic nailing ± radiotherapy. Mirels signs are a useful guide to fracture risk:

	1	2	3
Site	Upper limb	Lower limb	Peritrochanteric
Pain	Mild	Moderate	Functional
Lesion	Blastic	Mixed	Lytic
% shaft diameter	<1/3	1/3–2/3	>2/3

Total score: 7 = 5% fracture risk; 8 = 15% fracture risk; 9 = 33% fracture risk.
Mirels suggests fixation for score >9[1].

Reference

1 Mirels H. Metastatic disease in long bones. A proposed scoring system for diagnosing impending pathologic fractures. *Clin Orthop Relat Res.*1989;**249**:256–64.

Adjuvant therapy and palliative care in musculoskeletal malignancy

Chemotherapy

Chemical agents given systemically which preferentially kill tumour cells. Neoadjuvant (given prior to surgical resection) chemotherapy commonly used to reduce tumour mass and vascularity in osteosarcoma and Ewing's sarcoma. Restage post-therapy and assess tumour 'kill rate', which is prognostic for patient survival. Further chemotherapy can be given after surgery once soft tissues have healed. Complications include physeal damage, osteoporosis (OP), AVN, 2° malignancy and organ toxicity (heart, kidneys and nervous system).

Radiotherapy

Ionizing radiation causes damage by rupture of chemical bonds linking complex molecules and formation of free radicals which inhibit cell reproduction. Normal tissue has greater potential for recovery and repair than tumour cells. Can use preoperatively to reduce tumour mass or as adjuvant therapy to kill residual microscopic disease. Can dramatically reduce rates of local recurrence, facilitating limb salvage surgery. Complications include joint and soft tissue stiffness, inflammation of bladder, bowel and liver, hair loss and lymphoedema, 2° malignancy.

Palliative care

Care is best achieved in a multidisciplinary environment to address the patient's and relatives' physical and psychological needs. Radiotherapy and bisphosphonates may be indicated to reduce bone pain. Early introduction of opiate analgesia with appropriate antiemetics and aperients is important.

Congenital disorders

These are any abnormality or anomaly which is present at birth. The causes of congenital disorders may be genetic or environmental. Embryonic limb bud development occurs between the 4th and 8th intrauterine week, and insults at this critical time are responsible for some of these abnormalities. The cause of others remains unknown.

Orthopaedic congenital disorders may occur in isolation or be associated with other musculoskeletal anomalies, or with anomalies in other organ systems, e.g. the VACTERL association—**V**ertebral, **A**norectal, **C**ardiac, **T**racheo-o**e**sophageal, **R**enal and **L**imb abnormalities. Other syndromes include Holt–Oram (cardiac and upper limb defects) and thrombocytopenia–absent radius (TAR).

Upper limb disorders have an accepted classification system which can be a useful way of thinking about abnormalities in other areas also.

Classification of congenital upper limb abnormalities[1]

- Failure of formation of parts
- Transverse arrest—amputations occurring at any level
- Longitudinal arrest—radial, ulnar, central or segmental deficiencies
- Failure of differentiation (separation) of parts
- Soft tissue, e.g. arthrogryposis, Sprengel shoulder, absent muscles, simple syndactyly
- Skeletal, e.g. synostoses (elbow, forearm, carpus), complex syndactyly, clinodactyly
- Congenital tumorous conditions, e.g. arteriovenous malformations
- Duplication—of all or part of a limb (most commonly extra digits)
- Overgrowth—of all or part of a limb (e.g. hemihypertrophy, macrodactyly)
- Undergrowth, e.g. radial hypoplasia, brachydactyly
- Constriction ring syndromes
- Generalized disorders—chromosomal abnormalities or other causes.

Lower limb disorders—examples

- Developmental dysplasia of the hip (see 📖 p. 516)
- Proximal femoral focal deficiency (PFFD)
- Congenital knee dislocation
- Tibial bowing
- Congenital pseudarthrosis of the tibia
- Fibular hemimelia (see 📖 p. 527)
- Congenital vertical talus (see 📖 p. 538)
- Clubfoot (see 📖 p. 536)
- Metatarsus adductus (see 📖 p. 547).

Spine disorders—examples

- Congenital kyphosis or scoliosis—due to defects in segmentation, such as hemivertebrae
- Spina bifida
- Intraspinal abnormalities, e.g. Chiari malformation, tethered cord, diastematomyelia (split cord).

General disorders—examples

- Skeletal dysplasias, e.g. osteogenesis imperfecta, multiple epiphyseal dysplasia
- Progressive neuromuscular disease, e.g. muscular dystrophies
- Chromosomal abnormalities e.g. Down syndrome.

Reference

1 Swanson AB. A classification for congenital limb malformations. *J Hand Surg* 1976;1A:8–22.

Acquired disorders

These are disorders not present at birth, but that develop at some time thereafter (cf. Congenital disorders).

Use of a 'surgical sieve' facilitates thinking about the possible causes of acquired conditions. Below are the categories with some orthopaedic examples.

- Traumatic—fractures, tendon ruptures
- Infective—osteomyelitis, pyomyositis
- Neoplastic
  - Benign—osteoid osteoma, osteochondroma
  - Malignant—osteogenic sarcoma, chondrosarcoma
- Idiopathic—Paget's disease
- Metabolic—osteomalacia
- Iatrogenic—drug side effects, trochanteric bursitis after total hip replacement (THR)
- Degenerative—osteoarthritis, degenerative spondylolisthesis
- Vascular—Perthes disease
- Neurogenic—scoliosis in muscular dystrophy, CP
- Autoimmune—RA, lupus
- Drugs and alcohol—osteonecrosis of femoral head
- Inflammatory—RA.

Perioperative care

Pain control

Adequate pain control at rest is important on humane grounds, but also to reduce the stress response to injury or surgery and facilitate early motion, preventing unnecessary swelling and joint stiffness. Science of pain control would fill a larger text than this, but simple management measures include:

- Proper and early immobilization of fractures
- Elevation where possible to limit swelling
- Maintain mobility in arthritis to prevent stiffness-related pain
- Multidisciplinary approach—pain control nurse/team, physiotherapy
- Analgesic medication
  - Simple: NSAIDs, codeine phosphate, paracetamol
  - Opiates and opiate-like drugs, e.g. tramadol
- Local nerve blocks and regional anaesthetic techniques to pre-empt surgery
- Surgery
  - Joint replacement or arthrodesis.

Acute pain

Pain following surgery or trauma is managed as shown in McQuay[1]. Intermittent opioid injection titrated to pain is effective and safe (from respiratory depression) provided dose is titrated to effect (pain relief). Avoid pethidine as accumulation of its (toxic) metabolite may cause convulsions. In renal failure, less morphine will be required as its (active) metabolite will accumulate—again safe as long as dose titrated to effect. Patient-controlled analgesia with appropriate lockout is effective though can be problematic during sleep (give background infusion). Epidural infusion of opioid–local anaesthetic mixture is synergistic, allowing lower doses of each for equivalent analgesia.

Chronic pain

Same analgesics used in acute pain are effective in ~80% chronic sufferers. When conventional analgesics fail, unconventional analgesics may be indicated:

- Antidepressants (tricyclic antidepressants)—in lower dosage than for depression
- Anticonvulsants—trigeminal neuralgia, diabetic neuropathy, phantom limb pain
- Local nerve blocks—break the pain cycle
- Alternative treatments include transcutaneous electrical nerve stimulation[2], acupuncture and behavioural therapy.

References

1 McQuay H. Pain and its control. In: Bulstrode C, Buckwater J, Carr A, et al., eds. *Oxford Textbook of Orthopaedics and Trauma*. Oxford: Oxford University Press, 2002:415–24.
2 Melzack R, Wall PD. Pain mechanisms: a new theory. *Science* 1965;**150**:171–9.

Sedation

Sedation

Derivation from Latin *sedare* 'to settle'; involves administration of agents—analgesic and anaesthetic—usually to allow performance of a therapeutic procedure, e.g. fracture reduction, relocation of a dislocated joint. Implicit is patient's ability to maintain and protect own airway.

Pharmacokinetics and dynamics of the agents being used must be familiar to person administering them with appropriate monitoring to avoid potentially disastrous respiratory or cardiovascular complications. The effects of the agents administered often last well beyond the procedure for which they were given.

Only patients of ASA class I or II (see 📖 p. 95) appropriate for 'outpatient' sedation; all others require an anaesthetist in appropriate setting. As a minimum for sedation the following are required:
- No contraindications (see 📖 p. 95)
- Oxygen delivered at 15litres/min for at least 60min
- Suction
- Resuscitation equipment with full range of airway options and reversal drugs such as flumazenil (for midazolam) and naloxone (for opiates)
- Pulse oximetry
- ECG
- Non-invasive blood pressure (NIBP) monitoring.

Commonly used drugs

Midazolam (buccal, 0.5mg/kg up to max 8mg in children; parenteral, 2.5mg initial followed by titrated 1mg increments up to 10mg)

Advantages
- Quick onset with IV administration
- Amnesia.

Disadvantages
- Large dose may cause restlessness and confusion
- Caution in the elderly
- Synergistic with opiates for respiratory depression.

Propofol (parenteral 10–25mcg/kg/min)

Advantages
- Can be used to produce any level of sedation form drowsiness to general anaesthesia
- Short half-life with quick recovery.

Disadvantages
- Not readily available outside anaesthetic room
- Not suitable in children <3yrs.

Nitrous oxide 50%
- Easy to administer, analgesic, few side effects
- Rapid onset of action, quick recovery
- Avoid in pregnancy, lung disease, children with nasal blockage.

ASA (American Society of Anesthesiologists) classification of physical status

- Class I—normally healthy patient
- Class II—mild systemic disease
- Class III—severe systemic disease
- Class IV—severe systemic disease that is a constant threat to life
- Class V—Moribund patient not expected to survive without an operation.

Contraindications to sedation

- abnormal airway
- raised intracranial pressure (ICP)
- depressed conscious level
- history of sleep apnoea
- respiratory or cardiac failure
- neuromuscular disease
- bowel obstruction
- active respiratory tract infection
- allergy to sedative drug/previous adverse reaction
- child too distressed despite adequate preparation
- older child with severe behavioural problems (high failure rate)
- inadequate consent or informed refusal.

Local and regional nerve blocks

Use of local and regional anaesthetic techniques avoids the systemic effects of narcotics, potentially diminishes the stress response to surgery and can provide lasting postoperative pain relief with relatively low doses of local anaesthetic agent[1]. A peripheral nerve stimulator greatly facilitates performance of local nerve blocks.

Modes of administration:
- Local infiltration for limited wounds
- Haematoma block—injection into fracture haematoma
- Peripheral nerve block, e.g. brachial plexus, femoral nerve
- Regional—spinal or epidural anaesthesia.

Long-acting peripheral nerve blocks are not appropriate when assessment of limb function is important for diagnostic purposes, e.g. compartment syndrome.

Controlled hypotension secondary to sympathetic blockade with regional anaesthesia may reduce blood loss and aid postoperative recovery. Spinal or epidural anaesthesia reduces the prevalence of DVT after hip surgery by improving venous flow ± local fibrinolytic effect. It is also of benefit for patients with respiratory disease, but caution is required in patients with cardiac failure. Spinal, epidural or other anaesthesic route involving sympathetic blockade should be avoided in trauma patients with uncorrected or ongoing hypovolaemia.

Epidural anaesthesia

Can be used in isolation or combined with general anaesthesia for surgery on lower limbs. Administered as a single shot or continuous infusion via an epidural catheter (facilitating ongoing postoperative analgesia). Agents include local anaesthetics and opiates (fentanyl, diamorphine, clonidine).

Potential complications similar to spinal anaesthetic but may differ in time of onset and severity: postdural puncture headache (CSF leak through accidental dural puncture), epidural haematoma (rare unless clotting abnormality; avoid this route if INR >1.5 but probably safe up to this), epidural abscess (prompt recognition key; withdraw catheter, aspirate for sample and treat with antibiotics ± drainage).

Tips to reduce pain during local anaesthetic injection:
- Use smallest possible needle
- Inject slowly
- Warm anaesthetic to body temperature
- Avoid adrenaline.

Common anaesthetic agents and their dosage

Lidocaine dose: 3mg/kg without adrenaline, 7mg/kg with adrenaline
- Rapid onset in a few minutes with short duration of action.

Bupivacaine (Marcaine®) dose: 2mg/kg
- Narrow safety margin for (cardiac) toxicity (requiring prolonged CPR)
- Delayed onset but longer duration of action (up to 48h).

Prilocaine dose: 6mg/kg without adrenaline, 8.5mg/kg with adrenaline
- Agent of choice for IV regional anaesthesia (Bier's block)
- Similar pharmacokinetics to lidocaine but safer cardiac risk profile.

Ropivacaine dose: 3.5mg/kg
- Similar pharmacokinetics to bupivacaine, less cardiotoxic than bupivacaine
- Motor function blocked less than sensory.

EMLA®
- Mixture of 2.5% prilocaine and 2.5% lidocaine
- Used for topical anaesthesia prior to cannulation or injection in children.

Addition of adrenaline (epinephrine) yields
- Increased duration of block
- Greater safety margin as systemic absorption slowed
- Reduced surgical bleeding.

Note: avoid near end-arteries (terminal ischaemia) and use dilute solutions of <1:200 000. Solutions with adrenaline ARE more acidic so may be more painful to inject.

Reference
1 Fischer HBL, Pinnock CA. *Fundamentals of Regional Anaesthesia*. Cambridge: Cambridge University Press, 2004.

Prevention of DVT and PE

Thromboembolic disease (TED) refers to a group of disorders that can occur in either the arterial or venous system. In the orthopaedic patient venous thromboembolism is more common and it includes DVT and PE.

Incidence—epidemiology

- DVT after THR without thromboprophylaxis can be 15–50%
- DVT after total knee replacement (TKR) without thromboprophylaxis can be as high as 84%
- PE after THR or TKR without thromboprophylaxis is between 0.1 and 3.4%
- DVT rates after pelvic, acetabular or hip fractures vary from 20 to 60% and increase when surgery is delayed >2 days. Although symptomatic PE ranges from 2 to 10%, fatal PE occurs in 0.5–2%
- Rates are lower after spinal and foot/ankle surgery.

Virchow's triad

Three major factors that contribute to TED:
- Venous stasis (e.g. immobilization, limited ambulation)
- Endothelial injury (e.g. direct trauma, haematoma, tourniquet)
- Hypercoagulability (intrinsic factors, transient postoperative hypercoagulability).

Addressing these three factors is the basis of TED prevention techniques.

Prevention

Identify preoperative risk factors
- Proposed major surgery (especially pelvic), previous thromboembolism, advanced age, malignancy, obesity, varicose veins, congestive heart failure, pre-existing thrombophilia (e.g. antithrombin III deficiency, protein C or S deficiency, SLE or antiphospholipid syndrome).

Adjust intraoperative technique
- Regional anaesthesia
- Minimal soft tissue damage
- Meticulous haemostasis
- Compression devices for calves.

Postoperative measures
- Mechanical—TED stockings, pneumatic foot compression devices, early mobilization
- Chemical—aspirin, oral factor Xa inhibitors, oral direct thrombin inhibitors, LMWH, unfractionated heparin or warfarin. They all bear the risk of bleeding
- Combinations: better effects are achieved when mechanical and chemical means of prevention are combined.

For more information on DVT, see NICE guidelines (www.nice.org.uk).

Management of MRSA infections

'Meticillin-resistant *S. aureus*', but also resistant to all β-lactams and variable resistance to erythromycin, ciprofloxacin and trimethoprim. Usually treated with vancomycin, teicoplanin or rifampicin.

Typically *colonize* skin surfaces (especially wounds and ulcers), nose and throat.

Common sites of *infection*: wounds, implanted metalwork and prosthetic joints.

Prevention critical as treatment is potentially prolonged and expensive.

Prevention (infection control)

- Screen all patients (one of the few indications for superficial swabs) entering hospital and get previous admissions history. Isolate if MRSA positive or at risk, e.g. recent admission to another hospital
- Barrier nurse all MRSA-positive patients or possible carriers in a separate room in which visitors must wear apron/gloves and wash hands after every interaction with patient
- Have separate wards for patients admitted for elective procedures and screen them at preadmission clinic for MRSA. If swabs positive, attempt to eradicate infection at home with chlorhexidine washes and nasal mupirocin cream, then reswab. Some patients will remain carriers despite treatment; should be isolated and barrier nursed
- Staff should change uniforms/clothes at least every day.

Treatment

- For MRSA wound infection: debride, sample (deep specimens) and irrigate as for any infection
- Deep clean theatre after use and leave empty for 3h to allow sufficient air changes before using for another case
- All theatre staff to change clothing and shoes after case
- Give antibiotics postoperatively according to microbiology culture results and local guidelines, e.g. vancomycin. May require prolonged course.

Prevention of infection in orthopaedics and trauma

In a specialty built around the implantation of foreign materials, infection is a serious issue. Bacteria evolve many strategies to evade host immune systems when they colonize an implant, e.g. development of a 'glyco-calyx' (antiphagocytic capsule) or 'quorum sensing' to invoke a state of dormancy. Prevention is therefore paramount.

Definitions

- *Contamination*—presence of microorganisms in a host site (assumed sterile)
- *Colonization*—a non-invasive (but stable) association between pathogen and host
- *Infection*—pathological state in which pathogen multiplies within host tissues, usually some degree of damage exciting an inflammatory response.

Microorganisms which have contaminated an implant may form a stable and asymptomatic relationship (colonization) but later reactivate and become infective ('contingency loci').

Timeline of preventive measures

Identify and treat septic lesions, e.g. foot lesion or UTI. Treat prostatism before operation to reduce risk of urinary problems perioperatively).

Preoperative (prophylactic) antibiotics significantly reduce arthroplasty infection rates and a duration of 12h seems just as effective as 2 weeks[1]. One dose probably sufficient; see local policy for type and duration.

In a standard (Plenum—see opposite) operating theatre, 95% of wound contamination is from the air: keep operating time to a minimum, cover surgical instruments when not in use, minimize theatre traffic and operate in laminar flow (especially for arthroplasty). Use 4% chlorhexidine skin preparation with spirit in contact for 2min (95% reduction in skin bacteria). Wear disposable, non-woven gown ± exhaust suit (staff skin flora a significant contaminant).

Minimize the use of diathermy and suture material but ensure meticulous haemostasis and eliminate dead space. Observe theatre rituals: cover hair, face-mask, double gloving, properly laundered clothing.

Lidwell's MRC trial of 8000 patients in the 1980s demonstrated a 50% reduction in deep infection with ultraclean air ventilation and a further 25% decrease with prophylactic antibiotics (effects cumulative)[2]. Surgeon body exhaust suits and ultraclean air may decrease the rate towards 0.1%; ultraviolet (UV) irradiation may be a cheaper alternative in some institutions.

Important postoperative factors include:
- Postoperative antibiotics (short term)
- No-touch technique of wound dressing
- Inspection of wounds and prompt action for discharging (oozy) wounds
- Good general hygiene, in particular hand washing.

Theatre ventilation

- *Plenum* ventilation—air taken at roof level through high efficiency particulate air (HEPA) filter; humidified and warmed/cooled, positive pressure clean air pumped in at wall/ceiling level and diffuses out via vents just above floor level. Produces 150 bacterial colony-forming particles (bcp) per m³.
- *Laminar flow*. Entire body of air within defined space moves with uniform velocity in a single direction (vertical or horizontal). Reduces contamination to 30bcp/m³.
- *Exponential flow* (Howarth enclosure). Clean flow of air in shape of inverted trumpet to prevent entrainment. 'Ultraclean' air <10bcp/m³.

References

1 Pollard JP, Hughes SP, Scott JE, *et al.* Antibiotic prophylaxis in total hip replacement. *Br Med J* 1979;**1**:707–9.
2 Lidwell OM, Elson RA, Lowbury EJ, *et al.* Ultraclean air and antibiotics for prevention of postoperative infection. A multicenter study of 8,052 joint replacement operations. *Acta Orthop Scand* 1987;**58**:4–13.

Complications related to pathology

There is no operation, no matter how small, that does not go wrong from time to time for a reason not directly related to the actual procedure. However, many problems following orthopaedic surgery are predictable and potentially preventable. Elective surgery should be preceded by a visit to a preadmission assessment clinic where a suitably trained nurse or doctor can identify these risks and precautions be put in place or surgery delayed until the risks have been dealt with.

Common identifiable risks include:
- *Ischaemic heart disease:* MI within 6/12, poorly controlled angina, coronary artery bypass graft (CABG), arrhythmia; consider cardiac echo and cardiology opinion
- *Obesity:* increased anaesthetic risk due to difficult airway control, higher ventilation pressures and increased cardiac strain, increased wound infection rates; consider postponing surgery until body mass index (BMI) <30
- *Smoking:* pulmonary problems, delayed wound healing, delayed or non-union of fractures and osteotomies, failure of free muscle flaps; stop preoperatively if possible
- *Paget's disease:* increased risk of bleeding perioperatively and loosening of implants in the long term. Tight control with bisphosphonates preoperatively recommended
- *UTI:* increased risk of prosthetic infection, all patients should be screened preoperatively and all symptomatic UTIs treated prior to surgery. Catheterization for postoperative urinary retention must have antibiotic cover (consider suprapubic catheterization in males)
- *Peripheral vascular disease:* poor wound healing and infection common in foot surgery. Be cautious with tourniquet in severe arteriopathies
- *OP:* poor fixation in soft bone leads to high risk of implant loosening and cut-out. Careful choice of implant required
- *Bleeding disorders:* close cooperation with haematologists and blood bank required to cover even minor surgery with clotting factors, etc. Referral to specialist centres advised
- *Jaundice:* screen for ongoing hepatitis risk
- *Diabetes mellitus:* a perioperative sliding scale of insulin is recommended
- *Warfarin therapy:* if possible stop preoperatively. If significant risk of thrombosis (e.g. mechanical heart valve) then IV heparin cover is most controllable perioperatively
- *Previous DVT/PE, oral contraceptive pill, pelvic/hip surgery, underlying malignancy, obesity, thrombophilia:* higher risk of DVT/PE. NICE guidance recommends careful risk assessment for DVT risk and bleeding risk. Anticoagulants are only recommended when DVT risk is **not** outweighed by bleeding risk. LMWH or oral anticoagulants are started after surgery. The duration of prophylaxis is contentious but should cover the in-hospital period at least.

Complications related to treatment

Complications and **sequelae** result from procedures and add new problems to the underlying disease. Complications are differentiated from sequelae as unexpected events not intrinsic to the procedure. So for an arthroscopic meniscectomy, postoperative knee swelling would be a sequela but damage to the tibial artery would be a complication.

Failure is when the purpose of the procedure is not fulfilled—the knee still locks after the surgery.

The following grading system[1] for complications is helpful to grade severity and promote uniform reporting:

- **Grade 1**—alterations from the ideal operative or postoperative course which are non-life-threatening and cause no lasting disability
- **Grade 2**—potentially life-threatening complications without residual disability (a 'near-miss' incident) but may require additional treatment
- **Grade 3**—complications with residual disability
- **Grade 4**—deaths as a result of complications.

The common complications of orthopaedic and fracture surgery are:
- Wound infection; 0.5–1% in elective surgery, 20% in open fractures
- Respiratory infection and UTI, especially with immobility
- MI; most common cause of death after orthopaedic surgery
- Local neurovascular injury; especially radial and common peroneal nerve
- DVT; 40–60% in THR and TKR, mostly asymptomatic
- PE; 0.1% fatal in THR, higher in hip fracture surgery
- Compartment syndrome; usually after tibial fracture or forearm injury
- Bleeding; can be fatal after pelvic or major hip revision surgery
- Paralysis; uncommon after spine surgery
- Periprosthetic fracture; may be intraoperative or delayed
- Malposition of implants
- Malunion or non-union of fractures
- Joint stiffness; after trauma and elective surgery.
- Heterotopic ossification; especially around hip after pelvic fracture
- Chronic regional pain syndrome.

Reference
1 Clavien PA, Sanabria JR, Strasberg SM. Proposed classification of complications of surgery. *Surgery* 1992;**111**:518–26.

Fracture non-union[1,2]

Defined as the failure of biological union of fracture.

Delayed union describes slower fracture healing than expected, which may in turn progress to non-union. Long bone fracture non-union usually cannot be determined until 6–9 months postinjury. Approximately 2–5% of fractures become non-unions.

Hypertrophic non-union

Non-union secondary to mechanical instability of fracture; excessive motion prevents biological union. Characterized by hypertrophic bone ends, exuberant callus formation. Radiological 'elephant's foot' appearance of bone ends. Biologically active.

Seen classically in fractures mobilized too early, or with insufficient rigidity of fixation to allow union. Examples include metatarsal and metacarpal fractures, fractures treated by intramedullary nailing, ulnar nightstick fractures.

Treatment involves stabilization of the fracture (casting/bracing, off-loading (non-weightbearing), and/or rigid internal or circular external fixation. It is unnecessary to graft these non-unions or even open fracture gap surgically. Rapid progression to union is seen when these conditions have been met.

Atrophic non-union

Non-union due to lack of biological activity in fracture site. Most commonly seen in high-energy, open or infected fractures, in smokers and with use of NSAIDs.

Classical cause of failure of internal fixation. Most usually seen in midshaft humerus, clavicle and scaphoid fractures, and internally fixed tibial shaft fractures. Bone ends are usually sclerotic or osteopenic, without evidence of callus formation, and may taper into fracture site. Can occur with aggressive periosteal stripping during internal fixation.

Management strategies include surgical debridement of bone ends, autologous or allogeneic bone grafting (and possible use of bone morphogenic proteins). Rigid compression and stability, either with traditional compression plating or circular external fixation. This allows progressive distraction of an initially compressed non-union, according to the principles of distraction osteogenesis. The use of electric field induction has theoretical potential in management of atrophic non-union; however has not been conclusively proven to be of benefit.

Oligotrophic non-union

Non-union secondary to excessive fracture gap distraction, post-infection segmental defect, extruded fracture fragments or interposed avascular comminuted fragments. Most commonly seen in the tibia.

Minimal callus formation without hypertrophic bone ends, but biological activity present. Results from inability of biological effort to cross fracture gap. Cause of failure of bridge plating osteosynthesis.

Treatment is similar to atrophic non-union.

Fibrous union

Synonymous with non-union. Used to describe an asymptomatic non-union with dense fibrous tissue bridging the fracture and giving some stability. Expectant management may be applied.

Pseudarthrosis

End result of non-union; mobile non-union site develops synovial characteristics with membrane. May be subdivided into stiff (hypertrophic) or lax (atrophic) types. Often painless. May be the end result of multiply grafted non-union attempts, or recurrent infection, and, if asymptomatic, may be desirable to accept asymptomatic pseudarthrosis.

Management for symptomatic is that of atrophic non-union, with the addition of full surgical excision of synovial envelope. High risk of failure with grafted rigid internal fixation osteosynthesis. Preferred management is circular external fixation, with initial compression and subsequent distraction osteogenesis.

Infected non-union

Infection is a potent cause of non-union. The pattern may be atrophic or hypertrophic. These non-unions always have segments of non-viable bone with bacteria living in biofilms on dead bone.

Treatment is complex, requiring excision and sampling of all infected tissue, with reconstruction using external fixation (Ilizarov method). Prolonged specific antibiotic treatment may be indicated with systemic and local therapy.

Referral to a specialist centre with a multidisciplinary team is recommended.

References

1 Megas P. Classification of non-union. *Injury* 2005;**36** Suppl 4:S30–7.
2 Biasibetti A, Aloj D, Di Gregorio G, *et al.* Mechanical and biological treatment of long bone non-unions. *Injury* 2005;**36** Suppl 4:S45–50.

Biomaterials and implants

Biomechanics and biomaterials[1]

Orthopaedic surgeons need to understand some key properties and interactions of materials which are used as implants and occur naturally in the human form.

A biomaterial is something applied internally to a body part in order to enhance its function, e.g. joint replacement, internal fixation plate. The behaviour of biomaterials is best considered by looking at their physical properties.

Stress–strain curves

Stress is the force applied to a material per unit of cross-sectional area (units = N/m² = Pa). *Strain* is the ratio of the resultant change in length of that material to its original length (a proportion; therefore no units). When a material is stressed to failure, a plot of stress (*y*-axis) against strain (*x*-axis) will display an elastic phase over which the two values are directly proportional . The slope of this straight line part of the graph is *Young's modulus of elasticity* (E); the steeper the line, the stiffer the material. Elastic materials return to their original shape when deforming stress is removed.

With additional stress the material deforms permanently; this is the *plastic* phase. *Brittle* materials show little or no plastic deformation before they fracture, e.g. ceramics, bone cement, whereas ductile materials display large amounts of plastic deformation, e.g. metals.

Viscosity is the resistance of a fluid to shear. A *viscoelastic* material, such as a ligament or cartilage, combines the behaviour of an elastic solid and a viscous fluid. Critically, its deformation in response to load varies according to the rate of application of that load; at low strain rates it behaves as a viscous fluid with no elastic (all plastic) deformation; at high strain rates it behaves as an elastic (but brittle) solid. Injury to the ACL, for example, is therefore more likely at high rates of strain.

Other important viscoelastic properties are:
- *Stress relaxation*—with time a viscoelastic material held at constant length shows a reduction in internal stress (the principle behind serial splintage)
- *Creep*—the material progressively deforms under constant load (explaining why traction restores length and alignment to a fractured bone)
- *Hysteresis*—loading and unloading force–displacement curves follow different paths so, although the material returns to its original shape, energy is lost to the system as heat.

Tribology

The study of lubrication and wear (Greek *Tribos* = rub). Wear is the erosion of a solid surface by interaction with another. Lubrication is the introduction of various substances between sliding surfaces to reduce wear and friction.

The 3 main types of lubrication are:
- **Fluid-film**, which completely separates sliding surfaces
- **Boundary**, a failure of the fluid film completely to separate the surfaces so that the friction between them is determined by the properties of both the lubricant and the surfaces
- **Solid**, when liquid lubricants lack adequate resistance to load.

Different types of wear and lubrication relevant to orthopaedics include:

Wear
- *Adhesive*—bonds form between sliding surfaces so a thin film stripped off one material by a harder one, e.g. metal–polyethylene bearing in hip replacement
- *Abrasive*—surface roughness or asperities cause erosion, e.g. scratched metal bearing during implantation
- *Fatigue induced*—repetitive loading causes catastrophic failure by cracking and delamination, e.g. knee replacement with thin polyethylene insert
- *Third body wear*—small particles acting between sliding surfaces, e.g. cement particles or polyethylene debris.

Lubrication
- *Hydrodynamic*—surfaces moving above a critical speed entrain fluid which separates them (*fluid film lubrication*). This is the rationale behind large diameter bearing surfaces in hip replacement
- *Elastohydrodynamic*—deformation of moving articular surfaces, e.g. cartilage, separated by a thin layer of fluid
- *Squeeze film*—advancing joint surfaces separated by a fluid front squeezed out between them
- *Weeping*—fluid shifts from surfaces under load
- *Boosted*—concentrated pool of large molecules left behind in areas under contact; solvent (water) is driven into cartilage.

Reference
1 Ramachandran M, ed. *Basic Orthopaedic Sciences: The Stanmore Guide*. Stanmore: Hodder Arnold, 2006.

Implants[1]

Non-living objects inserted into the body to perform a specific function and intended to remain there for a significant period of time. The ideal implant should be biocompatible (inert, non-immunogenic, non-toxic and non-carcinogenic), have sufficient strength, be easily worked, free from corrosion, inexpensive and not affect subsequent imaging.

Implants are used to replace damaged or diseased structures, aid fracture healing or correct deformity.

Screws

Transform rotational force into compression between two or more surfaces. Screws have a head, shaft and thread. The profile of the thread determines the pull out strength (grip) of a screw. Bone screws, commonly made of stainless steel, are predrilled and tapped to cut a thread.

Plates

Stabilize bone fragments allowing early movement of muscles and joints. Compression at a fracture site encourages bone healing. Plate stiffness is predominantly related to thickness of the plate, but also to length.

Intramedullary nails

The tubular cross-section of long bones allows internal placement of a nail for stabilization after a fracture, osteotomy or for protection from an impending pathological fracture. Nail stiffness is proportional to diameter and inversely proportional to *working length* (greatest distance between points of bone contact or between locking screws). Locking screws primarily resist rotational deformation.

Joint replacements

Commonly made of stainless steel or cobalt chrome by casting from a mould. Joint replacements have a bearing surface where movement occurs, commonly metal on polyethylene. Metal on metal and ceramic bearings are alternatives with improved wear characteristics.

Failure of implants

- *Corrosion*: a chemical reaction where material is removed from an object
- *Fatigue*: cyclical or repetitive loading of a material below its ultimate stress
- *Wear*: the removal of material from solid surfaces by mechanical action.

See also Arthroplasty 📖 p. 164.

Reference

1 Miller M. *Review of Orthopaedics*, 5th edn, Phildelphia, PA: Saunders Elseviser.

Section 2

Anatomy and surgery

Anatomy

Head and neck anatomy[1]

Skull

The frontal, parietal and occipital bones make up the cranial vault; between these are the coronal, sagittal and lambdoid sutures. The skull base is made up of the sphenoid, petrous part of the temporal and the occipital bones. The cranium houses the brain, its meningeal coverings and the CSF in which the brain is suspended.

Skeleton of the cervical spine

The cervical vertebrae are specialized in a number of ways:
- There is no vertebral body to C1. Instead there is a narrow anterior arch behind which lies the odontoid process of C2 (the dens) which is stabilized by the alar, cruciate and transverse ligaments
- C2–C6: bifid spinous processes provide attachments for the ligamentum nuchae; the foramen transversarium transmits the vertebral arteries bilaterally. The lateral masses articulate through facet joints with vertebra above and below. The vertebral body has a small upward projection on each side (the uncus) which articulates with the inferior aspect of the vertebral body above (the uncovertebral joint)
- C7: has a large spinous process ('vertebra prominens'), the foramen transversarium does not transmit the vertebral artery at this level.

Cervical fascia

Beneath the skin is the superficial fascia and platysma muscle. The deep cervical fascia encases the major structures of the neck.
- the deep investing layer (the most superficial part, that splits to encase the sternocleidomastoid and trapezius muscles)
- the pretracheal layer (that splits to encase the thyroid gland)
- the prevertebral layer (which covers the prevertebral muscles, the cervical plexus and trunks of the brachial plexus)
- the carotid sheath (which contains the carotid arteries, internal jugular vein, the vagus nerve and ansa cervicalis—the cervical sympathetic trunk lies just posterior, on top of the prevertebral fascia.

Triangles of the neck

The main landmark is the sternocleidomastoid muscle which demarcates the anterior and posterior triangles.

The posterior triangle (between sternomastoid, clavicle and trapezius) contains:
- muscles: scalenes, levator scapulae, inferior belly of omohyoid
- vasculature: external jugular vein, occipital and transverse cervical arteries and, at the inferior margin, subclavian and suprascapular vessels
- nerves: accessory nerve, cervical plexus, brachial plexus, phrenic nerve
- lymphatics: lymph nodes (and at the inferior margin on the left side lies the thoracic duct).

The anterior triangle (between sternomastoid, mandible and midline) contains:

- midline structures: thyroid and parathyroid glands, hyoid bone, trachea and larynx, oesophagus and pharynx
- muscles: suprahyoid muscles, infrahyoid ('strap') muscles, omohyoid
- vasculature: common carotid with bifurcation into internal carotid and external carotid (and branches). Internal jugular vein (and branches)
- nerves: the hypoglossal and branches of glossopharyngeal and vagus nerves.

NB: the carotid sheath lies under cover of sternocleidomastoid and is therefore not included in the contents of the triangles of the neck.

Recurrent laryngeal nerve

Ascends in the tracheoesophageal groove and is at risk during anterior cervical surgery. A left-sided approach is said to be safer with regards nerve injury. On the right side the nerve is occasionally non-recurrent.

Reference

1 McMinn RMH, ed. *Last's Anatomy, Regional and Applied*, 9th edn. London: Churchill Livingstone.

Back anatomy

The spine comprises the vertebrae, neural tissue (spinal cord and spinal nerves) and their coverings, intervertebral discs, ligaments and muscles (Fig. 6.1). The vertebrae are stacked in a column which is straight when viewed in the coronal plane. There are physiological curvatures in the sagittal plane—cervical lordosis, thoracic kyphosis, lumbar lordosis. However, these curves are normally balanced so that the head is centred over the pelvis when viewed in both the sagittal and coronal planes.

Vertebrae

There are 7 cervical, 12 thoracic and 5 lumbar, a sacrum composed of 5 fused vertebrae and a rudimentary coccyx.

Main bulk is anterior (vertebral body) with an arch extending posteriorly forming the vertebral canal containing the neural elements. The arch comprises the pedicles (continuous with the body) and the inferiorly sloping laminae more posteriorly, which meet in the midline to form the spinous process. Below each pedicle, a spinal nerve root is transmitted via the intervertebral foramen. Superior and inferior articular processes from adjacent vertebrae articulate to form the facet joints. Transverse processes are large in the lumbar spine, smaller in the thoracic and cervical regions.

Neural elements and coverings

The spinal cord is continuous with the brainstem at the foramen magnum of the skull and runs caudally to L1 where it terminates as the conus medullaris. It is covered with dura mater, continuous with that of the brain. Outside of the dura is the epidural space; within it is the neural tissue bathed in CSF in the subarachnoid (spinal) space. Paired nerve roots branch off the spinal cord and exit through the intervertebral foramina. The nerve roots for segments below L1 are contained in the dural sac as the cauda equina.

Intervertebral discs

Secondary cartilaginous joints (symphyses) between vertebral bodies, composed of a fibrous ring (annulus fibrosus) and a gelatinous centre (nucleus pulposus). The annulus is made up of lamellae that are predominantly type I collagen. The fibres of one lamella run at an angle of 30° to its immediate neighbour. The nucleus contains proteoglycans that are strongly hydrophilic.

Ligaments

There are 3 ligaments that run the length of the spine—all in the midline:
• Anterior longitudinal ligament—anterior to vertebral bodies
• Posterior longitudinal ligament—immediately posterior to the vertebral bodies
• Supraspinous ligament—between the tips of the spinous processes.

Shorter ligaments—consistent paired ligaments between each vertebra:
• Interspinous ligament—between spinous processes
• Intertransverse ligament—between transverse processes
• Ligamentum flavum (yellow ligament)—between the laminae.

Muscles

Spinal movement is brought about by many different muscles, including those distant from the spine itself, e.g. rectus abdominis. Paraspinal musculature is composed of both flexors and extensors.
• The flexors are situated anterior to the vertebral bodies—longus colli from T4 to skull base; in the lumbar spine, psoas major acts as a powerful flexor
• Extensors—divided into superficial, intermediate and deep muscle groups, all supplied by posterior primary rami of the spinal nerves:
  • Superficial—the erector spinae muscle group: iliocostalis, longissimus and spinalis
  • Intermediate—the transversospinalis group: multifidus, levator costarum and the semispinalis capitis, cervicis and thoracis
  • Deep—intertransversalis, interspinalis and rotatores.

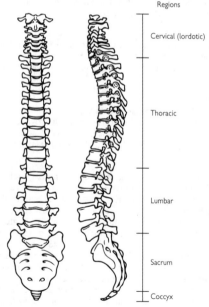

Regions

Cervical (lordotic)

Thoracic

Lumbar

Sacrum

Coccyx

Fig. 6.1 Anatomy of the spine.

Anatomy of the shoulder girdle

The upper limb, shoulder girdle, arm, forearm, wrist, and hand, is attached to the body by one bone, the clavicle, and muscles (Fig. 6.2).

Embryology

Upper limb bud appears at ~24 days, formed from ectoderm and mesoderm from C5 to T1. Longitudinal growth is governed by the apical ectodermal ridge and the postaxial border (ulnar side) defined by the zone of polarizing activity.

Biomechanics

Rotation occurs around the humeral head. Due to large lever arm, lifting even small masses can create large forces within the GHJ making it equivalent to a weight-bearing joint. Only 1/3 of the humeral head is in contact with the glenoid. Stability is enhanced by static constraints (capsule, ligaments, labrum, negative intra-articular pressure, surface adhesion) and dynamic constraints (muscles).

Sternoclavicular joint (SCJ)

The proximal end of the clavicle articulates with the sternum. It is a synovial joint with an intervening fibrocartilage disc.

Clavicle

Stabilizes upper limb to axial skeleton. Muscle attachments include sternocleidomastoid, pectoralis major (clavicular head) and subclavius. Anterior and posterior divisions of the brachial plexus pass deep to it, as do the subclavian vessels.

Acromioclavicular joint (ACJ)

The distal end of the clavicle articulates with the acromion. The joint is a synovial joint with intervening fibrocartilage disc. It allows a small amount of rotation of shoulder girdle on long axis of clavicle. Stabilized by intrinsic (acromioclavicular) and extrinsic (coracoclavicular) ligaments.

Scapula

Parts of the scapula are: body; spine; acromion; neck; glenoid fossa. The rotator cuff muscles arise from the posterior (supraspinatus, infraspinatus, and teres minor) and anterior (subscapularis) aspects of the body. Muscle attachments to or those crossing the scapula stabilize it to the thorax (rhomboids major and minor, pectoralis minor, levator scapulae, seratus anterior, latissimus dorsi, and trapezius). The deltoid muscle arises from the spine of the scapula and acromion in addition to the clavicle. It gives the shoulder its rounded shape. The coracoid is palpable just medial to the GHJ line and distal to the ACJ. It serves as origin or insertion point for 3 muscles (pectoralis minor, coracobrachialis, short head of biceps) and 3 ligaments (coracoclavicular, coracohumeral, coracoacromial). The brachial plexus and subclavian vessels are immediately medial to the coracoid.

Proximal humerus

The proximal humerus consists of an articular surface which meets the shaft at the anatomical neck, the surgical neck is more distal; the greater tubercle (supraspinatus, infraspinatus, and teres minor muscles attached here), lesser tubercle (subscapularis attached here) and the intertubercular groove (long head of biceps tendon runs along this groove).

Glenohumeral joint (GHJ)

During movement at the GHJ the stabilizers of the shoulder keep the humeral head opposed to the glenoid surface.

- Abduction—deltoid (axillary nerve) and supraspinatus (suprascapular nerve)
- Adduction—latissimus dorsi (thoracodorsal nerve), pectoralis major (medial and lateral pectoral nerves) and cuff muscles except supraspinatus
- Flexion—deltoid (axillary nerve), biceps (musculocutaneous nerve) and pectoralis major (lateral pectoral nerve)
- Extension—latissimus dorsi (thoracodorsal nerve), deltoid (axillary nerve) and triceps (radial nerve)
- External rotation—supraspinatus, infraspinatus (suprascapular nerve) and teres minor (axillary nerve)
- Internal rotation—subscapularis (subscapular nerves), pectoralis major (medial and lateral pectoral nerves), and teres major (lower subscapular nerve).

Blood supply of humeral head

- Anterior and posterior circumflex humeral arteries from the third part of the axillary artery anastomose around the neck of the humerus
- Intramedullary supply from the humerus.

Blood supply can be disrupted with anatomical neck fracture and may result in osteonecrosis.

For further reading, see Moore and Dalley[1].

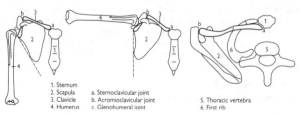

1. Sternum
2. Scapula
3. Clavicle
4. Humerus

a. Sternoclavicular joint
b. Acromioclavicular joint
c. Glenohumeral joint

5. Thoracic vertebra
6. First rib

Fig. 6.2 Anatomy of the shoulder girdle.

Reference

1 Moore KL, Dalley AF. Upper limb. In: *Clinically Orientated Anatomy*. Philadelphia, PA: Lippincott Williams and Wilkins, 1999:664–830.

Anatomy of the elbow

Biomechanics

The elbow (Fig. 6.3) can be thought of in terms of the:

- Humeroulnar joint (HUJ). Trochlea of humerus articulates with the trochlea notch of the ulna
- Radiocapitellar joint (RCJ). Capitellum of humerus articulates with radial head
- Proximal radioulnar joint (PRUJ). Proximal radius articulates with ulna.

With the elbow extended there is valgus angulation called the carrying angle. Greater in women than men (15 vs 10°). Biceps and brachialis act to flex the elbow at a mechanical disadvantage due to the lever arm effect of the forearm. The ulnar collateral ligaments stabilize the elbow medially and the radial collateral ligaments stabilize the joint laterally.

Ossification centres

Useful to estimate age of a child. They appear in the following order (approximate age)—capitellum (1yr), radial head (3yrs), medial epicondyle (5yrs), trochlea (7yrs), olecranon (9yrs) and lateral epicondyle (11yrs).

Surface landmarks

Bony landmarks

- Lateral epicondyle of the humerus—from the anterior surface arise the extensor tendons of the forearm and hand
- Medial epicondyle—forearm and hand flexors arise from here
- Olecranon of ulna—posteriorly providing the insertion for triceps.

With the elbow flexed to 90° these three points above form an isosceles triangle. With the elbow fully extended they line up in the transverse plane.

Anterior structures

From medial to lateral the following structures cross in front of the elbow: (i) flexors of wrist and hand, (ii) median nerve, (iii) brachial artery, (iv) biceps tendon, (v) lateral cutaneous nerve of the forearm (terminal cutaneous sensory branch of the musculocutaneous nerve), (vi) brachialis tendon, (vii) radial nerve (posterior interosseous and superficial branches), (viii) brachioradialis and (ix) common extensors. The ulnar nerve passes behind the medial epicondyle in a groove.

Elbow joint

Stabilized by static and dynamic constraints.

Static

- Capsule
- Ligaments—medially the anterior band of the medial collateral ligament is the most important restraint to valgus force. Laterally the lateral ulnar collateral ligament is important, and loss may result in posterolateral instability. The radial head is constrained by the annular ligament
- Bony architecture—stability provided by congruency. Fractures of the radial head may contribute to valgus instability.

Dynamic

- Common flexor origin
- Common extensor origin
- Instability may occur if these are avulsed traumatically
- Anconeus helps prevent posterior subluxation of the radial head.

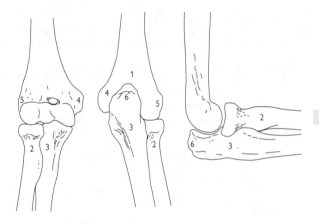

1. Humerus
2. Radius
3. Ulna
4. Medial epicondyle
5. Lateral epicondyle
6. Olecranon

Fig. 6.3 Arm and elbow anatomy.

Anatomy of the forearm

Flexors in the forearm. Muscles controlling elbow movements (Fig. 6.4):
• Biceps—flexion and supination
• Brachialis—flexion
• Triceps—extension
• Pronator teres—flexion and pronation.

These can be thought of in three layers from superficial to deep.
• Superficial (lateral to medial)—pronator teres, flexor carpi radialis (FCR), palmaris longus (PL) and flexor carpi ulnaris (FCU)
• Middle layer—FDS
• Deep layer (proximal to distal)—FDP, flexor pollicis longus (FPL) and pronator quadratus (PQ).

Extensors in the forearm

In addition to brachioradialis and supinator, the extensor compartment includes the following muscles.
• Extensor carpi radialis longus and brevis (ECRL and ECRB)—supplied by the radial nerve though the brevis is occasionally supplied by the posterior interosseous nerve (PIN)
• Extensor digitorum (ED), extensor carpi ulnaris (ECU), extensor indicis (EI), extensor digiti minimi (EDM), and extensor pollicis longus (EPL) which are supplied by the PIN.

Course of the major nerves

• Radial nerve—formed from the posterior cord of the brachial plexus. Passes through the triangular interval bounded by triceps long head, humeral shaft and teres major. Then winds around back of humerus in spiral groove to pierce the lateral intermuscular septum. Enters the forearm anterior to the lateral epicondyle, passes between brachialis and brachioradialis and splits to form PIN and superficial branch. PIN pierces two heads of supinator and travels in the extensor compartment terminating at wrist. Superficial branch travels deep to brachioradialis
• Median nerve—from the medial and lateral cords of the plexus. Accompanies the brachial artery in the arm, crosses the antecubital fossa then passes between the two heads of pronator teres. In the forearm it lies deep to FDS before entering the carpal tunnel superficial to the flexor tendons. The anterior interosseous nerve (AIN) is given off at the elbow and accompanies the equivalent artery
• Ulnar nerve—from the medial cord of the plexus. Passes from anterior to posterior through the medial intermuscular septum then behind the medial epicondyle. It then passes between two heads of FCU into the forearm where a dorsal branch is given off before the nerve enters Guyon's canal.

Range of movements of the elbow

Flexion is from −5° to 150°. Pronation 80° and supination 90°.

For further reading, see Moore and Dalley[1].

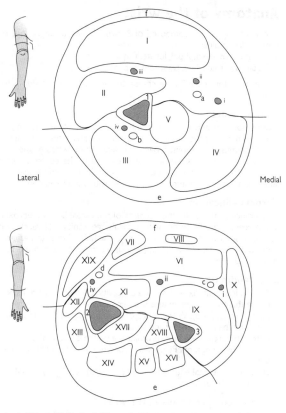

1. Humerus 2. Radius 3. Ulna

I) Biceps II) Brachialis III) Lateral head of triceps IV) Long head of triceps
V) Medial head of triceps VI) Flexor digitorum superficialis VII) Flexor carpi
radialis VIII) Palmaris longus IX) Flexor digitorum profundus X) Flexor carpi
ulnaris XI) Flexor pollicis longus XII) Extensor carpi radialis longus
XIII) Extensor carpi radialis brevis XIV) Extensor digitorum communis
XV) Extensor digiti minimi XVI) Abductor pollicis longus XVII) Extensor carpi ulnaris XVIII) Extensor pollicis longus XIX) Brachioradialis
a) Brachial artery b) Deep brachial artery c) Ulnar artery d) Radial artery
e) Extensor compartment f) Flexor compartment i) Ulnar nerve ii) Median
nerve iii) Musculocutaneous nerve IX) Superficial branch of radial nerve

Fig. 6.4 Upper limb—transverse sections.

Reference

1 Moore KL, Dalley AF. Upper limb. In: *Clinically Orientated Anatomy*. Philadelphia, PA: Lippincott Williams and Wilkins, 1999:664–830.

Anatomy of the wrist

The wrist (Fig. 6.5) is composed of 8 carpal bones, arranged in 2 rows. From radial to ulnar:
- Proximal row—scaphoid, lunate, triquetrum, pisiform
- Distal row: trapezium, trapezoid, capitate, hamate.

There are 6 dorsal and 2 volar compartments that contain tendons to the hand.

Biomechanics

Interosseous ligaments (e.g. the scapholunate ligament) are vital in guiding the movements of the carpal bones relative to each other. The action of particular muscles on joint movement depends on whether the tendon passes in front of (flexion) or behind (extension) the centre of rotation of that joint, not on the position of the muscle. Forearm pronation and supination occur by rotation of the radius around the fixed ulna.

Carpal ossification

Appearance of the ossification centres of the carpal bones (approximate age in years) is useful to estimate a child's age: capitate (1 year), hamate (2yrs), triquetrum (3yrs), lunate (4yrs), scaphoid (5yrs), trapezium and trapezoid (5–6yrs). The pisiform (9yrs) is a sesamoid bone in the tendon of the FCU.

Bony landmarks

- Anatomical snuffbox—This is the concavity formed, with extension of the thumb, between extensor pollicis longus (EPL) and extensor pollicis brevis (EPB). Within this space can be palpated the radial artery overlying the radial styloid and scaphoid waist
- Lister's tubercle—is a bony prominence on the dorsum of the distal radius. The tendon of EPL passes around the ulnar border using it as a pulley
- Ulnar head—(distal end, radial head proximal) sits slightly dorsally relative to the distal radius.

Extensor compartments of the wrist

The extensor tendons at the distal radius/ulna run deep to the extensor retinaculum in six distinct compartments. From radial to ulnar these are:
- First—abductor pollicis longus (APL) and extensor pollicis brevis (EPB)
- Second—extensor carpi radialis longus and brevis (ECRL and ECRB)
- Third—EPL
- Fourth—extensor indicis (EI) and extensor digitorum (ED)
- Fifth—extensor digiti minimi (EDM)
- Sixth—extensor carpi ulnaris (ECU).

Where two extensor tendons act on a finger (EI and EDM) the ED tendon is located on the radial side.

The carpal tunnel

A fibro-osseous tunnel whose boundaries are the carpal bones with the transverse carpal ligament (TCL) forming the roof. The TCL is attached to the hamate and pisiform and the scaphoid tubercle. It contains the tendons of FDS and FDP within synovial sheaths, tendon of the FPL and the median nerve. The motor branch of the median nerve to the thenar muscles may pass through the TCL.

Guyon's canal

The canal lies between the pisiform and hook of hamate. The floor is the TCL with the roof being the volar carpal ligament (VCL). Contains the ulnar nerve and artery.

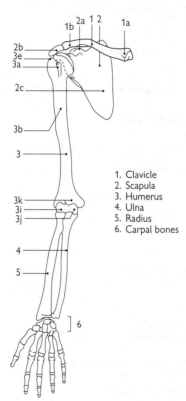

1. Clavicle
2. Scapula
3. Humerus
4. Ulna
5. Radius
6. Carpal bones

Fig. 6.5 Anatomy of the upper limb.

Anatomy of the hand

The hand is composed of 5 metacarpals and 14 phalanges (Fig. 6.6). The bony architecture is complex. It can be divided into:
- Volar (palmar) aspect—contains muscles, flexor tendons, and digital nerves
- Dorsal aspect—contains muscles and extensor tendons/mechanisms.

Flexor zones
- Zone 1—over the middle phalanx, FDP tendon only
- Zone 2—'no-man's land'. FDS and FDP within their flexor sheath. Distal to distal palmar crease
- Zone 3—Distal to carpal tunnel
- Zone 4—Within the carpal tunnel
- Zone 5—Forearm.

For the thumb there are 4 zones, with T-1 being distal to the IPJ, T-2 distal to the MCPJ, T-3 being the thenar eminence, and T-4 is within the carpal tunnel.

Innervation of the hand
Median nerve
- Sensory—palmar skin of radial three and a half digits
- Motor—lateral two lumbricals, opponens pollicis, abductor pollicis brevis and flexor pollicis brevis. Remember 'L.O.A.F.'.

Ulnar nerve
- Sensory—Ulnar one and a half digits
- Motor—Remaining intrinsic muscles of the hand, i.e. those intrinsic muscles not innervated by the median nerve.

Radial nerve
Remaining dorsal skin, particularly over the anatomical snuff box.

Movements of the fingers
The complexity of movements depends on the fine balance between the intrinsic muscles of the hand and the more powerful extrinsic muscles from the forearm which act on the hand.

Movements of joints of the fingers
Metacarpophalangeal joints: flexion—intrinsics. Extension—ED. Abduction—dorsal interosseii. Adduction—palmar interosseii.

Proximal and distal interphalangeal joints: extension—intrinsics. Flexion—PIPJ by FDS, DIPJ by FDP.

Movements of joints of the thumb
Flexion at MCPJ is by FPB and at the IPJ is by FPL. Extension at MCPJ is by EPB and at the IPJ by EPJ. Other movements are provided by the thenar muscles. Axis of thumb movement is rotated by 90°.

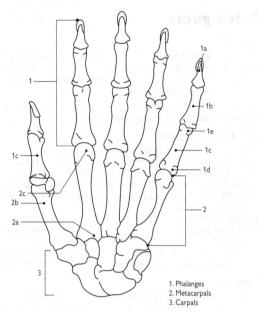

1. Phalanges
2. Metacarpals
3. Carpals

Fig. 6.6 Anatomy of the hand.

Pelvic girdle

Bones
The pelvic girdle is composed of two innominate bones and the sacrum. Each innominate bone comprises three united bones: the ischium, ilium and pubis. These meet in the cup-shaped acetabulum and unite here by a triradiate cartilage after puberty.

The orientation of the pelvis in the upright adult is such that the ASIS and symphysis pubis lie in the same coronal plane.

Joints and ligaments
Viewed from above, the pelvis makes an obvious ring structure, and strong connecting joints form the articulations between its individual component bones. Supporting ligaments further strengthen the complex.
- SIJs—strong synovial joints which allow very little motion. The joint is surrounded by a strong posterior ligament complex and weaker anterior ligaments
- Pubic symphysis—connects the two sides of the pelvis anteriorly
- Sacrococcygeal joint—a symphysis which allows flexion and extension
- Sacrospinous and sacrotuberous ligaments—help form the greater and lesser sciatic foramen. The former transmits the sciatic nerve and piriformis muscle and the latter the short external rotators of the hip.

Muscles
The pelvic girdle is an important site of origin and insertion (on both its internal and external surfaces) of muscles governing hip and truncal stability. The pelvic floor is a muscular sheet intrinsic to the pelvis, on which lie the pelvic viscera. Integrity (or otherwise) of this is an important factor predicting haemorrhage in pelvic fractures.

Nerves
- The **lumbar plexus** is formed in the psoas muscle, from the anterior rami of L1–L4 nerve roots. Important branches are the lateral femoral cutaneous, the femoral and the obturator nerves
- The **sacral plexus** is formed from the anterior rami of L4–S4 and is found in the pelvis, on the piriformis muscle anterior to the sacrum. It gives rise to the sciatic nerve, superior and inferior gluteal nerves, the posterior cutaneous nerve of the thigh, the pudendal nerve, the pelvic splanchnic nerves and individually named branches to quadratus femoris, obturator internus, and piriformis.

Vessels
- External iliac arteries—transit the pelvis for supply to the lower limbs
- Internal iliac arteries—the main supply to the pelvic viscera and the gluteal region. The largest branch, the superior gluteal artery, exits the pelvis via the greater sciatic foramen to supply the buttock
- Pelvic veins—are numerous and form large plexuses which eventually become confluent and drain to the internal iliac veins, but communication also exists to the vertebral venous plexuses.

Anatomy of the lower limb: overview

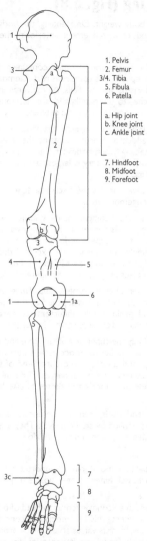

1. Pelvis
2. Femur
3/4. Tibia
5. Fibula
6. Patella

a. Hip joint
b. Knee joint
c. Ankle joint

7. Hindfoot
8. Midfoot
9. Forefoot

Fig. 6.7 Anatomy of the lower limb.

Anatomy of the lower limb: thigh, knee, and leg (Fig. 6.8)

Accounts for 10% body weight. On standing, the body centre of gravity passes behind the axis of hip movement, anterior to the knee and ankle.

Thigh

Anterior thigh—the flexor compartment containing the femoral nerve and vessels. Quadriceps femoris comprises rectus femoris, vastus medialis, vastus lateralis and vastus intermedialis. All converge into the quadriceps tendon which attaches to the patella and is continuous with the patellar ligament. Action—flexion of the hip and extension of the knee. Sartorius.

Femoral triangle—boundaries: inguinal ligament, medial sartorius and medial border of adductor longus. Contains the femoral nerve, artery, vein and canal containing lymph nodes/fat. Vein, artery, and nerve (medial to lateral). *Profunda femoris* artery is largest branch—important in blood supply to the hip joint.

Greater saphenous vein—pierces the fascia lata 4cm inferolateral to pubic tubercle to enter the femoral vein.

Medial thigh—Adductor compartment—gracilis superficial, adductor longus, and adductor brevis deeper. These muscles arise from pubic rami. Adductor magnus is the deepest adductor and arises from the ischial tuberosity. *Nerve supply*—obturator nerve except adductor magnus which is partly innervated by the sciatic nerve inferiorly. *Adductor hiatus* is where the femoral artery passes en route to the popliteal fossa.

Posterior thigh—Extensor compartment. *Gluteal muscles.* Gluteus maximus (hip extensor) forms the bulk and is supplied by the inferior gluteal nerve. Gluteus medius and minimus (hip abductors) converge on the greater trochanter of the femur and are supplied by the superior gluteal nerve.

Piriformis muscle—Only the superior gluteal nerve and vessels enter from the pelvis above it; all else below. *Sciatic nerve* enters below to piriformis, deep to hamstrings, and divides at the upper end of the popliteal fossa into the tibial and common peroneal nerves. Piriformis along with obturator internus, quadratus femoris and tensor fasciae latae contribute to lateral rotation.

Hamstrings—Semi-tendonosis, semi-membranosis and biceps femoris span hip and knee (supplied by sciatic nerve). They arise from the ischial tuberosity. Action: hip extension and knee flexion.

Knee

Tibiofemoral and patellofemoral joints. Supported by collateral and cruciate ligaments. Synovial hinge joint—capsule replaced anteriorly by patella complex.

Ligaments: LCL—lateral epicondyle femur to head of biceps (resist varus). Medial collateral ligament (MCL)—medial epicondyle to inferior to medial condyle of tibia. Resists valgus strain. ACL—front of upper tibia to inside of lateral condyle femur—resists anterior displacement of tibia on femur. PCL—posterior tibia to medial condyle femur—resists posterior displacement.

Menisci—C-shaped cartilaginous structures. Medial meniscus attached to the MCL (not lateral meniscus). As the medial menisci are less mobile—more likely to be injured.

Bursae—suprapatellar, semi-membranosus, prepatellar.

Movements: flexion—hamstrings, gastrocnemius, popliteus. Extension—quadriceps femoris. Medial rotation of tibia—semi-membranosus and semi-tendinosus. Lateral rotation—biceps femoris.

Popliteal fossa—diamond shaped. Boundaries—biceps femoris (common peroneal nerve behind and lateral), semi-membranosus, lateral head of gastrocnemius, plantaris and medial gastrocnemius. Structures—superficial to deep (tibial nerve, popliteal vein, popliteal artery). Tibial nerve runs between heads of gastrocnemius, deep to soleus supplies all the calf muscles dividing into the medial and lateral plantar nerves. Common peroneal nerve winds around neck of the fibula, divides into superficial peroneal nerve (sensory/peroneii) and deep peroneal nerve (extensor muscles/1st web space skin).

Leg

Compartments of the leg

- Anterior—tibialis anterior, extensor digitorum longus, extensor hallucis longus, extensor digitorum brevis, extensor hallucis brevis
- Posterior
  - Superficial: soleus and gastrocnemius
  - Deep: flexor hallucis longus, tibialis posterior, flexor digitorum longus
- Lateral—Peroneus brevis and peroneus longus.

For further reading see Moore and Dalley[1].

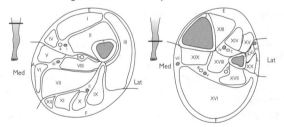

1. Femur 2. Tibia 3. Fibula

I) Rectus femoris II) Vastus medialis III) Vastus lateralis IV) Sartorius V) Adductor longus
VI) Gracilis VII) Adductor magnus VIII) Adductor brevis IX) Gluteus maximus X) Biceps femoris
XI) Semitendinosus XII) Semimembranosus XIII) Tibialis anterior XIV) Extensor hallucis longus
XV) Extensor digitorum XVI) Soleus XVII) Flexor hallucis longus XVIII) Tibialis posterior
XIX) Flexor digitorum longus XX) Peroneus longus XXI) Peroneus brevis a) Femoral artery
b) Profunda femoral artery c) Anterior tibial artery d) Peroneal artery e) Posterior tibial artery
i) Femoral nerve ii) Sciatic nerve iii) Obturator nerve iv) Deep peroneal nerve v) Tibial nerve
vi) Superficial tibial nerve vii) Saphenous nerve

Fig. 6.8 Lower limb—transverse sections.

Reference

1 Moore KL, Dalley AF. Lower limb. In: *Clinically Orientated Anatomy*. Philadelphia, PA: Lippincott Williams and Wilkins, 1999:503–663.

Anatomy of the lower limb: ankle and foot

Ankle

Joint situated between lower tibia, fibula and talus. It has a capsule that is reinforced by the medial deltoid ligament and lateral ligamentous complex comprising anterior and posterior talofibular and calcaneofibular ligaments.

Structures entering the foot posterior to the medial malleolus are, from medial to lateral, tibialis posterior, flexor digitorum longus, the tibial nerve, the posterior tibial artery, and flexor hallucis longus.

Movements

Dorsiflexion—tibialis anterior, extensor hallucis longus, extensor digitorum longus, and peroneus tertius.

Plantiflexion—gastrocnemius, soleus, tibialis posterior, flexor hallucis longus, flexor digitorum longus, peroneus longus and peroneus brevis.

Stability

- Bony—talus stabilized between tibia and fibula
- Ligamentous complexes—deltoid ligament stabilizes the ankle medially preventing abduction, and the lateral complex prevents adduction. Rotatory stability is conferred by alignment of the talus in the mortise and the collateral and syndesmosis ligaments. The syndesmosis consists of anterior and posterior tibiofibular and interosseous ligaments.

Foot

Hindfoot The bones of the hindfoot are the calcaneus and talus.

Subtalar joint

The talocalcaneal joint allows supination and pronation of the hindfoot. There are three articular facets between the talus and calcaneus—anterior, middle and posterior. The most important ligaments are the interosseous ligament in the sinus tarsi canal and medial ligament (deep portion of the deltoid ligament). The calcaneofibular ligament stabilizes the subtalar joint laterally.

Midfoot The bones of the midfoot are the navicular, cuboid and three cuneiforms.

Midtarsal joints—talonavicular and calcaneocuboid joints
Movements

These movements are primarily those of:
- Inversion—tibialis anterior, tibialis posterior
- Eversion—peroneus longus and brevis.

Stability

The bifurcate ligament, consisting of the plantar calcaneonavicular (spring) ligament and calcaneocuboid ligament, contributes to the stability of the joints between the hindfoot and midfoot. The spring ligament is situated between the sustentaculum tali of calcaneus and the navicular. The talonavicular joint is a ball and socket type joint that allows gliding and rotatory movements. The head of the talus articulates with the calcaneus and navicular bones and is supported by the spring ligament. The calcaneo-cuboid joint is saddle shaped and allows some abduction and adduction. Stability is conferred by the shape of the joint and the long and short plantar ligaments.

Forefoot The bones of the forefoot are the metatarsals and phalanges.

Tarsometatarsal, metatarsophalangeal, and interphalangeal joints

Movements

The forefoot can be flexed and extended, and there is a small amount of adduction, abduction, and circumduction.

Stability

The tarsometatarsal joints are stabilized by dorsal, plantar, and interos-seous ligaments. The second and third metatarsals are attached to the respective cuneiforms by strong ligaments limiting movements at these joints, whereas the first, fourth, and fifth metatarsals are more mobile. The metatarsophalangeal joints are condylar joints that allow flexion, extension and some abduction, adduction, and circumduction, whereas the interphalangeal joints are hinge joints and only allow flexion and extension. The metatarsophalangeal and interphalangeal joints are stabi-lized by their capsules and collateral and plantar ligaments.

Plantar aponeurosis—arises from the medial and lateral tubercles of the calcaneus, divides into 5 slips, one for each toe, and fuses with the fibrous flexor sheaths and metatarsophalangeal joint capsules. It contributes to the stability of the longitudinal arch of the foot.

Sole of the foot muscle layers:

- 1st layer—abductor hallucis, abductor digiti minimi, flexor digitorum brevis
- 2nd layer—lumbricals, quadratus plantae
- 3rd layer—flexor hallucis brevis, adductor hallucis, flexor digiti minimi brevis
- 4th layer—dorsal and plantar interossei.

Innervation of the foot

Sensory

- Dorsum—superficial and deep fibular nerves
- Sole—medial plantar nerve (medial three and a half toes and medial sole) and lateral plantar nerve (lateral sole and lateral one and a half toes)
- Medial side of foot as far as the metatarsal head—saphenous nerve
- Heel—calcaneal branches of the tibial and sural nerves.

Motor

The medial plantar nerve supplies the abductor hallucis, flexor digitorum brevis, flexor hallucis brevis and the first lumbrical muscle. The lateral plantar nerve supplies all the other muscles of the sole.

For further reading see Moore and Dalley[1].

Reference

1 Moore KL, Dalley AF. Lower limb. In: *Clinically Orientated Anatomy*. Philadelphia, PA: Lippincott Williams and Wilkins, 1999:503–663.

Nervous system

The nervous system is categorized anatomically into:
- Central nervous system—brain and spinal cord
- Peripheral nervous system—all other neural tissue.

It can also be categorized functionally into:
- Somatic nervous system—under conscious control
- Autonomic nervous system.

Somatic nervous system

The cerebrum consists of two cerebral hemispheres which consist of grey matter (cell bodies), white matter (axons) and CSF-filled lateral ventricles. The surface folds (sulci) and prominences (gyri) create a consistent surface map of various functional centres. The central sulcus lies between the precentral and postcentral gyri, which control motor and sensory function, respectively. The axons which connect these centres to their target skin and muscle locations mostly cross in the brainstem or spinal cord, such that the left motor and sensory functions of the body are controlled mostly by the right side of the brain, and vice versa.

Damage to the motor part of the CNS manifests itself clinically as an UMN dysfunction, whereas damage to the motor part of the peripheral nervous system manifests itself as LMN dysfunction.

Autonomic nervous system

The autonomic nervous system controls smooth and cardiac muscles as well as glandular function. It is not under voluntary control. It consists of the sympathetic system and the parasympathetic system.

Sympathetic nervous system

Preganglionic fibres are located between T1 and L2, and they synapse in paravertebral ganglia using the neurotransmitter acetylcholine. The postganglionic axons then distribute to the glands or body walls, using noradrenaline at the axonal endplate. The sympathetic innervation of skin and blood vessels uses acetylcholine at the endplate.

Parasympathetic nervous system

The parasympathetic nervous system does not innervate the skin or extremities. Preganglionic fibres are located in the brainstem in cranial nerve nuclei and from S2–S4. The vagus nerve contains parasympathetic nerves which supply the respiratory tract, heart, and gastrointestinal organs. The S2–S4 preganglionic axons supply the pelvic organs. The splenic flexure of the large bowel divides vagus-supplied organs from those innervated by the sacral parasympathetic nerves.

The vascular system

Arterial system

Major arteries are often given different names as they pass anatomical landmarks, for example:

Upper limb
- The subclavian artery changes name to the axillary artery in the axilla at the outer border of the 1st rib
- The axillary artery changes name to the brachial artery at teres major muscle border
- The brachial artery keeps its name until it bifurcates into the radial and ulnar arteries at the elbow.

Lower limb
- The external iliac artery changes name to the femoral artery at the inguinal ligament in the groin
- The femoral artery changes name to the popliteal artery when it leaves the adductor hiatus in the distal thigh to enter the popliteal fossa
- The popliteal artery keeps its name until it bifurcates into the anterior and posterior tibial arteries at the soleus.

Venous system

The venous system is anatomically divided into
- Superficial venous system
- Deep venous system.

In the lower limb, the short and long saphenous veins constitute the superficial venous system, while the femoral vein and its tributaries constitute the deep venous system.

The external vein is renamed the femoral iliac vein when it crosses the inguinal ligament and is renamed the popliteal vein when it enters the popliteal fossa. The popliteal vein receives tributaries from the anterior and posterior tibial veins and the short saphenous vein. These three veins constitute the deep veins of the calf (the 'calf pump').

The venous flow is maintained by one-way valve systems and muscle contractions, which squeeze the deoxygenated toward the heart. The superficial venous system and deep venous system communicate via perforating veins, which are also valved. Competent valves prevent blood from flowing from deep to superficial veins; incompetent valves do not prevent this, resulting in expanded or varicose veins.

Gait in children and adults

In normal gait there is a complex coordination of movement and muscular contraction involving the lower limb, pelvis, and spine as well as secondary movements of the upper limbs. This is most often disturbed in neurological disorders, commonly CP.

Phases: the foot is either on the floor (stance phase, 60% of gait cycle) or in the air (swing phase, 40%). Stance begins with 'initial contact' which is normally a 'heel strike', but in CP, for example, with a tight or overactive tendo-achilles and an equinus foot, initial contact will be with the forefoot. Next is a 'loading response' as the foot comes flat and takes weight; eccentric (paying out) contraction of the calf muscles decelerates the body and brings its centre of mass in front of the knee joint which passively extends. If the knee is fixed in flexion, this cannot occur and the quadriceps will need to be active throughout stance phase which is inefficient. A brief period of double limb support follows (10% of cycle) as the opposite foot strikes the ground before the calf muscles contract concentrically (pulling up) to plantar flex the ankle and generate 'heel rise' and 'toe-off' into the swing phase.

Gait analysis: walking is too complex a cycle to analyse effectively by simple observation. At its simplest level, a video recording of the individual walking is taken from in front and the side and played back repeatedly. Markers placed on the limbs and girdles can be tracked by special sensors to record displacements in time and space (kinematics). Surface electrodes record muscle contractions and forces generating movement (kinetics). This information is plotted against normal patterns of displacement and muscle activity. Calorimetry or measurement of oxygen consumption can be used to assess the energy cost of walking.

This information can be analysed against the 5 prerequisites for normal gait described by Gage[1]:
• Stability in stance
• Foot clearance in swing
• Adequate step length
• Ability to preposition the foot prior to initial contact and loading
• Energy efficiency over the whole cycle.

This can be used to inform appropriate intervention. A muscle which is overactive can be lengthened and one which is firing out of phase can be transferred. Rotational deformity can be addressed by corrective osteotomy. The holistic information provided by gait analysis facilitates a complete prescription for primary and secondary abnormalities at multiple levels. This avoids the 'Birthday syndrome' described by Mercer Rang; when a procedure at, for example, the ankle, uncovers a problem at the knee and subsequently the hip, all of which lead to separate interventions during a child's development.

Reference
1 Gage JR. Gait analysis: an essential tool in the assessment of cerebral palsy. *Clin Orthop Rel Res* 1993;**288**:126–34.

Surgical approaches

Surgical principles

Effective operative orthopaedics only became possible in the last hundred or so years with the advent of the '3 amigos': anaesthesia, asepsis (and later antibiotics), and X-rays. Modern orthopaedics has seen the rise of joint replacement and endoscopic reconstructive surgery, heavily backed by huge industrial players, with the future containing sophisticated outcomes analysis and increased genetic understanding of orthopaedic disorders.

Why think? Why not try the experiment? John Hunter

Orthopaedic surgery can be distilled into two main objectives: to ease pain and restore function. However, any intervention carries the risk of complications, which can be devastating and irreversible, and an economic cost. Before listing a patient for surgery the clinician must be certain that all available non-operative measures have been exhausted and there is a reasonable base of evidence for the intervention proposed. Computers and the internet bring this evidence base to the clinician's fingertips in the workplace; there is no longer any place for experimental surgery in our day to day practice.

Orthopaedic surgeons are part of a multidisciplinary team including nurse specialists, physiotherapists, orthotists, occupational therapists, pain specialists. Look especially to these colleagues for alternative treatments when the risk:benefit ratio of surgery is high, but also involve them at an early stage in your operative scheduling to ensure resources are used efficiently.

Good surgeons know how to cut; great surgeons know when to cut

If surgery is indicated, the doctrine of informed consent requires us to impart sufficient and appropriate information to each individual patient such that they can make up their own minds on whether to proceed. Some patients will ask what you would do; be frank—it's not paternalistic to offer an opinion. In fact it's what you have been trained to do and often what patients want to do.

The difference between an efficient surgeon and a slow one is knowledge of anatomy

Read up all you can about a procedure before undertaking or assisting at it. Above all know the anatomy, internervous planes[1] and structures at risk. Once in the operating theatre pay great attention to sterility, handle soft tissues with respect and be meticulous with haemostasis to avoid infection. If you are assisting, imagine you are doing the procedure yourself to anticipate the next step and maintain concentration.

Reference

1 Hoppenfeld S, deBoer P. *Surgical Exposures in Orthopaedics. The Anatomic Approach*, 3rd edn. Philadelphia, PA: Lippincott Williams and Wilkins, 2003.

Preoperative planning

Patient factors have been optimized and consent obtained through the preadmission clinic. Patient side marked, blood ordered.

A preoperative plan is the strategy for your tactics on the day. It includes organizing and disposing staff (appropriate assistance, anaesthetist competent to perform blocks, radiographer for image intensifier), in correct setting (laminar flow theatre for joint arthroplasty) with the requisite materials and equipment (range of implant sizes, allograft, special drills, saws, or reamers). Orthopaedics is a highly technical specialty requiring early forward surgical planning.

Consider also potential problems that may arise intraoperatively and the additional plans and equipment which may become necessary.

Below are some examples of planning techniques:

Hip arthroplasty

Use of templates supplied by the implant manufacturer facilitates:
- Determination of leg length for equalization
- Selection of correct cup size and position
- Planning of femoral neck cut and sizing/position of femoral stem.

Trauma

Can trace fracture fragments on overlays of radiograph to plan reconstruction and placement of screws/plates (manufacturer templates available). Check for mechanical axis correction with hip, knee, and ankle square to ground at end of intended reduction and fixation.

Be familiar with your local system of external fixation for emergent treatment of open fractures and those with significant vascular injury.

Limb deformity correction

Planning traditionally done on printed films with a pencil and 'linefinder' ruler and protractor[1]. Software packages available to assist planning on-screen with digital imaging systems.

Aim to identify site(s), level and magnitude of deformity to plan corrective osteotomy(ies). In simple terms:
- Identify mechanical axis of leg (line drawn from centre of femoral head to centre of ankle joint on a long leg AP film). This should pass through the centre of the knee joint; if not there is mechanical axis deviation
- Draw in anatomic (along centreline of bone) or mechanical (from centre of joint above to centre of joint below) axes for femur and tibia and measure the angle they form with the joints. If these are different from the opposite (assumed normal) side or expected normal values there is deformity in that bone
- Where axes drawn relative to joints within that bone (which should be collinear) intersect, this marks the level of the deformity. The angle of intersection is the magnitude of the deformity.

Reference

1 Paley D. *Principles of Deformity Correction*. Belin: Springer, 2005.

Principles of wound care

The frequency of disastrous consequences in compound fractures contrasted with the complete immunity to life or limb in simple fractures is one of the most striking as well as melancholy facts in surgical practice.

Lister, 1867

A wound closed by apposition of its skin edges heals by primary intention; one which is left open heals by secondary intention.

Phases of wound healing (some overlap):
- Inflammatory 0–5 days
- Proliferation 3–14 days
- Maturation 7 days to 1yr.

Clean wounds

Close surgical incisions with sutures or staples, keep clean and dry, minimize stress (can add Steri-Strips™ to prevent spreading) and pressure on the area.

Clean with sterile water and cover only if likely to become contaminated. Time suture removal by site: face 5–7 days, limbs 10–14 days, trunk 10 days.

Contaminated wounds

Debride (with or without preoperative radiograph or USS) to ensure all foreign material removed. Irrigate thoroughly with solution of chlorhexidine in saline. Leave open with a saline-soaked gauze wick or pack. Check tetanus status, administer prophylactic antibiotics tailored to likely contaminants.

Plan second look at 48h ± further debridement and irrigation. If clean at this stage can appose skin edges with interrupted sutures.

Infected wounds

Unless obviously superficial, plan to debride, irrigate and take deep samples for bacteriology prior to starting antibiotics. Leave wound open unless over a joint or prosthesis, 2nd look at 48h. If infection involves a prosthesis then thorough debridement is mandatory with exchange of modular components, e.g. polyethylene insert in knee replacement.

General

All staff must wash hands between patients and wear gloves when inspecting and changing wound dressings. Discourage patients from touching the wound. Optimize patient factors to help wound healing:
- Good blood sugar control
- Stop smoking
- Elevate limb to reduce swelling
- Supplemental oxygen
- Complete antibiotic course.

Surgical approaches to the cervical spine (anterior approach to the lower cervical spine)

Anatomy

Allows exposure to anterior aspect of vertebral bodies from C3–T1. The recurrent laryngeal nerve is the most important structure at risk—it is less at risk on the left as it ascends between trachea and oesophagus, having branched off the vagus nerve at the level of the arch of the aorta. The right recurrent laryngeal nerve runs alongside the trachea after looping around the right subclavian artery. It crosses from lateral to medial in the lower part of the neck and can be vulnerable. Personal preference as to which side to use.

Positioning

Preoperative planning

Under general anaesthetic, patients placed in a supine position with extension of the neck. Head ring or Mayfield clamp used to support the head and nasogastric tube inserted to enable identification of the oesophagus. Level checked with radiographs. Patient's head turned away from the planned incision. Head of the table elevated 30° to reduce bleeding.

Incision

An oblique skin crease incision is made at correct level (landmarks are: mandible C2 level, hyoid C3 level, thyroid C5 level and cricoid C6 level). Incision extended from the midline to the anterior border of sternocleidomastoid.

Surgical approach (Fig. 7.1)

Superficial

Transverse incision made from the anterior border of the *sternocleidomastoid* to midline and carried down through the platysma muscle and fascia. The platysma muscle is elevated and cut in line with the incision or split with fingers in the line of fibres.

Deep

The sternocleidomastoid is retracted laterally and sternohyoid and sternothyroid muscles medially. Omohyoid lies over carotid sheath divided as necessary. Carotid artery palpated and a plane is developed between the medial edge of the carotid sheath and the midline structures (thyroid, trachea and oesophagus), dividing through pretracheal fascia. Cervical vertebrae are covered by longus colli muscle and prevertebral fascia. Anterior longitudinal ligament is cut in midline.

Damage

Risk of injury to the recurrent laryngeal nerve, sympathetic chain and thoracic duct (on the left). The cervical sympathetic chain is anterior to the *longus capitis* muscle and lateral to the *longus coli*. The left recurrent laryngeal nerve is protected during a left-sided approach as it runs between the trachea and the oesophagus.

Posterior approach to the cervical spine

Position

Prone position with the head and neck in neutral position, supported on a head ring or held in a Mayfield clamp.

Approach

A midline incision is performed. Ligamenum nuchae is then divided in the midline. The superficial layer and the intermediate layer of paraspinal muscles are then divided (splenius, semispinalis, and longismus coli) and reflected laterally. The erector spinae muscles are retracted laterally using a Cobb elevator. A laminectomy is performed to access the spinal canal.

Dangers

During surgery the erector spinae muscles should not be dissected laterally beyond the facets to avoid denervation of posterior cervical muscles. Superiorly the vertebral artery is at risk, especially where it leaves the foramen transversarium and tracts medially to pierce the atlanto-occipital membrane. Protection should be given to the greater occipital nerve C2 and the third occipital nerve C3.

For further reading see Hoppenfeld and deBoer[1].

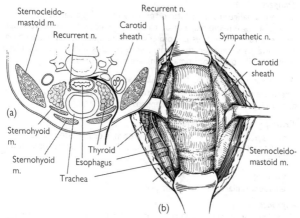

Fig. 7.1 Anterior cervical approach.

Reproduced from Bulstrode et al., *Oxford Textbook of Orthopaedics and Trauma*, with permission from Oxford University Press.

Reference

1 Hoppenfeld S, deBoer P. *Surgical Exposures in Orthopaedics. The Anatomic Approach*, 3rd edn. Philadelphia, PA: Lippincott Williams and Wilkins, 2003.

Surgical approaches: approaches to the lumbar spine

Posterior approach to the lumbar spine

Positioning

The patient is placed in a prone position on a Montreal mattress or on all fours with hips and knees flexed at 90° to prevent excessive pressure on the chest wall and minimize the increase in intra-abdominal pressure, which decreases bleeding during surgery.

Approach

A straight midline incision is made over the vertebrae that need to be exposed. The lumbar fascia is divided. The paraspinal muscles are innervated segmentally and therefore the approach to the spine is an internervous plane. The paraspinal muscles can be mobilized from the sides of the laminae. A laminotomy or laminectomy can then be performed to access the spinal canal. The approach can be extended proximally or distally along the entire spine. As no nerves cross the midline, the nerve supply of the paraspinal muscles is safe.

Dangers

There is a danger to the posterior primary rami of the segmental nerves. Loss of a single nerve may not be clinically significant as the nerve supply to the paraspinal muscles is from several levels. Segmental vessels from the aorta pass between the transverse processes and if cut may bleed profusely. The posterior primary rami are close to these vessels.

Anterior approach to the lumbar spine

There are two approaches to the anterior lumbar spine—transperitoneal approach and the retroperitoneal approach.

Transperitoneal approach

Provides access from L1 to S1. The approach is usually used for fusion of L5 to S1 and occasionally L4 to L5. The umbilicus lies approximately at the level of L3.

Positioning

The patient is placed in the supine position.

Approach

A midline longitudinal approach skirting the umbilicus is made to just above the umbilicus. The internervous plane between the two recti is developed. The incision is deepened to expose the peritoneum, which is incised. Bowel and the bladder are retracted and the posterior peritoneum can then be incised at the level of the sacral promontory. The aortic bifurcation is exposed and the median sacral artery ligated and divided. The L5/S1 disc space can then be identified.

Dangers

Injury to the superior hypogastric plexus that overlies the L5 lumbar vertebrae.

Retroperitoneal approach

Provides access from L1 to S1.

Positioning

Patient is placed in a lateral position, usually right side down. It is preferable to approach from the left as it is easier to mobilize the aorta.

Approach

An oblique incision is made extending from the border of the 12th rib to the lateral border of the rectus abdominal muscle. The muscles of the anterior abdominal wall are then divided (external, internal oblique, and the transversus abdominis). The retroperitoneal space is exposed by developing a plane between the peritoneum and wall of the abdomen, revealing the psoas major with the overlying genitofemoral nerve. The segmental vessels can then be ligated and the aorta mobilized. The sympathetic chain is also mobilized.

Dangers

Sympathetic chain which lies between the vertebral body and the psoas major can be damaged. The ureter can also be damaged as it lies on the psoas fascia over the transverse processes.

Surgical approaches: shoulder

Anterior approach (deltopectoral)

Indication: shoulder replacement, open stabilization, some fractures.

Position: deckchair (45° reclined), arm draped free.

Incision: from coracoid process to a point just lateral to axillary fold.

Dissection: identify the groove between the deltoid muscle (axillary nerve supply) and the pectoralis major (pectoral nerves). Isolate and retract the cephalic vein in this interval (usually laterally as most tributaries drain here). Develop the deltopectoral groove and identify the conjoint tendon (short head of biceps and coracobrachialis). Retract this medially ± partial tenotomy (protecting underlying musculocutaneous nerve just below coracoid origin). Front of the shoulder joint is covered by subscapularis (with overlying bursa); externally rotate shoulder, divide tendon at insertion into lesser tuberosity (insert stay sutures for later repair). Dissect off underlying capsule, then incise to expose GHJ.

Risks: musculocutaneous nerve and brachial plexus, also axillary nerve passes posteriorly under lower border of subscapularis tendon (bleeding from the circumflex vessels which accompany the nerve is a warning sign).

Posterior approach

Indication: rarely used; posterior instability, tumour excision, tendon transfer.

Position: lateral.

Incision: along scapular spine.

Dissection: between teres minor (axillary nerve supply) and infraspinatus (suprascapular nerve).

Risks: axillary nerve; stay above teres minor to avoid in quadrilateral space.

Lateral approach to the rotator cuff

Indication: cuff repair, reattachment greater tuberosity fracture.

Position: as for deltopectoral.

Incision: just lateral to edge of acromion; transverse heals better, longitudinal allows better access.

Dissection: split deltoid in line of its fibres to expose subacromial bursa (often thickened) which covers superior aspect of the rotator cuff (supraspinatus and infraspinatus).

Risks: axillary nerve passes forwards 5cm distal to tip of the acromion (do not extend incision beyond this), adherent to the deep surface of deltoid.

Arthroscopy portals

Position: deckchair (head on a ring mounted off the table to facilitate access), or lateral with arm traction (weights from a drip stand attached to table).

Incision: stab with small blade, 1 thumb's width below and medial to the posterolateral corner of the acromion in the palpable 'soft spot'. Aim a blunt trocar anteriorly towards the coracoid to access the GHJ, withdraw and aim superiorly under the acromion for the subacromial bursa (sweep the trocar side to side within bursa to clear a space). Further portals can be placed laterally (through deltoid for viewing or passing shavers into subacromial space) or anteriorly (under direct arthroscopic vision or using a 'switching stick' railroading technique).

Surgical approaches: arm

Anterior approach

Indication: humeral fracture, osteotomy, excision of infected bone or tumour.

Position: supine, arm outstretched on armboard.

Incision: from coracoid process, distally in deltopectoral groove then following lateral border of biceps.

Dissection: proximally, dissect deltopectoral groove as for anterior approach to shoulder, expose humeral shaft by incising periosteum lateral to pectoralis major insertion. Distally, incise deep fascia lateral to biceps, identify brachialis and separate medial two-thirds (musculocutaneous nerve supply) from lateral third (radial nerve). In practice, exploring the interval between biceps and brachialis is reasonable if care taken to protect the musculocutaneous nerve (lies on the brachialis, terminal sensory branch the lateral cutaneous nerve of the forearm).

Risks: musculocutaneous nerve, radial nerve (stay subperiosteal on humerus to avoid it posteriorly proximally and laterally distally).

Posterior approach

Indication: as for anterior.

Position: lateral, arm over well-padded bolster support.

Incision: longitudinal in posterior midline down to olecranon.

Dissection: expose triceps aponeurosis distally; identify and divide its (superficial) lateral and long heads more proximally. Deep to these is medial head below the spiral groove of humerus; the marker for the radial nerve and profunda brachii artery. Identify and protect these, then expose bone subperiosteally to avoid damage to ulnar nerve medially.

Risks: radial and ulnar nerves.

Lateral approach to distal humerus

Indication: fixation lateral condyle fracture, tennis elbow (ECRB) release.

Position: supine, arm across chest.

Incision: over lateral supracondylar ridge.

Dissection: between triceps and brachioradialis (both supplied by radial nerve but well proximal).

Risks: radial nerve (pierces lateral intermuscular septum in distal third of arm; do not extend above this).

Surgical approaches: elbow

Lateral approach

Indication: radial head fracture, supracondylar fracture (with medial displacement of distal fragment disrupting soft tissue envelope laterally).

Position: supine with armboard, forearm pronated to protect PIN.

Incision: curvilinear, centred over the epicondyle towards dorsal ulna.

Dissection: identify the origins of ECRL, ECU and ECRB (deeper); underneath them is the elbow joint capsule. In supracondylar fracture proximal fragment may buttonhole through brachialis, in which case dissection simply follows haematoma.

Risks: PIN if incision taken too far distally (beyond annular ligament), or from retractors. Minimize posterior dissection to preserve vascularity of capitellum.

Posterior approach

Indication: distal humeral fracture.

Position: prone (intubated) with forearm hanging over end of armboard.

Dissection: dissect out and pass soft loops around ulnar nerve medially, then transverse or chevron osteotomy of olecranon 2cm from tip. Excellent exposure but osteotomy intra-articular; fix with screw or tension band wire technique.

Risks: ulnar nerve, radial nerve above distal third of humerus.

Anterior approach

Indication: rarely used, best done with plastic or vascular surgeon for supracondylar fracture with injury to brachial artery (remember distal fasciotomy). Also for repair biceps avulsion, exploration of lacerations.

Position: supine, arm extended on armboard.

Incision: longitudinal with gentle 'S' curve over the elbow flexion crease.

Dissection: identify and protect lateral cutaneous nerve of forearm between biceps and brachialis. Then incise bicipital aponeurosis—beware brachial artery (with vein and median nerve medially) is directly underneath. Radial nerve crosses in front of elbow joint also between brachialis and brachioradialis.

Risks: above-named nerves and vessels.

Surgical approaches: forearm

Anterior approach to the radius (extensile approach of Henry)

Indication: fracture, excision of infected bone or tumour, osteotomy.

Position: supine with armboard, forearm supinated.

Incision: along a line from lateral to the biceps tendon proximally to radial styloid distally.

Dissection: palpate the 'mobile wad of 3'—brachioradialis, ECRL, and ECRB. Develop plane between this and FCR (protect superficial radial nerve (SRN) underneath brachioradialis). Retract radial artery medially. Detach supinator, pronator teres, and FDS to expose bone proximal to distal.

Risks: PIN in proximal third—pierces supinator to enter posterior compartment of forearm.

Posterior approach to the radius (Thomson)

Indication: as for anterior (allows plating of fracture on tension side of bone).

Position: supine with armboard, forearm pronated.

Incision: along a line from lateral epicondyle to Lister's tubercle at wrist.

Dissection: between ECRB (radial nerve supply) and extensor digitorum communis (EDC) proximally and EPL distally (both PIN). Identify and protect PIN emerging 1cm proximal to distal end of supinator, then detach this and more distally lift off APL and EPB (retract either side) to access bone.

Risks: PIN preservation is the key to this approach.

Approach to the ulna

Indication: as for approaches to radius.

Position: supine with arm pronated across chest.

Incision: along subcutaneous border of ulna.

Dissection: through plane between the ECU and FCU (some fibres running between them need to be divided).

Risks: stay subperiosteal to avoid ulnar nerve.

Surgical approaches: wrist and hand

Volar approach to the carpal tunnel

Indication: decompression of median nerve, flexor tenosynovectomy, drainage of sepsis, repair of tendon lacerations.

Position: supine, armboard, forearm supinated.

Incision: longitudinal, from intersection of Kaplan's cardinal line (from 1st web space runs medial parallel to palmar wrist crease) and another line extending from radial border of ring finger up to wrist crease.

Dissection: careful dissection of superficial fat and palmar fascia, ideally with loupe magnification, to avoid palmar cutaneous branch of median nerve. Expose and incise transverse carpal ligament (flexor retinaculum), biased ulnarwards to protect motor branch of the median nerve (course displays several anatomical variants).

Risks: superficial palmar arch, stay proximal to Kaplan's line.

Volar approach to the distal radius

Indication: fractures, excision of infected bone or tumour.

Position: supine, armboard, forearm supinated.

Incision: longitudinal over tendon of FCR.

Dissection: incise FCR tendon sheath, retract it medially and radial artery laterally. Through FCR bed is pronator quadratus; detach from its radial insertion and reflect medially to access distal radius and radiocarpal joint (including proximal pole of the scaphoid).

Risks: median nerve and palmar cutaneous branch, radial artery.

Dorsal approach to the distal radius

Indication: tendon repair or transfer, tenosynovectomy, fractures, ulnar head excision.

Position: supine, armboard, forearm pronated.

Incision: longitudinal, midway between radial and ulnar styloid processes, in the line of 3rd metacarpal.

Dissection: sharp through superficial fat to expose extensor retinaculum; lift as an ulnar-based flap (and replace deep to the tendons if rheumatoid disease) or incise between 3rd and 4th dorsal compartments to expose dorsal aspect of distal radius.

Approach to the flexor tendons

Indication: tendon and nerve repair, release Dupuytren's contracture, drainage sepsis.

Position: supine, armboard with a 'lead hand' to hold the fingers extended.

Incision: zig-zags in fingers between flexion creases, extended onto the palm as necessary.

Dissection: full thickness flaps reflected to expose flexor tendon sheaths.

Risks: neurovascular bundles at lateral border of flexor sheaths, separated from volar subcutaneous flap by a thin layer of fibrous tissue.

Surgical approaches: hip and femur

Lateral approach (multiple variations and eponyms)

Indication: hip replacement and hemiarthroplasty for fractured femoral neck.

Position: lateral, or supine with sandbag under affected side (so buttock hangs free).

Incision: longitudinal, centred over greater trochanter, incision based two-thirds proximal, one-third distal to trochanter.

Dissection: cut fascia lata in line of incision, incise trochanteric bursa to define gluteus medius tendinous insertion into greater trochanter. Detach its anterior half to two-thirds, leaving a cuff to repair, and continue distally into origin of vastus lateralis to expose neck and proximal femur. Externally rotate hip and incise underlying gluteus minimus to expose thick capsule of hip joint.

Risks: superior gluteal nerve between gluteus minimus and medius 3–5cm above greater trochanter; do not split above this.

Posterior approach

Indication: as for lateral.

Position: lateral.

Incision: as for lateral approach, but flex hip up 90° during skin incision so that it curves posteriorly with hip extended.

Dissection: incise the fascia lata, proximally split gluteus maximus in the line of its fibres (beware bleeding from avulsed vessels). Expose short external rotators (piriformis, obturator internus and gemelli), place a curved Mayo scissors under them and detach close to femoral insertion (internally rotate hip to put muscles on stretch, insert stay suture for later repair, stay out of quadratus femoris to reduce bleeding). Thus the capsule is exposed.

Risks: sciatic nerve lies in fat on short external rotators; reflect these back with stay suture to protect it.

Anterior approach (Smith-Peterson)

Indication: open reduction late presenting developmental dysplasia of hip (DDH), drainage hip sepsis.

Position: supine, sandbag under affected side.

Incision: from ASIS 2 finger-breadths below iliac crest, parallel to it and curving medially over anterior inferior iliac spine (AIIS).

Dissection: develop plane between sartorius and tensor fasciae latae (TFL), rectus femoris lies in base; detach from origin on AIIS to expose hip capsule. Sharply incise and split the iliac apophysis down to bone to expose subperiosteally the inner and outer tables of the pelvis and superior capsule. Reflected head of rectus femoris can be followed around superior capsule.

Risks: lateral cutaneous nerve of the thigh, usually lies alongside sartorius so identify and retract medially with muscle. Ascending branch of medial circumflex artery lies distally in TFL/sartorius interval, needs to be coagulated to control bleeding.

Lateral approach to femur

Indication: fracture fixation, excision of infected bone or tumour, osteotomy.

Position: supine ± sandbag under affected side so patella points anteriorly.

Incision: longitudinal following the line of the femoral shaft.

Dissection: split fascia lata in line with incision, split vastus lateralis muscle in line of its fibres or lift anteriorly and dissect off the lateral intermuscular septum to reveal the femoral shaft.

Risks: arterial perforators in lateral intermuscular septum which may retract into muscle if divided, causing troublesome bleeding. Try to identify and coagulate first.

Surgical approaches: knee and tibia/fibula

Medial parapatellar approach
Indication: joint replacement, arthrotomy.

Position: supine.

Incision: midline longitudinal from above patella to tibial tubercle.

Dissection: incise quadriceps tendon in the midline and skirt medial border of patella and patellar tendon. Evert patella and flex knee 90° to expose joint.

Arthroscopy portals
Position: supine, with knee able to flex over side or end of table and a post or leg holder to facilitate valgus stressing.

Incision: with knee flexed identify soft spot between inferolateral border of patella and lateral femoral condyle. Insert small blade through capsule (point cutting edge away from meniscus), then trocar and sweep up into suprapatellar pouch with knee going into extension. Then flex knee again, insert arthroscope and view medial compartment; pass a white needle into this compartment through medial soft spot (adjust according to angle of attack for anticipated procedure) and follow with blade and probe.

Anterior approach to tibia
Indication: excision of infected bone or tumour, osteotomy.

Position: supine.

Incision: longitudinal, 1cm lateral to anterior border of the tibia.

Dissection: elevating skin flaps exposes subcutaneous border of tibia; elevate or detach origin of tibialis anterior muscle to expose lateral surface of bone.

Risks: long saphenous vein runs up medial side of calf; identify and preserve.

Approach to the fibula
Indication: osteotomy, harvest for vascularized graft, fracture fixation.

Position: supine with sandbag under ipsilateral buttock.

Incision: longitudinal, just posterior to the fibular shaft, from lateral malleolus to fibular head then curving gently backwards in line with the biceps tendon.

Dissection: develop plane of the intermuscular septum between the peronei (peroneal compartment) and soleus (posterior compartment). Expose bone subperiosteally.

Risks: common peroneal nerve; runs behind biceps femoris tendon to wind around neck of fibula. Identify it under the tendon and retract gently forward by releasing the fibres of peroneus longus which cover it on the fibular neck.

Surgical approaches: ankle

Approach to medial malleolus
Indication: fracture, osteotomy to expose tibiotalar joint.

Position: supine.

Incision: curvilinear over anterior aspect of medial malleolus.

Dissection: dissect directly onto bone to expose malleolus; deltoid ligament fans out below this and can be split (repair later) to expose joint capsule.

Risks: identify and protect the long saphenous vein and saphenous nerve in superficial fat.

Approach to lateral malleolus
Indication: fracture.

Position: supine, sandbag under ipsilateral buttock.

Incision: directly over the bone, or slightly posterior to avoid prominent scar.

Dissection: through superficial tissues to expose bone, then subperiosteal on the fibula.

Risks: short saphenous vein and sural nerve posteriorly.

Posteromedial approach to ankle
Indication: posterior malleolar or triplane fracture, clubfoot open release, tendon repair, lengthening or transfer.

Position: supine with hip flexed and externally rotated, or prone.

Incision: midway between tendo-achilles and posterior border of medial malleolus.

Dissection: sharply dissect to and incise flexor retinaculum. Identify flexor hallucis longus (FHL), the only muscle here (see opposite) that still has fibres at this level, and retract medially or laterally to expose joint capsule.

Risks: posterior tibial artery and nerve in front of FHL; identify and protect.

Anterior approach to ankle joint
Indication: arthrotomy, fixation tibial pilon fractures.

Position: supine.

Incision: longitudinal, midway between malleoli.

Dissection: preserving branches of superficial peroneal nerve, identify and incise extensor retinaculum in interval between EHL and extensor digitorum longus (EDL). Mobilize and retract neurovascular bundle medially with EHL, incise periosteum of distal tibia and capsule to expose the joint.

Risks: deep peroneal nerve and anterior tibial artery.

Tendons passing behind medial malleolus from anterior to posterior

- Tom (tibialis posterior)
- Dick (flexor digitorum)
- And (neurovascular bundle)
- Harry (hexor hallucis longus—'beef to the heel')

Surgical approaches: foot

Lateral approach to os calcis

Indication: calcaneal fracture fixation.

Position: supine, sandbag under ipsilateral buttock.

Incision: use the 'extended lateral approach' of Eastwood[1]: a proximal posterior midline incision meets a distal incision passing directly posteriorly from the 5th metatarsal base just above the specialized weight-bearing skin of the sole.

Dissection: subperiosteal dissection onto the os calcis allows a flap to be retracted anteriorly containing skin and soft tissue including the peroneal tendons, sural nerve and posterior peroneal artery.

Risks: poor wound healing and sural nerve damage; use the approach described above to preserve vascularity and minimize risk of sural nerve damage.

Dorsomedial approach to 1st MTPJ

Indication: bunionectomy and hallux valgus correction, 1st metatarsal fusion.

Position: supine.

Incision: dorsomedial over 1st MTPJ, preserving superficial sensory nerve branches.

Dissection: expose joint via a racket-shaped capsulotomy flap to facilitate reefed closure (capsulorrhaphy).

Risks: damage to tendon of EHL in lateral aspect of wound.

Reference

1 Eastwood DM, Atkins RM. Lateral approaches to the heel: a comparison of two incisions for the fixation of calcaneal fractures. *The Foot* 1992;**2**:143–7.

Total hip replacement

Pioneered in Britain by Sir John Charnley (1911–1982, Manchester), a brilliant engineer and surgeon, whose entry in 'Who's who?' famously reads 'Recreation—other than surgery, none'. He almost abandoned arthroplasty when his original metal on Teflon© bearing failed after initial good clinical results; he walked away when a technical representative first demonstrated polyethylene (for use in gears) to him. His workshop manager put it through mechanical testing anyway and, 2 days later, when it showed minimal wear, Charnley realized 'we were on again'.

Hip replacement gives reliable pain relief and improved function for osteoarthritis and inflammatory arthritis. Worldwide 400 000 hips are replaced annually, 85% for osteoarthritis and 70% for >65yr olds. Expect survival at 10yrs of 90–95% falling to 85% at 20yrs[1].

Indications

Cardinal indication is pain, also loss of function and stiffness. Untreated sepsis is a contraindication; young age, medical or psychiatric disease and obesity relatively so.

Symptoms of dull ache usually in groin radiating down thigh to knee; buttock and below-knee pain may be from spine. Use of a stick, difficulty tying shoelaces, maximal analgesia are good indications that replacement is reasonable.

In younger, active patients revision surgery more likely so consider alternatives such as arthrodesis, acetabular osteotomy (e.g. Ganz) or augmentation (e.g. Chiari). Exception; the young patient with juvenile inflammatory arthropathy for whom arthroplasty greatly improves quality of life with reasonable survival[2].

Choice of implant

Surface replacement uses large head, metal on metal articulation; imparts stability and potentially excellent wear characteristics. Conserves femoral bone but not acetabular, which is generally the problem side. Risk of femoral neck fracture.

Stemmed (total) hip replacement has longer term data but variations abound: cemented/uncemented/hybrid fixation of implants to bone; metal on polyethylene/metal/ceramic or ceramic on ceramic bearings, etc. Choose one with proven registry survival unless part of proper trial.

Risks

- Infection (2%) and dislocation (3%)
- Aseptic loosening (osteolysis secondary to polyethylene wear particles)
- Leg length discrepancy (15%)
- Persistent pain or otherwise dissatisfied (1%)
- Nerve or vessel damage (0.1%)
- DVT, fatal PE (<0.1%).

References

1 Schulte KR, Callaghan JJ, Kelley SS, *et al.* The outcome of Charnley total hip arthroplasty with cement after a minimum 20 year follow-up. *J Bone Joint Surg Am* 1993;**75**:961–75.

2 Wedge J, Cummishmey D. Primary arthroplasty of the hip in patients who are less than 21 years old. *J Bone Joint Surg Am* 1994;**76**:1732–4.

Arthroscopy

Literally 'joint viewing', this is one of the great advances of the modern era of orthopaedics. Initially a diagnostic tool (and one of the earliest surgical procedures in this guise), now the basis of a huge range of reconstructive procedures.

Thus we can reconstruct the ACL through the arthroscope with small, supplementary incisions, and the results of arthroscopic surgery for anterior shoulder instability now approach those of the open procedure. We can visualize the more challenging joint surfaces of the hip (deep joint with difficult access) and wrist (small joint). Recovery times and surgical insult of arthroscopic compared with open surgery are significantly reduced.

As the need for direct diagnostic visualization has receded with the advent of MRI, the therapeutic possibilities have grown. The downside is that it is more difficult for trainees to learn the triangulation and visual–spatial skills required in the absence of simple diagnostic cases.

Equipment
- Telescope
  - Usually rigid with fibreoptic illumination
  - Passed through sheath or cannula inserted into joint with a trocar
  - Saline infused to distend and visualize the joint
  - Can obtain a number of views by rotating the arthroscope or using an arthroscope with lenses angled at 30° or 70°. Choice depends on joint and work being done
  - Camera
  - Now almost always linked to a television screen for ease of viewing by operator and assistants
- Hand instruments
  - Probe, punch, scissors, grabber, suture passer, etc.
- Power instruments
  - Shaver—soft tissue or bone cutting with suction to remove debris
  - Electrosurgery—for haemostasis and to cut or vaporize tissue.

Examples of joint-specific procedures
- **Knee**—menisectomy or repair for meniscal tear, removal of loose bodies (e.g. osteochondritis dissecans (OCD)), lateral retinacular release (for patellar maltracking), debridement (for OA), synovectomy (for RA), microfracture or fixation of osteochondral defect
- **Shoulder**—arthroscopic subacromial decompression (for impingement), rotator cuff repair
- **Ankle**—cheilectomy (excision osteophyte) or debridement (for OA or 'footballer's ankle'—impingement from anterior osteophytic rim).
- **Elbow**—removal of loose body or osteophyte, synovectomy
- **Wrist**—diagnostic mainly, but also for assistance of percutaneous scaphoid fracture fixation
- **Hip**—visualization and debridement of labral tear.

Arthroplasty

Surgical reconstruction or replacement of a malformed or degenerated joint.

The earliest arthroplasties, usually around the hip joint, involved simple excision of the articulating surface(s)[1]. In 1827, Barton performed a sub-trochanteric osteotomy below an ankylosed hip which went on to form a mobile, if rather unstable, fibrous pseudarthrosis. Ollier described various forms of interposition arthroplasty in 1885 using a variety of tissues and materials; this remained an accepted treatment for elbow arthritis until quite recently, but the results are generally poor.

In the early 20th century there was a flurry of interest in joint trans-plantation, recovering articular surfaces from cadavers, old dislocations and lesser joints such as the toes. The modern era of prosthetic joint reconstruction began in the 1930s with the mould arthroplasty of Smith-Peterson, using glass and then cobalt chrome cups interposed between the femoral head and acetabulum. The development of Charnley's THR is detailed in total hip replacement on 📖 p. 161. In the new millennium, there is barely a joint in the body for which a prosthetic articulation has not been designed.

Indications

Primarily pain resistant to simpler forms of treatment, though function often improved by restoration of joint motion and muscle lever arms.

Cautions

Young or active patients; increased demands in terms of load and longevity.

Neurological imbalance predisposing to dislocation.

Contraindications

Current or recent sepsis of the joint to be replaced.

General considerations

- Biomechanics
- Correct selection and orientation of components to restore offset (for muscle function) and reduce risk of dislocation
- Materials
  - See 📖 Chapter 5, p. 107
- Fixation
  - Cement (polymethylmethacrylate) as a grout (space filler between bone and prosthesis) rather than glue
  - Uncemented implants
  - Porous materials promote bony ingrowth for biological fixation
  - Need initial fixation by 'press fit' or interference whilst biology takes its time
  - Hydroxyapatite coating promotes bony on-growth
  - Screws can also be used for initial stability, e.g. uncemented hip cup

- Design
  - Total replacement (both joint surfaces) or hemi-arthroplasty
  - Hinge (elbow) with varying degrees of constraint
  - Resurfacing or stemmed femoral components in hip and shoulder arthroplasty
  - Mobile or fixed bearing knee joints which may retain or substitute for the (posterior) cruciate ligaments.

Long-term considerations

- Infection—a disaster; can occasionally clear if early diagnosis and aggressive debridement, but usually requires (staged) exchange of implant
- Loosening—septic or aseptic
- Wear particles—metal ions currently topical as produced in massive volumes with big head metal-on-metal hip resurfacing; an operation recommended for younger, active patients, but ions can cross the placenta and long-term effects unknown
- Implant failure—corrosion, fracture, excessive wear of articulation
- Dislocation.

Reference

1 Rang M. *The Story of Orthopaedics.* W.B. Saunders, 2000.

Tendon repair

General guidelines on which lacerations to repair and how:
- <25% simply resect any oblique flap to ensure free-running tendon
- <50% use a running peripheral suture only
- >50% use a core suture in addition to a continuous peripheral one.

Explore any pain or restricted motion with suspected tendon injury; risk delayed tendon rupture or triggering otherwise.

Tendon structure
- Consist of type I collagen fibres and tenocytes in fascicles (long spiralling bundles) within endotenon
  - Tenocytes include synovial cells and fibroblasts
  - Blood vessels and nerves within tendon unit
- Fibrous epitenon covers the above elements, continuous with mesotenon (contains arterial supply to tendon, also referred to as vinculae)
- Tendon within synovial lined sheath at sites of excursion over joints, e.g. ankle and wrist/hand
- Tendon shape and size depend on site and the functional requirements
- Musculotendinous units arranged in pairs around joints so each has at least one antagonist muscle
- Tendons are strong structures—capable of withstanding significant loads in tension.

Tendon repair
Strength of repair is proportional to the number of (equally tensioned) core strands and the calibre/characteristics of the suture used. Non-absorbable braided (strong and inelastic) suture best for core, e.g. Ticron® with a Teflon coating to facilitate sliding. The running epitendinous suture should be a smooth monofilament such as Prolene® which stretches but also slides.

Core suture configurations and circumferential running suture applied to round tendons; flat ones repaired with simple, square or mattress-type sutures. Various core suture placement techniques described; all designed to prevent direct pull out through the striated structure, e.g. Bunnel, Kessler, Strickland.

Delayed repair can be very difficult with retraction of muscle/tendon and degeneration of tendon tissue. Can augment repair or use suitable graft; otherwise consider an appropriate transfer.

Healing
- 1 week—inflammatory response and phagocytosis
- 3 weeks—fibroblastic proliferation and synthesis of new collagen. Vascularity re-established. Repair is weakest at this point generally
- 8 weeks—longitudinal, mature collagen fibrils present, but adhesions will have developed unless motion before this point.

Rehabilitation

Controlled stressing of repaired tendons promotes healing/remodelling and maintains joint nutrition and cartilage viability. Specific regimes described, e.g. Sheffield splint for tendo-achilles repair, Belfast regime for hand flexor tendons. Extension block splints are useful after flexor repair; prevent eccentric contraction against extensor stretch but allow controlled tendon excursion.

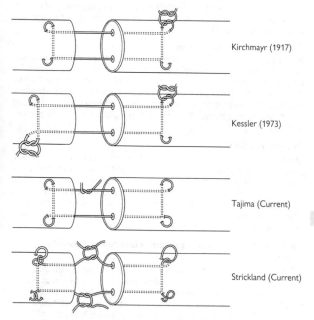

Kirchmayr (1917)

Kessler (1973)

Tajima (Current)

Strickland (Current)

Fig. 7.2 Illustration of the original Kirchmayr flexor tendon core suture of 1917, and its more recent modifications.

Reproduced from Bulstrode et al., *Oxford Textbook of Orthopaedics and Trauma*, with permission from Oxford University Press.

Soft tissue reconstruction and microvascular surgery

Principles of soft tissue management are:

To prevent further injury

Resuscitation, reduction of deformity and early skeletal stabilization (external fixation rapid and effective), emergency management of vascular injury and compartment syndrome, avoid further contamination and desiccation (cover wound).

'Debridement' or 'wound excision'

An open wound inevitably colonizes with bacteria which will rapidly become invasive and pathological. 'Debridement' means literally to unbridle or release the soft tissues for lavage of contamination and bacterial colonies. Important principle is to excise non-viable tissue which will otherwise be the breeding ground for subsequent infection. Assess tissue and muscle viability by four 'Cs': contractility, colour, consistency, capacity to bleed.

Reconstruction

Options depend on extent of tissue deficit at end of adequate wound excision; will often require a '2nd look' in theatre at 48h to reappraise zones of equivocal viability. Where primary closure is not possible, application of a suction sponge (vacuum) dressing has become popular to maintain closed coverage, reduce local oedema and remove residual bacteria. Application after first debridement may lead to excessive blood loss and use in very deep wounds may irritate local nerves.

Reconstructive ladder if primary closure not possible or safe:

- Delayed 1° closure—at 2nd look; suture line must be tension free
- Healing by secondary intention—allow wound to heal by granulation from base and wound edge contraction; cosmesis generally poor
- Split skin grafting—requires appropriate bed of vascularized tissue; will not take on bone, cartilage or tendon unless periosteum, perichondrium or paratenon intact
- Full thickness or composite grafts
  - **Local flaps**—cutaneous, fasciocutaneous, myofascial block of tissue rotated on its vascular pedicle from local site into defect, e.g. gastrocnemius muscle flap to cover exposed bone in open tibial fracture, then cover with split skin graft from thigh
  - **Free flaps**—block of tissue from remote donor site. Vascular pedicle divided and anastomosed to appropriate vessel at recipient site, e.g. gracilis and latissimus dorsi flaps.

Ideally replace losses with like tissue. Cover should be durable, protect underlying structures, and have minimal donor site morbidity. If flap coverage is required following an open fracture, muscle is preferable for excellent blood supply: nutrient factors, stem cells, and antibiotic delivery.

Microvascular surgical technique

Surgical procedures involving structures so small that magnification is required. Microscope provides 16x to 40x magnification, cf loupes (worn like spectacles) up to 5x. Essential for structures <2mm diameter. Most microscopes are diploscope or triploscope with additional ports for assistant and a television screen. Specialized microsurgical instruments used and nylon sutures from 9.0 to 12.0.

Replantation

Definition

Surgical reattachment of a traumatically amputated digit or limb.

Involves shortening and stabilization of bone followed by extensor and flexor tendon repair, arterial microvascular anastomosis, nerve repair, finally vein anastomosis and closure.

Considerations

Anticipated function should exceed that of prosthesis or amputation, and difference worth risk, time and expense.

Injury mechanism important (clean and sharp better than crush).

Factors important in decision making:
- age
- severity of injury
- level of amputation
- warm ischaemic time (up to 6h, 12h if cooled)
- multiple or bilateral amputations
- segmental injuries to amputated part
- co-morbidity and rehabilitation potential
- economic factors.

Initial care of amputated part

Rinse gently with sterile saline, then either wrap in saline-soaked gauze and place in plastic bag or immerse in saline in bag, then place bag on ice to cool to 4°.

See Fractures, p. 396, for Gustilo and Anderson fracture classification.

Section 3

Adults

Adult orthopaedics

Rheumatoid arthritis

RA is a chronic, systemic inflammatory disease affecting the synovial joints and extra-articular system.

Epidemiology

Affects 1–3% population. Most common in young females (30–50yrs).

Aetiology

Uncertain but related to T cell-mediated immune response. The inflammatory response is directed against synovium initially; later cartilage and bone. Human leukocyte antigen (HLA) DR4 and HLA DW4 linked.

Clinical

Often insidious onset of generalized joint aches and stiffness. Swollen, painful and stiff hands and feet usually worse in the morning. Progressive symmetrical symptoms, often with fatigue, malaise and anorexia.

Less common presentations include:

- Relapsing and remitting arthritis of different large joints (palindromic)
- Persistent monoarthritis (often of knee)
- Systemic illness with minimal joint involvement
- Vague limb girdle discomfort
- Sudden onset widespread arthritis.

Articular examination

- Small joint swelling, esp. MCPJ, PIPJ, wrist
- Later ulnar deviation and volar subluxation at MCPJs
- Boutonniere and swan neck deformities of fingers and Z-thumbs
- Wrist subluxation and prominence of ulnar head (piano key)
- Extensor tendon rupture and muscle wasting
- Similar changes in feet—claw toes and hallux valgus
- Larger joint involvement
- Atlanto-axial joint subluxation occurs and can threaten the spinal cord.

Extra-articular examination

- Rheumatoid nodules
- Anaemia
- Lymphadenopathy
- Vasculitis
- Multifocal neuropathies, carpal tunnel syndrome
- Episcleritis, scleritis, keratoconjunctivitis, Sicca syndrome
- Pericarditis
- Pulmonary fibrosis
- OP
- Amyloidosis
- Felty's syndrome—splenomegaly and neutropenia
- Sjogren's syndrome—autoimmune exocrinopathy associated with RA.

Investigations

X-ray findings (initially normal radiographs):

- Periarticular erosions
- Soft tissue thickening

- Juxta-articular osteopenia
- Loss of joint space
- Subluxed or dislocated joints
- Protrusio acetabuli.

Blood tests

No test is specific for the disease:
- Rheumatoid factor (RhF)—(+)ve in 80% (non-specific—may be positive in other disease including Sjogren's syndrome, sarcoid and SLE).
- Increase in CRP and ESR.
- Antinuclear antibody (ANA) (+)ve in 30%.

Joint fluid assay

Confirms inflammatory arthritis, but is non-specific.

Diagnostic criteria (American Rheumatism Association)

- Morning stiffness (>1h for >6 weeks)
- Joint swelling
- Nodules
- Positive laboratory tests
- Positive radiographic findings.

Management

Early care can prevent complications. It should include:

Non-operative treatment

- Exercise
- Physiotherapy and occupational therapy
- Orthoses
- *Medical treatment*—NSAIDs, antimalarials, disease-modifying agents (methotrexate, sulfasalazine, gold and penicillamine), steroids and cytotoxic drugs. Tumour necrosis factor (TNF) inhibitors (infliximab).

Operative options

Surgery to improve function and reduce pain and swelling. Options include synovectomy, soft tissue realignment and arthroplasty (see 📖 p. 164). Synovectomy reduces pain but does not halt radiographic progression, delay need for arthroplasty or improve joint range of movement. Soft tissue realignment has limited indication. All patients need a full clinical assessment of the cervical spine and cervical radiographs because of the risk of cervical instability (up to 90% of patients with RA) prior to anaesthesia.

Treatment goals are

- Control destructive synovitis
- Reduce pain
- Maintain joint function
- Prevent deformity
- Treatment in a multidisciplinary setting.

Systemic lupus erythematosus

Definition
SLE is a chronic autoimmune disease characterized by ANAs and vasculitis. It can affect any part of the body but major target organs are the skin, joints, bone marrow, kidneys and brain.

Epidemiology
More common in people of non-European descent. Incidence is 3.5–7.6 per 100 000. Nine times more common in women (12–25yrs).

Aetiology
Associated with HLA DR2 and HLA DR3. SLE runs in families, but no single gene cause has been identified. Environmental triggers are thought to initiate or exacerbate SLE and include: medications (antibiotics, antidepressants), UV radiation, sex hormones and stress.

Clinical
Patients commonly present with fatigue, malaise, joint pains, myalgias and fever.

Musculoskeletal (most common >80%): Arthralgia, myalgia, myositis and proximal myopathy. Arthritis affects mainly PIPJs and MCPJs, the carpus and knees. Rheumatoid-like pattern but is typically less destructive. There may be periarticular and tendon involvement. Progressive deforming arthropathy (10–15%) is due to capsular laxity (Jaccoud's arthropathy). Aseptic bone necrosis, especially if treated with high dose steroids.

Skin (30%): Photosensitive, butterfly, malar rash (over nasal bridge and spreading to cheeks), scarring alopecia, livedo reticularis (net-like blush), Raynaud's, purpura, oral ulceration, urticaria and conjunctivitis. In 'discoid' lupus there are 3 stages of the rash: stage 1 erythema; stage 2, pigmented hyperkeratotic oedematous papules; stage 3, atrophic depressed lesions.

Central nervous system: depression, psychosis, fits, hemi- or paraplegia, cranial nerve lesions, cerebellar ataxia, chorea and meningitis occur in SLE. Headaches are common.

Renal: painless haematuria or proteinurea. Lupus nephritis may lead to oedema, hypertension and renal failure.

Pulmonary: pleurisy, pneumonia, obliterative bronchiolitis, fibrosing alveolitis, oedema pleuritis, pleural effusion, pneumonitis, pulmonary hypertension or pulmonary haemorrhage.

Cardiovascular: pericarditis and endocarditis (Libman–Sacks: non-infective) or myocarditis.

Blood: normochromic, normocytic anaemia, haemolysis (rare), leukopenia, lymphopenia and thrombocytopenia. Splenomegaly.

Diagnosis

Blood tests
- Typically positive for ANA and HLA DR3
- High titre anti-DNA antibodies
- 40% RhF positive
- Low complement levels—better marker than ESR for disease activity.

Clinical diagnostic criteria Four or more of the following findings initially or serially on two occasions:
- Serositis
- Oral ulcers
- Arthritis
- Photosensitivity
- Blood disorder
- Renal disorder
- ANA positive
- Neurological disorder
- Immunological disorder (anti-DNA antibody, anti-Smith antibody, false-positive syphilis test or LE cells)
- Discoid rash.

Management

Non-operative treatment: management of SLE is symptomatic. Medical options include: supportive care, lifestyle changes, medication with disease-modifying drugs (methotrexate, cyclophosphamide, azathioprine). Immunosuppressive drugs (steroids), analgesics and NSAIDs.

Operative options: splinting not usually successful. Fusions of small joints and arthroplasty for large joints can be successful.

Drug-induced lupus

Isoniazid, hydralazine, procainamide, chlorpromazine and anticonvulsants may induce lupus.

Pulmonary disease and rashes are common. Renal and CNS effects are rare.

Antiphospholipid syndrome

Features are arterial or venous thromboses, thrombocytopenia, stroke, migraine, myelitis, MI, multiinfarct dementia and recurrent miscarriages, with SLE. There are antiphospholipid antibodies (anticardiolipin antibodies or 'lupus anticoagulant') present in the blood.

Outcome

SLE has a relapsing, remitting course with mortality related to renal disease.

For further reading see Bulstrode et al.[1].

Reference

1 Bulstrode C, Buckwater J, Carr A, et al., eds. *Oxford Textbook of Orthopaedics and Trauma.* Oxford: Oxford University Press, 2002.

Scleroderma (systemic sclerosis)

A condition in which there is progressive fibrosis and tightening of the skin. There is excessive collagen deposition and small vessel obliteration resulting in tissue ischaemia and atrophy.

This pathological process may extend beyond the skin to involve other organs. This is referred to as systemic sclerosis.

It affects females more than males and mainly in the 4th and 5th decades.

Diagnostic criteria for scleroderma (systemic sclerosis)

Proximal skin scleroderma or any of two findings:
- Sclerodactyly
- Digital pitting scars
- Pulp loss
- Bibasilar lung fibrosis.

Other clinical features of systemic sclerosis

- Raynaud's phenomenon
- Calcinosis—common at tips of fingers
- Telangiectasia
- GI tract hypomobility, pseudo-obstruction, malabsorption (secondary to bacterial overgrowth) and oesophageal involvement resulting in reflux and dysphagia
- Renal involvement—causes severe hypertension and renal impairment or failure
- Myocarditis and myositis
- Joint stiffness and contractures.

CREST syndrome (**C**alcinosis of subcutaneous tissues, **R**aynaud's phenomenon, disordered o**E**sophageal motility, **S**clerodactyly and **T**elangiectasia) is a form of the disease with a more benign course.

Investigations

No single test. It is primarily a clinical diagnosis.

Blood:
- Increase in ESR and immunoglobulins
- ANA positive (>50%)
- Scl 70 antibodies in progressive systemic sclerosis
- Anticentromere antibodies in CREST.

Radiology: subcutaneous calcinosis. Barium swallow or oesophageal manometry used to assess oesophageal dysfunction.

Management

- Symptomatic support
- Medical:
  - D-Penicillamine may delay progression of disease
  - Raynaud's: heated gloves and calcium channel blockers
  - Critical ischaemia of digits: IV iloprost and antibiotics if infected

- Oesophageal disease: H_2 antagonists, proton pump inhibitors and motility stimulants
- Malabsorption: antibiotics
- Renal hypertension: ACE inhibitors
- Surgical:
  - Refractory Raynaud's—periadventitial digital sympathectomy
  - Proximal IPJ deformity with dorsal skin ulcer—arthrodesis
  - Calcific deposits—may need to be excised
  - Refractory finger tip ulcers—conservative tip amputation.

Prognosis

Approximately 75% survival at 5yrs. Better prognosis with CREST variant.

For further reading, see Callan and Wordsworth[1].

Reference

1 Callan M, Wordsworth P. Inflammatory connective tissue disease and vasculitis. In: Bulstrode C, Buckwater J. Carr A, et al., eds. *Oxford Textbook of Orthopaedics and Trauma.* Oxford: Oxford University Press, 2002:1393–4.

Polyarteritis nodosa

Necrotizing vasculitis causing aneurysms of medium sized arteries.

Affects males more than females (4:1), classically middle-aged men.

Incidence

Approximately 1 per million per year.

Clinical features

- General: fever, malaise, weight loss and arthralgia
- Renal: hypertension, haematuria, proteinuria, renal failure and intrarenal aneurysm are found. Renal failure is the main cause of death
- Cardiac: cardiac disease is the second biggest cause of death. Coronary arteritis and infarction. Hypertension and heart failure. Pericarditis. Childhood version (Kawasaki's disease): coronary aneurysms
- Pulmonary: focal pulmonary infiltrates
- Neurological: mononeuritis, mononeuritis multiplex, sensorimotor polyneuropathy, fits, hemiplegia and psychoses
- GI: abdominal pain (infarction) and malabsorption because of chronic ischaemia and GI bleeding
- Associated with hepatitis B infection
- Skin: urticaria, purpura, infarcts, livedo reticularis, nodules and gangrene
- Eyes: scleritis
- Genitals: testicular infarction
- Blood: increased white cell count (WCC), eosinophilia, normochromic normocytic anaemia, increased ESR, increased CRP. Antinuclear cytoplasmic antibody (ANCA) may be positive.

Diagnosis

Clinical diagnosis supported by renal or mesenteric angiography or kidney/skin biopsy to demonstrate focal vasculitic process affecting medium sized arteries.

Check for hepatitis B surface antigen.

Treatment

Treat hypertension.

High dose prednisolone then cyclophosphamide.

Prognosis

Without treatment most patients affected die within 2–5 years. With treatment survival is much better (approximately >70% at 10yrs).

For further reading, see Callan and Wordsworth[1].

Reference

1 Callan M, Wordsworth P. Inflammatory connective tissue disease and vasculitis. In: Bulstrode C, Buckwater J, Carr A, et al., eds. *Oxford Textbook of Orthopaedics and Trauma.* Oxford: Oxford University Press, 2002:1393–4.

Polymyositis and dermatomyositis

Insidious symmetrical proximal muscle weakness resulting from muscle inflammation.

Most common in 6th decade.

Clinical features

Musculoskeletal

- Proximal myopathy—progressive and symmetrical
- Polyarthralgia.

Skin

- Skin involvement variable
- Heliotrophic rash (purplish rash of eyelids) with periorbital oedema
- Scaly erythematous rash on extensor surfaces of elbows, knees and fingers
- Raynaud's phenomenon.

Gastrointestinal: dysphagia.

Respiratory: dysphonia, lung involvement, respiratory weakness.

Cardiovascular: MI (rare).

Other

- Retinitis
- Cancer risk: with increased age there is a higher probability that myositis is associated with an underlying malignancy, usually adenocarcinoma of breast or lung. The malignant disease is usually apparent and an extensive search for occult malignancy unjustified.

Diagnosis

Increase in creatine phosphokinase (CPK) levels, increase in ESR, EMG changes and abnormal muscle biopsy (pathognomonic inflammatory response).

Autoantibodies: those individuals with anti-Jo-1 antibodies characteristically suffer from pulmonary fibrosis in association with myositis.

Treatment

Rest, steroids (prednisolone) and immunosuppressive agents (azathioprine and methotrexate). Skin condition may respond to antimalarials.

For further reading, see Callan and Wordsworth[1].

Reference

1 Callan M, Wordsworth P. Inflammatory connective tissue disease and vasculitis. In: Bulstrode C, Buckwater J, Carr A, et al., eds. *Oxford Textbook of Orthopaedics and Trauma.* Oxford: Oxford University Press, 2002:1393–4.

Ankylosing spondylitis—pathology

Definition

AS is a chronic systemic inflammatory arthropathy of unknown aetiology which principally affects the axial skeleton.

Epidemiology

Incidence is 0.1–0.3%. In HLA B27-positive patients, incidence increases 100-fold. <5% of those who are HLA B27 positive have AS. Incidence increases 20-fold in first-degree relatives. Usually manifests in the 3rd or 4th decades of life. Sex distribution is 3:1 male to female.

Pathophysiology

Inflammatory arthropathy affecting synovial and fibrous joints. The SIJs are affected in all patients. Inflammatory process leads to joint destruction and ankylosis.

Clinical features

Onset is insidious and course characterized by flares and remissions. Inflammation seen in ligaments, capsules and subchondral bone. It is an axial arthritis, but girdle joints (hips and shoulders) are affected in 20%. Patients often have early morning stiffness which improves during the day. May be sacroiliac tenderness, decreased spinal mobility, flattening of the lumbar spine and flexion contraction of hips. Extra-articular manifestations include: aortic insufficiency, conduction defects, decreased chest expansion, uveitis (25%), Achilles tendonitis, plantar fasciitis.

Investigations

Blood tests: HLA B27, ESR.

Radiology: X-rays show squaring of vertebral bodies in early stages; syndesmophytes, spinal fusion (bamboo spine) and osteopenia seen late. Bone scan shows increased uptake in SIJs. MRI shows inflammation in ligaments, capsule and subchondral bone of the SIJs.

Management

Non-operative treatment: exercise is the mainstay of treatment and is aimed at maintaining flexibility. Educate patient about disease. Multidisciplinary care (GP, rheumatologist, opthalmologist, physiotherapist, occupational therapist, orthopaedic surgeon) needed. NSAIDs are the most common type of drug used. Secondary drugs include corticosteroids, sulfasalazine, pamidronate and TNFα blockers.

Operative options: surgery is reserved for complications—fixation of spinal fractures, correction of spinal deformity and hip replacement.

Complications: spinal fractures especially of cervical spine after minor trauma. A high risk of death after cervical spine fracture.

For further reading see Bulstrode et al.[1] and Maddison et al.[2].

References

1 Bulstrode C, Buckwater J, Carr A, et al., eds. *Oxford Textbook of Orthopaedics and Trauma.* Oxford: Oxford University Press, 2002.
2 Maddison PJ, Isenberg DA, Woo P, et al., eds. *Oxford Textbook of Rheumatology.* Oxford: Oxford University Press, 2004.

Psoriatic arthritis

Definition
Psoriatic arthritis is an inflammatory arthritis associated with psoriasis.

Epidemiology
Psoriasis is common, affecting 2% of the Caucasian population, and 10% may develop an arthropathy. Sex distribution is equal male to female. Usually seen at 30–50yrs in patients with known psoriasis, but may occur in childhood.

Aetiology
Psoriasis, 50% association with HLA B27, and there is often a strong family history of arthritis in a third of cases.

Clinical
Presentations of psoriatic arthritis:
- Asymmetrical oligoarthritis affecting finger joints—sausage finger and toes (70%)
- Symmetrical polyarthritis including RA (15%)
- Distal interphalangeal joint arthritis with nail changes (5%)
- Arthritis mutilans with severe deformities secondary to osteolysis of affected joints (5%)—associated with sacroiliitis and widespread skin disease
- Spondyloarthritis presenting as sacroiliitis and/or spondylitis (5%).

Clinical features in keeping with psoriasis, but nail changes (pitting, ridging, onycholysis) are more common in those with psoriatic arthritis (70% vs 30%) than those without.

Investigations
Radiology: X-ray changes include erosions and ankylosis of joints.

Management
Treatment is aimed at control of psoriasis and protection of joints.

Non-operative treatment: medication includes NSAIDs, immunosuppressive drugs (methotrexate, sulfasalazine, azathioprine) and analgesics. Joints are injected with steroids or with gold. Antimalarial therapy is sometimes used. Splints are important in managing joint pain and deformities.

Operative options: reconstruction of joints helps preserve function.

Complications
Destruction of joints, and ankylosis.

For further reading see Bulstrode *et al.*[1] and Maddison *et al.*[2].

Reactive arthritis (Reiter's syndrome)

Definition
Reactive arthritis is an aseptic inflammatory arthritis associated with urogenital, ocular, mucocutaneous and musculoskeletal infections.

Epidemiology
Seen in young sexually active adults, mostly men, but may be underdiagnosed in women due to subclinical *Chlamydia* infections.

Incidence
Affects whites more than other racial groups. 70% associated with HLA B27.

Aetiology
Follows 2 weeks after urethritis, cervicitis or diarrhoea. Associated with Crohn's disease. Triggering infections include *Chlamydia*, *Shigella*, *Salmonella*, *Camplyobacter*, *Yersinia*, *Giardia lamblia* and *Cryptosporidium*.

Clinical
Asymmetrical, oligoarticular arthritis (90% have peripheral joint involvement) and dactylitis (tenosynovitis leading to sausage fingers). Skin lesions include psoriasiform lesions (keratoderma blenorrahagica), circinate balanitis, small oral ulcers and opacity and thickening of nails.

May have urethritis, conjunctivitis, uveitis, erythema, photophobia or diarrhoea. Systemic disease with fever and malaise. The triad of arthritis, urethitis and conjunctivitis is present in <1/3 patients initially. History, especially the sexual history, is very important in making the diagnosis.

Investigation
- Rule out septic arthritis by joint aspiration
- Blood tests unhelpful, but ESR and CRP useful to monitor disease progression
- *Imaging:* sacroiliitis on MRI. Later joint destruction with recurrent disease.

Management
Non-operative treatment: Treatment is aimed at eradicating the infection and relieving symptoms. NSAIDs, steroids and methotrexate used. Joint injections with corticosteroids suppress synovitis and prevent irreversible joint damage. Temporary splinting during acute phase, physiotherapy and exercise are necessary to preserve muscle strength and flexibility.

Usually resolves in 3 months but can become recurrent and up to 40% of patients have recurrent symptoms at 15yrs. Antibiotic treatment of the sexual partner may prevent reinfection; long-term sequelae with recurrence.

Operative options: Arthroplasty occasionally needed.

Complications

Joint destruction, sterility.

For further reading see Bulstrode et al.[1] and Maddison et al.[2].

References

1 Bulstrode C, Buckwater J, Carr A, et al., eds. *Oxford Textbook of Orthopaedics and Trauma.* Oxford: Oxford University Press, 2002.
2 Maddison PJ, Isenberg DA, Woo P, et al., eds. *Oxford Textbook of Rheumatology.* Oxford: Oxford University Press, 2004.

Enteropathic arthritis

Definition
Enteropathic arthritis is arthritis complicating IBD.

Epidemiology
It affects ~10% of patients with IBD and is twice as common in patients with Crohn's disease as in those with ulcerative colitis.

Clinical
Enteropathic arthritis may present as a spondyloarthropathy or as a peripheral arthritis. The spondyloarthritic form is unlikely to progress. The peripheral arthritis form may be more aggressive but does not usually destroy joints.

Spondyloarthritis: sacroiliitis is common with Crohn's disease and ulcerative colitis. There is a clear relationship between bowel disease flare-ups and arthropathy. 60% association with HLA B27.

Peripheral arthritis
- Type 1: pauciarticular with acute short-lived attacks often related to IBD activity. Associated with HLA B27
- Type 2: polyarticular with persistent symptoms less related to IBD attacks. Associated with HLA B44.

Investigations
Radiology: MRI useful for identifying isolated sacroiliitis.

Management
The spondyloarthritic form and type 1 peripheral form respond to control of IBD. Type 2 peripheral form is more likely to lead to joint deformity. Simple analgesics, intra-articular steroids, systemic steroids, sulfasalazine are used. NSAIDs may not be well tolerated with IBD. Anti-TNF therapy may successfully treat arthropathy and IBD.

For further reading see Bulstrode et al.[1] and Maddison et al.[2].

References
1 Bulstrode C, Buckwater J, Carr A, et al., eds. *Oxford Textbook of Orthopaedics and Trauma*. Oxford: Oxford University Press, 2002.
2 Maddison PJ, Isenberg DA, Woo P, et al., eds. *Oxford Textbook of Rheumatology*. Oxford: Oxford University Press, 2004.

Behcet's disease

Definition
Behcet's disease is a recurrent systemic vasculitis of unknown aetiology.

Epidemiology
Prevalence is 0.3 per 100 000 in Northern Europe, rising to 5 per 100 000 in Turkey. In Japan prevalence is 10 in 100 000. Onset is usually between 20 and 40yrs of age.

Aetiology
The cause is unclear but it is thought to be due to an abnormal response to herpes and streptococcal infections. It is associated with HLA B51.

Pathophysiology
The main histological finding is a widespread vasculitis.

Clinical
Recurrent aphthous ulcers (often the first sign) is universal, large oro-genital ulcers, skin lesions (erythema nodosum, acne and ulcers) seen in up to 80%, eye disease (uveitis, retinal vasculitis) seen in 50%, neurological (pyramidal and cerebellar signs, dementia, and psychiatric problems) seen in 10%, thrombophlebitis seen in 25%.

Joint involvement is common with mono- or oligoarticular synovitis (may last several weeks).

Diagnosis requires recurrent oral ulceration, and two of the following: recurrent genital ulceration, eye lesions, skin lesions, positive pathology test (a pin-prick develops a pustular response in 24–48h).

Investigations
Blood test to include FBC and inflammatory markers. In Behcet's disease the ESR and CRP are elevated, and there is often a chronic anaemia.

Management
Steroids in the acute phase, azathioprine for eye disease and cyclophosphamide for arterial disease. Ciclosporin A is the drug of choice in the treatment of severe uveitis of Behcet's disease. Thalidomide is used to treat orogenital ulcers.

For further reading see Bulstrode et al.[1] and Maddison et al.[2]

References
1 Bulstrode C, Buckwater J, Carr A, et al., eds. *Oxford Textbook of Orthopaedics and Trauma*. Oxford: Oxford University Press, 2002.

2 Maddison PJ, Isenberg DA, Woo P, et al., eds. *Oxford Textbook of Rheumatology*. Oxford: Oxford University Press, 2004.

Musculoskeletal aspects of haemophilia

Epidemiology

X-linked recessive genetic disorder affecting 1:10 000 live male births, 1/3 due to new sporadic mutation. Affects factor VIII (classic/A) or factor IX (Christmas/B).

History and examination

Familial cases present due to family history; sporadic cases present with spontaneous bleeds and bruising, and prolonged bleeding with injury, surgery or dental extractions. Exclude non-accidental injury (NAI).

Bleeding risk related to factor levels: normal clotting if >50%; prolonged surgical bleeding if 5–25%; bleeds with minor injuries if 1–5%; spontaneous bleeds if <1%.

Musculoskeletal features

- Joint bleeds produce synovitis and angionogenesis (increasing likelihood of re-bleed). Recurrent haemarthroses cause a destructive arthropathy and fibrosis, producing stiff, painful joints
- Subperiosteal and intraosseous bleeds form encapsulated haematomata (pseudotumour), with local pressure effects and pathological fracture
- Muscle bleeds carry the acute risk of compartment syndrome and nerve compression. Recurrent bleeds produce fibrosis and contracture
- Surgery in specialist centres only due to requirement for factor cover (with potential antibodies) and risk of viral infections (HIV; hepatitis B/C).

Treatment

- Self-administered factor therapy with prodromal symptoms to abort bleeds; 20IU/kg to achieve factor levels 30–50% of normal
- Physiotherapy and splintage to mobilize gently after acute bleeds settle
- Low-dose prednisolone with factor prophylaxis after bleeds
- Synovectomy (chemical, radioisotope or surgical) if joint salvageable
- Osteotomy or arthroplasty with factor cover—risk of infection high, especially in HIV-positive patients.

Prevention

- Primary prevention—treatment ×2–3/week before bleeds start until skeletal maturity
- Secondary prevention—treatment after onset of bleeds to stop synovitis progression
- Achieve and maintain factor levels to prevent spontaneous bleeds.

Pigmented villonodular synovitis

Definition
Benign neoplasia of synovial joints (PVNS) and tendon sheaths (giant cell tumour of tendon sheath (GCTTS)).

Symptoms and signs
- **Localized** form creates a solitary nodular lesion, with mechanical symptoms—locking/catching in joints (generally the knee); painless slow-growing mass with cortical erosion in 10% in tendon sheaths (usually in hand, adjacent to IPJs)
- **Diffuse** form is more aggressive, giving rise to recurrent haemarthrosis with associated pain, stiffness and deformity. This form is locally invasive.

Investigations
- Plain films—look for bony erosion
- MRI—define nature and extent of disease.

Treatment
Localized
- Marginal excision (arthroscopic if intra-articular) with potential for recurrence if incompletely excised.

Diffuse
- Marginal excision, but with recurrence in up to 45%
- Total synovectomy, but tends to recur if extra-articular invasion
- Intra-articular or external beam radiotherapy for refractory cases
- Arthrodesis and total synovectomy for recurrent or aggressive diffuse disease
- Arthroplasty with synovectomy at the knee.

Osteoarthritis

A disorder of synovial joints characterized by focal articular cartilage degeneration, irregular regeneration and remodelling of subchondral bone.

Epidemiology

Osteoarthritis is very common (12% prevalence in those aged 25–74; radiographic OA in hand joints in 80% of those >70). While prevalence increases with age, osteoarthritic joints differ from those affected by normal age-related change.

Cartilage property	Age related	Osteoarthritis
Collagen	Content relatively unchanged	Arrangement disordered; content decreases
Proteoglycan synthesis	Reduced	Increased
Water content	Decreased	Increased
Modulus of elasticity	Increased	Decreased

Causes

- Primary (idiopathic)
- Secondary—biomechanical (instability/incongruity); biochemical (e.g. Gaucher's disease); congenital (e.g. DDH; epiphyseal dysplasias); osteochondritides; osteonecrosis; crystal deposition.

Pathophysiology

Cartilage loss can be viewed as an imbalance between synthesis and degradation. Initially there is oedema and softening of cartilage due to molecular degradation, but no macroscopic disruption. There is a variable repair response from chondrocytes but disease progression leads to macroscopic disruption of the architecture and eventually exposure of subchondral bone. Other changes such as bone remodelling, synovitis and osteophyte formation are secondary to the changes in the articular cartilage.

Risk factors

- Age
- Familial tendency
- Sex—females more likely to develop OA
- Obesity
- Racial differences, e.g. hip OA more common in white Europeans.

Classifications

- Radiographic—Kellgren and Lawrence: (i) minimal osteophytes; (ii) osteophyte; (iii) joint space narrowing; (iv) subchondral sclerosis
- Arthroscopic—Outerbridge: (i) soft/swollen cartilage; (ii) fissuring <1/2 inch; (iii) fissuring >1/2 inch; (iv) full thickness cartilage loss
- Histological—Mankin and Buckwalter: (i) matrix breakdown; (ii) matrix regeneration; (iii) cartilage loss.

Symptoms and signs

- Presence of radiographic OA changes does not necessarily imply symptoms, although the proportion who are symptomatic increases with radiographic severity. Up to 2/3 with radiographic changes may be asymptomatic in population screening studies
- Most present with **pain**, **stiffness** and **functional loss**
- Symptoms tend to increase stepwise from occasional, activity related (especially on initiation—'start-up') to a constant background rest pain with activity-related exacerbations
- Affected joints tend to be swollen and stiff due to osteophytes, capsular thickening and effusion. Tenderness and crepitus appear in advanced cases.

Differential diagnosis

- Monoarticular—acute trauma; septic arthritis; crystal synovitis
- Polyarticular—reactive arthritis; inflammatory arthritis.

Treatment

- Weight loss, exercise for range of motion preservation and muscle strengthening
- Lifestyle changes avoiding high load-bearing activity
- Cushioned footwear to reduce impact pain in lower limb joints
- Sticks, crutches
- Splints for ankle and wrist flare ups
- Simple analgesics, compound analgesics
- NSAIDs as second-line drugs.

Surgery

- Arthroplasty is a highly successful treatment for severe OA in the knee and hip. It is also indicated in the ankle and shoulder.
- Arthrodesis is effective in the ankle and DIPJs of hand and foot, and in the spine.
- Osteotomy, cartilage transplantation and joint distraction have limited indications.

Aseptic bone necrosis

Death of bone due to ischaemia. Lesions adjacent to articular surfaces are termed AVN, and those in the diaphysis bone infarcts.

Epidemiology

Mostly in under 50s; slight male preponderance; usually idiopathic; 50–80% bilateral.

Causes

- Vascular microemboli (sickle cell; haemoglobinopathies; polycythaemia; decompression nitrogen emboli; fat emboli in pancreatitis)
- Mechanical interruption (trauma)
- Infection
- Drugs (corticosteroids, alcohol)
- Radiation or autoimmune vasculitis
- Diabetes mellitus and Gaucher's disease.

Clinical features

Lesions seen on the convex side of articulations. Most found in the femur (head and medial condyle), humeral head and talus. Less often seen in the lunate (Kienböck's)—see 📖 p. 297, capitellum (Panner's disease), metatarsal head (Freiberg's in the 2nd) and scaphoid (Preiser's disease if spontaneous).

Bone resorption prior to re-formation leads to weakening of the bone, with microfractures forming and propagating, leading to subchondral collapse. The overlying cartilage, nourished by the synovial fluid, survives until degenerative changes follow due to joint incongruence.

Symptoms and signs

Pain (particularly nocturnal) and joint irritability ± effusion.

Investigations

Earliest radiographic changes seen on MRI (areas of low signal on T1; 'double line sign' on T2). Isotope scanning is less reliable; cold spot with a 'hot' front of revascularization. Later changes on plain radiographs (osteopenia and osteosclerosis; later subchondral fracture and collapse (crescent sign)).

Treatment

Depends on site and stage (Table 8.1). Remove avoidable risk factors. Offload joint to prevent collapse while healing occurs, decompression of the lesion by drilling (alone or with revascularization) or osteotomy, and salvage procedures for 2° osteoarthritis.

Table 8.1 Association Research Circulation Osseous classification (ARCO)

Stage	Symptoms	Imaging	Treatment
0	None	Normal MRI, isotope scan and plain films. Histological chance finding	Expectant; address avoidable risk factors
1	Minimal	Positive MRI; normal plain radiographs	Expectant; offload/rest
2	Moderate	Osteosclerosis and osteopenia	Rest; consider decompression/osteotomy
3	Severe	Subchondral fracture (crescent) and collapse	Decompression/osteotomy
4	Severe; of degenerative arthritis	Secondary OA	Salvage

Crystal arthropathies

Definition
Precipitation of inorganic crystals within the synovial fluid of a joint, combined with minor trauma, can induce an inflammatory reaction associated with pain, effusion, heat and decreased range of motion.

Gout
Gout is a disorder of purine metabolism. Uric acid is produced from xanthine by xanthine oxidase and, in gout, serum uric acid levels are raised (hyperuricaemia). Hyperuricaemia is common and often asymptomatic. Patients with gout may have normal serum uric acid levels.

Epidemiology
Gout is present in 1% of the population. More common in blacks than whites. Presents more commonly in men than women.

Clinical
History
Patients present with painful swollen joints, commonly the small joints of the extremities. An acute monoarthritis is the initial presentation in 90%. Previous gout attacks may have occurred. Conditions associated with high cell turnover, e.g. some malignancies, may result in hyperuricaemia. This can be exacerbated when chemotherapy is given to treat such conditions. Patients should have prophylaxis against hyperuricaemia.

Examination
Look for other signs of gout inflammation: swelling, erythema, warmth and tenderness. Clinical findings of acute gout may be indistinguishable from acute cellulitis. Tophi on extensor surfaces such as elbows and the ears, can be confused with rheumatoid nodules. Presence of tophi suggests longstanding hyperuricaemia.

Investigations
Bloods—FBC, electrolytes and serum uric acid.

Aspiration of the joint effusion—fluid is sent for microscopy and microbiological culture. Diagnosis confirmed with presence of strongly birefringent, needle-shaped crystals in the fluid examined with polarized light microscopy.

Radiology: X-rays—may show erosions of bone slightly away from the articular surface.

Differential diagnosis
Includes septic arthritis, pseudogout, RA and trauma.

Management
Non-operative treatment:
Acute episodes—NSAIDs such as diclofenac (drugs of choice) or colchichine 1mg stat followed by 500mcg up to every 4h. Colchicine has side effects (diarrhoea, myopathy and neuropathy) and total dose is limited. To prevent recurrent attacks—allopurinol, initial dose 100mg daily. Allopurinol should not be started during an acute episode but should be delayed for 2–3 weeks.

Operative options:

Joint reconstruction may become necessary. Tophi can be excised if problematic but healing may be prolonged.

Pseudogout (calcium pyrophosphate deposition disease)

Definition

Pseudogout is an inflammatory arthropathy caused by deposition of calcium pyrophosphate dihydrate.

Clinical

May present in a similar fashion to gout though large joints are more commonly affected. Most common joint affected is the knee. Examination of the joint reveals OA with superimposed synovitis.

Investigations

Radiology: X-rays—may show chondrocalcinosis—mineralization within fibrocartilage structures such as the menisci of the knee. This finding may be present in a number of conditions and is not diagnostic nor always symptomatic.

Joint aspiration fluid examined as for gout. Calcium pyrophosphate crystals are rhomboid in shape and weakly birefringent under polarized light.

Management

The treatment is essentially symptomatic with analgesics and NSAIDs. Painful joint effusions can be washed out arthroscopically.

Calcium hydroxyapatite deposition

Crystals of calcium hydroxyapatite are the major mineral content of bone. They can be deposited in other tissues such as tendons. If present in the synovial fluid they can lead to an erosive arthritis that can be rapidly progressive and mistaken for collapse of an osteonecrotic bone.

Differential diagnoses

A number of differential diagnoses must be considered when managing a joint affected by a crystal arthropathy including:

• RA—may start as a large joint monoarthropathy
• Seronegative arthritis
• Acute septic arthritis—fluid from joint aspirations should be sent for culture and sensitivity testing. Consider gonococcus in a sexually active younger patient
• Reactive arthritis—joint swelling can occur in response to a systemic condition.

Osteochondroses

Definition

A heterogeneous group of disorders, many bearing eponymous names. Many were first described soon after the invention of radiographs for viewing the skeleton. Causes include traction on apophyses of immature skeletons, osteonecrosis of bones with a fragile vascular supply or repeated microtrauma.

Pathology

The underlying pathology is poorly understood, but stress on the affected areas contributes to the development of degenerative changes or osteonecrosis followed by regeneration or recalcification.

Groups

a. Articular osteochrondoses (joint space involved)

- Panner's disease
- Legg–Calve–Perthes disease (see 📖 p. 520)
- Köhler's disease
- Freiberg's disease (see 📖 p. 194)
- Kienbock's disease.

b. Monoarticular osteochondroses

- Sinding–Larsen–Johanssen disease (SLJ; see 📖 p. 336)
- Osgood–Schlatter disease (OS; see 📖 p. 336)
- Sever's disease.

c. Epiphyseal osteochondroses

- Scheuermann's disease
- Blount's disease (also affects metaphysis) (see 📖 p. 528)

Panner's disease (humeral capitellum)
- Lateral elbow pain and stiffness with capitellar tenderness
- Usually found in boys 5–12yrs old
- May lose pronation and supination
- X-rays—irregular capitellum (early); radiolucent areas (later) appearance of capitellum normal after 1–2yrs
- Symptomatic treatment—rest, analgesia, physiotherapy.

Kienbock's disease (lunate)
- Affects adults in third and fourth decades
- Can develop after single, severe compressive forces or repetitive loading
- Pain over dorsum of wrist and stiffness
- X-ray findings depend on stage of the disease—normal architecture; increased density; fragmentation; osteoarthritic changes of the wrist
- Surgical treatment—depends on stage of disease and ulnar variance.

Köhler's disease (navicular)
- May be due to a vascular problem
- Affects children aged 2–10yrs old
- Presents with an antalgic limp and tenderness over navicular bone
- X-rays show sclerosis and fragmentation of the ossific nucleus
- Treatment is rest, avoidance of excessive weight bearing, and analgesia
- Pain may require 6 weeks' immobilization in a short walking cast if severe
- Chronic problem, usually resolves in 2yrs.

Sever's disease (calcaneum)
- Occurs in children aged 10–15yrs
- May be bilateral
- Heel pain aggravated by exercise, dorsiflexion of the ankle
- X-rays, sclerosis and fragmentation of calcaneal apophysis
- Managed by avoiding repetitive injury and protecting heel with a heel cup
- Rest, ice packs, NSAIDs and physiotherapy useful.

Scheuermann's disease (thoracolumbar spine)
- Defect in secondary ossification centres of vertebrae
- Occurs in adolescents and is more common in boys
- Activity-related pain and deformity are common presenting symptoms.
- Findings include increase in kyphosis (>40°), stiffness. Cardiorespiratory and neurological problems are rare
- Thoracolumbar standing X-rays: wedging (≥5° in at least 5 adjacent vertebrae are pathognomonic of Scheuermann's disease), increased kyphosis, loss of disc space height, irregular endplates and Schmorl's nodes
- Mild disease—observe and manage symptoms with rest and postural exercises. NSAIDs may be useful in alleviating pain
- More severe disease—spinal orthoses and surgery to be considered with progressive deformity, intractable pain or neurological deficit (fusion with or without decompression).

Osteochondritis dissecans

An idiopathic condition which results in detachment of fragments of cartilage and varying amounts of subchondral bone. Aetiology is unknown but may be:
- Vascular—end arterioles in the epiphysis are disrupted resulting in an area of necrosis which becomes detached with trauma
- Traumatic—recurrent microtrauma, possibly due to generalized laxity, leads to the detachment. This is distinct from an acute osteochondral fracture which is a different entity
- Abnormal ossification of the epiphysis—an area close to the cartilage ossifies earlier than the rest and becomes the focus of stresses.

Disorders of matrix

- Matrix deposition—osteogenesis imperfecta
- Inadequate matrix resorption—Paget's disease, osteopetrosis
- Insufficient matrix turnover—osteoporosis.

Osteogenesis imperfecta

An inherited defect in type I collagen synthesis, which is predominantly found in bone. Four types (Sillence classification):

- autosomal dominant (AD) inheritance, blue sclerae, deafness. IA = teeth involved—dentinogenesis imperfecta; IB = teeth uninvolved
- autosomal recessive (AR), lethal, blue sclerae
- AR, short stature with multiple fractures at birth
- AD inheritance, normal sclerae. IVA = dentinogenesis imperfecta, IVB = teeth uninvolved.

Clinical features

Fragility fractures, short stature, scoliosis, ligamentous laxity, basilar invagination causing spasticity and apnoeic spells. Fractures less frequent following puberty.

Investigations

Radiology—these show generalized osteopenia with thin cortices and healing fractures of varying ages. Wormian bones seen on skull X-ray.

Differential diagnosis

- NAI
- Juvenile OP (self-limiting disease).

Principles of management

- Protect child from fractures
- Aim to avoid radiographic diagnosis of clinically suspected fractures and immobilize affected bone as for normal fractures
- With multiple long bone fractures, the child may benefit from intramedullary rods with multiple osteotomies (Sofield–Miller procedure)
- Severe scoliosis requires instrumented fusion surgery as bracing is ineffective.

Paget's disease (osteitis deformans)

A metabolic disease of unknown aetiology, which is characterized by abnormal bone remodelling and greatly increased bone turnover. Altered osteoblastic and osteoclastic activity results in coarse trabeculae in weakened, hypervascular bone, which is prone to pathological fracture.

Epidemiology

- More common in UK, USA and Australia
- M:F = 2:1
- 5th decade—0.5% of UK population.

Clinical features

- Asymptomatic in most people
- Degenerative joint disease

- Cranial nerve compression from enlarged skull bones, e.g. VIII nerve compression in petrous temporal bone causes deafness
- High output cardiac failure
- Bowed tibiae
- Bone pain.

⚠ 1% risk of sarcomatous change—beware of unrelenting localized pain, rapid X-ray progression or soft tissue mass.

Investigations
- X rays—bony expansion, with remodelled cortices and coarse trabeculae. The matrix is both porotic and sclerotic. Can mimic metastases, but they do not usually expand bone
- *Bone scan*—useful to determine whether monostotic or polyostotic disease. Increased uptake in affected bone
- *Blood tests*—raised ALP
- *Urine tests*—raised urine hydroxyproline indicates increased bone turnover.

Management
Simple analgesics for bone pain. Bisphosphonates may reduce disease progression and reduce hypervascularity of affected bone before surgery. Osteotomy or joint replacement may be needed.

Osteoporosis
A quantitative reduction in bone mass, i.e. reduced overall bone density.

Epidemiology
Groups at risk:
- Northern European females
- Smokers
- Low BMI
- Low mobility
- Poor dietary intake of calcium and vitamin D
- Endocrine disorder; hypothyroidism, steroid use, Cushing's syndrome.

75% of Caucasian females at risk of osteoporotic fracture at age >50yrs.

Clinical features
- Insufficiency fractures, especially spine, with progressive kyphosis.
- Neck of femur and distal radius fractures after low-energy falls.

Investigations
- DEXA scan (dual-energy X-ray absorptiometry)
- Investigations to rule out other causes of OP, e.g. TFT.

Management
- Prevention of bone loss and stimulation of bone regeneration.
- Bone loss inhibitors—diphosphonates/bisphosphonates, phosphate
- Bone regenerators—oestrogen, calcium, vitamin D and strontium.

Disorders of cells

Hyperparathyroidism

Primary hyperparathyroidism

Common, with a prevalence of ~1 in 1000. Usual underlying cause is a parathyroid adenoma secreting inappropriately high levels of parathyroid hormone (PTH). Clinical features are those of hypercalcaemia:

- Bone disease—Brown tumours, fracture, osteopenia, deformity
- Renal stones
- Pancreatitis, peptic ulcer disease
- Psychological disturbance
- Proximal myopathy.

In addition to radiographs, take blood for PTH, vitamin D, Ca^{2+}, PO_4^- levels. Management is surgical parathyroidectomy.

Secondary and tertiary hyperparathyroidism

Conditions which cause hypocalcaemia result in sustained stimulation of the parathyroid glands, and PTH is secreted to correct the serum calcium levels (secondary hyperparathyroidism). Serum calcium may be normal, as the parathyroid glands are functioning appropriately. Management is to treat the underlying cause (e.g. renal failure, vitamin D deficiency).

If an autonomous parathyroid adenoma develops after a prolonged period of secondary hyperparathyroidism, raised calcium levels may develop; this is termed tertiary hyperparathyroidism (treatment is parathyroidectomy).

Cushing's syndrome

Caused by an excess of circulating glucocorticoid hormones.

Aetiology

- Steroid treatment, e.g. autoimmune disease
- Adrenal tumour
- Pituitary tumour, with excessive adrenocorticotrophic hormone (ACTH) stimulating the adrenals. This is true Cushing's disease
- Ectopic ACTH production from, for example, bronchial carcinoma.

Clinical features

- Central obesity, purple striae
- Hyperglycaemia
- Hypertension
- Myopathy
- Immunosuppression
- Psychological disturbance—euphoria/depression
- OP
- AVN of bone.

Diagnosis

- High serum cortisol levels
- 24h urine collection to determine cortisol excretion
- Insulin tolerance test
- Low-dose dexamethasone suppression test.

Management
- Treatment of the cause, e.g. removal of adrenal or pituitary tumour (transphenoidal hypophysectomy)
- Medical management, e.g. metyrapone (blocks cortisol synthesis).

Acromegaly
Excessive growth hormone production from a pituitary tumour.

Clinical features
- Large hands and feet
- Skull hypertrophy
- Macroglossia
- Diabetes mellitus
- Hypercalcaemia
- Hyperphosphataemia.

Diagnosis
- Oral glucose tolerance test
- Growth hormone serum assay, but growth hormone secretion is episodic; therefore, may obtain false-negative result.

Management
- Transphenoidal resection of pituitary tumour
- Bromocriptine inhibits growth hormone production in acromegaly.

Mucopolysaccharidoses
A group of inherited lysosome storage disorders, resulting in stunted growth and caused by hydrolase enzyme deficiencies.

The 4 principal types are:
- Hurler's syndrome
- Hunter's syndrome
- Sanfilippo's syndrome
- Morquio's syndrome.

Diagnosis
Urinary excretion of glycosaminoglycans.

Treatment
Difficult. Includes enzyme replacement therapy and bone marrow transplant.

Disorders of mineralization

Disturbances of bone mineralization are consequences of altered mineral homeostasis. The three main bone minerals are calcium, phosphate and magnesium. These are regulated by three hormones (vitamin D, PTH and calcitonin) which act on three organs—bone (mineral reservoir), intestine (dietary mineral absorption) and kidney (mineral excretion)—to achieve homeostasis.

Osteomalacia

Incomplete osteoid mineralization following physeal closure. Osteomalacia is a qualitative bone mass deficiency, as opposed to OP, which is a quantitative bone mass deficiency.

Causes

- Inadequate dietary intake of vitamin D (fish, fortified margarine), calcium (renal osteodystrophy) or phosphorus
- Inadequate mineral gut absorption/kidney reabsorption
- Excessive mineral excretion
- Insufficient exposure to UV light→7-dehydrocholesterol in skin remaining as an inactive vitamin D precursor
- Genetic
  - vitamin D-resistant rickets (**most common cause of rickets. AKA hypophosphataemic rickets/phosphate diabetes**)
  - Fanconi syndrome
  - hypophosphatasia
- Drugs—phenytoin, phosphate-binding antacids, chronic alcoholism.

Clinical features

Muscle weakness (proximal myopathy), diffuse bone pain, tiredness, enlarged joints from metaphyseal flaring, pathological fractures. In childhood rickets, bowed legs, costochondral junction enlargement (rickety rosary) and thoracic lateral indentation (Harrison's sulcus).

Investigations

- Blood tests—check calcium ($\leftrightarrow$ or $\downarrow$), phosphate (usually $\downarrow$) and ALP concentrations ($\uparrow$ in vitamin D-resistant rickets, $\downarrow$ in hypophosphatasia)
- Urine tests—urinary calcium. If family history of hypophosphataemia check for presence of urinary phosphoethanolamine
- X rays—osteopenia, coarse trabeculae, Looser's zones (pseudofractures—these are radiographically evident osteoid seams). In childhood osteomalacia (= rickets), most changes occur in developing bone at the provisional zone of calcification in the physis, so X-rays show widened, irregular, cupped growth plates, which may slip and deform, resulting in bowed legs and protrusio acetabuli.

Treatment

Dependent on underlying cause. Usually involves dietary supplements of vitamin D, calcium and phosphorus. Treatment of vitamin D-resistant rickets is high dose vitamin D and phosphorus.

Renal osteodystrophy

Renal disease results in inadequate urinary phosphate excretion and insufficient hydroxylation of vitamin D into its active metabolite. There may also be a metabolic acidosis, which inhibits bone mineralization. The reduced vitamin D levels result in reduced intestinal calcium absorption. Low serum calcium stimulates PTH (secondary hyerparathyroidism) to release calcium from bone reservoirs (as it cannot enable intestinal calcium absorption due to lack of active vitamin D).

Clinical features

Muscle weakness due to hypocalcaemia, diffuse bone pain, kidney stones, insufficiency fractures, carpal tunnel syndrome. Patients in chronic renal failure are prone to amyloidosis, which also causes joint pains.

Investigations

- Blood tests—low serum calcium, high serum phosphate, high PTH levels
- X rays—subperiosteal bone resorption, especially in phalanges, generalized osteopenia, ectopic soft tissue calcification, osteitis fibrosa cystica, bony sclerosis, as PTH stimulates osteoblastic as well as osteoclastic activity, Brown tumours (lytic lesions caused by collections of overactive osteoclasts resorbing bone).

Management

Reversal of chronic renal failure.

Joint infections

The most common cause of septic arthritis in the UK is *S. aureus* (70%). Other pathogens such as streptococci or *Haemophilus influenzae* (in children) and *Neisseria gonorrhoea* (sexually active adults) should be considered. Infection, proteolytic enzymes and loss of nutrition cause irreversible damage to cartilage within 48h.

Presentation
- *Pain;* rapid onset, constant
- *Swelling* (effusion)
- *Warmth*
- *Loss of movement;* joint often rigid with severe pain on any attempt at movement
- *Fever;* often quite unwell by 48h from onset of symptoms.

Differential diagnosis
- *Irritable hip* (reactive arthritis)
- *Perthes*
- *Trauma:* fracture or soft tissue injury may cause haemarthrosis or effusion (check clotting if minimal trauma)
- *Crystal deposition:* gout (uric acid), pseudogout (calcium pyrophosphate), acute calcific tendonitis in shoulder
- *Monoarticular presentation:* RA, seronegative arthritis (Reiter's, psoriasis), SLE
- *Other:* PVNS, primary or secondary tumour, effusion reactive to nearby osteomyelitis, overlying soft tissue swelling (bursitis, tendonitis, cellulitis).

Investigation
- *Blood test:* FBC, ESR, CRP, uric acid, blood culture, clotting, rheumatoid immunology
- *X-ray:* ? fracture, chondrocalcinosis, erosions
- *Joint aspiration:* aseptic technique, microscopy for crystals, cells, organisms and fluid for culture and antibiotic sensitivities. Note— presence of white (pus) cells in aspirate indicates inflammatory response but not necessarily infection.

Treatment
- *Early washout*: open or arthroscopic. Take multiple specimens for microbiology and histology. Repeat washout for re-accumulation as required
- *Antibiotics*: initial IV therapy (once specimens taken), agents tailored to organism and sensitivities in culture, 2 week IV course usual, followed by 4 weeks oral therapy.

Complications
- *In children:* AVN, joint subluxation/dislocation, growth disturbance
- *Adults:* secondary osteoarthritis, persistent or recurrent infection.

Osteomyelitis: overview

Infection in bone can present acutely, subacutely (Brodie's abscess) or in various chronic forms. Bacteria enter bones via the bloodstream (acute haematogenous), through penetrating injury (trauma, surgery) or from contiguous spread from nearby soft tissue infection or ulceration. Abscess formation in bone causes disturbance of the microcirculation and infarction. Infarcted bone (*sequestrum*) may become separated and walled off in a cavity, rendering it unreachable by host defence/repair mechanisms and impervious to antibiotic penetration. Pus lifting the periosteum causes new bone formation (*involucrum*). Pus tracking to the surface through a *cloaca* in the cortex may cause soft tissue swelling and induration before discharging as a *sinus*. This discharge, along with antibiotics, may relieve symptoms temporarily, but bacteria retained in dead bone or sequestra may reactivate at any time, frequently giving a cyclical pattern of pain, swelling, fever, discharge and resolution.

Presentation
- Pain; continuous, throbbing, often worse at night
- Fever
- General malaise
- Swelling and induration of soft tissues
- Discharging sinus or ulcer (may be able to probe to bone)
- *Marjolin's* ulcer seen in chronic sinuses (squamous carcinoma).

Investigation
- Bloods: FBC, ESR, CRP, glucose, U&E, LFT, blood cultures
- Plain X-ray: disturbed bony architecture, cloaca, lytic cavities, sclerotic dead bone/sequestrum, periosteal reaction, loosening of metalwork
- MRI: most useful for delineating extent of soft tissue and medullary involvement
- Biopsy: if diagnosis in doubt or tissue samples required to direct antibiotic suppression therapy. Bone biopsy with US, X-ray or CT guidance.

Classification (Cierny et al.[1])
Bony involvement
- Type I   Medullary: acute haematogenous
- Type II   Superficial: cortical
- Type III Localized: both cortex and medulla involved but continuous segment of uninvolved bone remains
- Type IV Diffuse; no uninvolved bone in continuity, e.g. infected non-union.

Host type
- Type A   Healthy
- Type B   Local or systemic compromise, e.g. smoker, diabetic, extensive scarring or poor vascularity
- Type C   Severe compromise or treatment worse than disease.

Reference
1 Cierny G, Mader J, Penninck J. A clinical staging system for adult osteomyelitis. *Contemp Orthop* 1985;**10**:17–37.

Osteomyelitis treatment[1]

Non-operative

Acute haematogenous disease responds to appropriate IV antibiotics; manage operatively if USS or MRI demonstrates an abscess/subperiosteal collection or failure to respond to non-operative treatment. Duration of IV therapy controversial, tailor this and step-down to orals according to clinical response and infective load.

In established or chronic osteomyelitis, suppressive antibiotics may be used to control symptoms in those with minimal or infrequent symptoms, when cure is unlikely or when treatment deemed worse than the disease (type IV disease in type B/C host).

Operative treatment of chronic osteomyelitis

Principles

- *Debridement:* lay open sinuses and fully expose diseased segment
- *Excision:* remove all dead/devitalized tissue, cut back to healthy bone in all directions (punctuate bleeding of cut surface), send multiple specimens for culture
- *Irrigate:* saline/water/0.05% aqueous chlorhexidine
- *Stabilize:* if large or segmental resection, with external or occasionally internal fixation
- *Dead space management:* large voids filled with blood act as a perfect culture medium. Avoid by filling dead space with antibiotic-loaded carrier (e.g. $CaSO_4$ or PMMA (polymethylmethacrylate) antibiotic beads) and/or muscle flap (muscle helps deliver systemic antibiotics). Bone transport or second stage bone graft for large defects
- *Antibiotics:* usually 6 week IV (home IV therapy if possible) followed by 3 months oral. Combination therapy tailored to cultures.

Outcome

- Expect 90–95% disease arrest
- Disease can recur at any stage; walled off nests of bacteria can reactivate many years after initial infection.

Reference

1 Lazzarini L, Mader T, Calhoun J. Osteomyelitis in long bones. *J Bone Joint Surg Am* 2004;**86**:2305–18.

Tumours—general principles

- Primary benign lesions may be latent (inactive, sclerotic), active (sclerotic and lytic, often symptomatic) or aggressive
- Most malignant tumours of the musculoskeletal system are metastases particularly from breast, bronchus, thyroid, renal and prostate primaries; the lesions may appear sclerotic, lytic or mixed
- Primary malignant lesions may be low or high grade lesions, arising from connective tissue cell lines (sarcomas—forming bone, cartilage or fibrous tissue) or non-connective tissues (reticuloendothelial system and haemopoietic cells).

History and examination

- Assess the presenting symptoms, and look for symptoms from other 'occult' lesions. Past history of malignancy or radiation exposure is important
- Local examination should determine the nature and site of any mass, whether distal nerve function has been affected (from compression or invasion), whether regional lymph nodes are involved and if other sites are involved (1° or 2°).

Differential diagnosis

Lesions that may 'mimic' bone tumours include reactive tissues to infection or fracture, bone islands and aneurysmal bone cysts.

Symptoms and signs

Bone tumours may present with **pain** (a deep ache, especially nocturnal), a **mass**, following a **pathological fracture**, functional **loss** (especially with pathological fractures) or as an **incidental finding**.

Investigations

Imaging should be undertaken before biopsy to minimize artefact.

Local diagnosis and staging

Plain radiographs will usually give a small differential diagnosis. Assess:

- Patient age
- The bone involved and the site within the bone (epiphysis, metaphysis or diaphysis; central or eccentric)
- Number of lesions. NB: the whole bone should be imaged
- The matrix (contents) of the lesion—is it chondroid (stippled, rings and arcs), osteoid (solid, cloudy, ivory) or a clear, fibrous appearance?
- Margin of the lesion—well defined or indistinct zone of transition?
- The response of the surrounding bone—lytic, blastic or mixed?
- MRI will determine the anatomical extent of the lesion (which compartments involved) and whether skip lesions are present.

Distant dissemination

Plain film skeletal survey or radioisotope scans will assess if multiple bony sites are involved. Lung and liver metastases can be assessed by CT scan.

Tissue diagnosis

- Ideally, undertaken by the team responsible for definitive care as using inappropriate biopsy techniques may prevent potential limb salvage
- The principle is to obtain sufficient tissue to reach a diagnosis of the nature and grade of the lesion via a safe route, minimizing contamination (by passing through compartments that are already involved and careful haemostasis) and fracture risk (by sampling soft tissues where possible)
- Samples can be obtained by needle with or without image guidance (aspiration cytology or core biopsy), or by a planned open approach
- Excision biopsy is reserved for lesions with benign MRI characteristics that are superficial and <5cm diameter. Send samples for both histology and microbiology.

Treatment

Metastases

- Treatment is aimed at alleviating symptoms and restoring function
- Pathological fractures of long bones should be stabilized and given local radiotherapy if appropriate
- Prophylactic fixation (usually intramedullary nailing) may be used in some circumstances. The scoring system of Mirels[1] can be used to predict the likelihood of fracture; this considers the site, size, matrix and pain from the lesion
- Chemo- or radiotherapy treatment may be used ± surgery.

Malignant primary bone tumour

- The main treatment goal is survival, with functional limb salvage a secondary goal
- Most plans include *en bloc* resection with an adequate tissue margin in combination with neoadjuvant and/or adjuvant chemo- or radiotherapy
- Tumour biology and systemic treatments will determine survival; resection margins will determine local disease control
- Neoadjuvant chemotherapy (given before surgery) may address systemic disease, shrink and define the tumour margins and give prognostic information from the tumour 'kill' rate seen histologically in the resection specimen
- Resection margins are planned after re-staging. The resection may be intralesional (leaving macroscopic disease), marginal (probably leaving microscopic disease) or wide (removing a cuff of 'normal' tissue, to remove the reactive zone); a radical resection (compartment and its fascia excised) or an amputation.

Reference

1 Mirels H. Metastatic disease in long bones. *Clin Orthop Rel Res* 1989;**249**:256–64.

Adult tumours—images

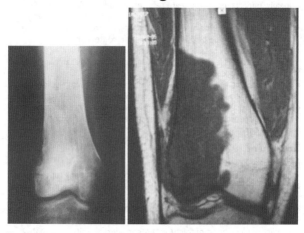

Fig. 8.1 Osteosarcoma of the femur.
Reproduced from Bulstrode et al., *Oxford Textbook of Orthopaedics and Trauma*, with permission from Oxford University Press.

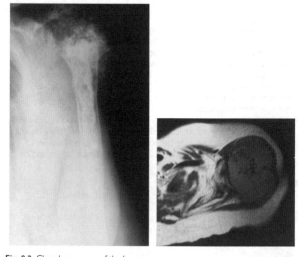

Fig. 8.2 Chondrosarcoma of the humerus.
Reproduced from Bulstrode et al., *Oxford Textbook of Orthopaedics and Trauma*, with permission from Oxford University Press.

Adult tumours—bone forming

Benign

Osteoid osteoma

Small, benign tumours presenting with pain, especially at night, characteristically eased by aspirin. This can cause a limp (with disuse muscle atrophy) or tenderness depending on the site. CT or MRI will usually confirm the diagnosis.

Treatment can be symptomatic (NSAIDs to control pain) with a high recurrence risk, or ablative. Radiofrequency ablation is less invasive than excision, but does not yield a specimen if the diagnosis is in doubt.

Osteoblastoma

Larger lesion with more aggressive appearances that may mimic osteosarcoma both radiologically and histologically. Presents with pain of an insidious onset. Aggressive lesions should be excised with an adequate margin; latent or active lesions can be treated with intralesional excision if a recurrence rate of up to 20% is acceptable.

Malignant

Osteosarcoma

A tumour of the young adult at metaphyseal sites of rapid growth. Metastases are present at diagnosis in 10–20% (40% micro-metastases) and determine survival.

Primary osteosarcoma is seen in 10–20yr olds, with a genetic link to Li–Fraumeni syndrome, retinoblastoma and familial. Lesion may be:
- Central (classical)—high grade lesions breach the cortex, creating a Codman's triangle with a soft tissue mass with sunburst mineralization on plain films. Low grade lesions rarely breach the cortex
- Telangiectatic—little mineralization in the osteoid, so appears lytic and expansile on plain films. May present with pathological fracture
- Surface—parosteal with marked bone formation and a mass; less aggressive (so may not need neoadjuvant chemotherapy). Periosteal have a larger cartilage element with sunburst spicules
- Multicentric—synchronous appearance of primary osteosarcoma at multiple sites.

Secondary osteosarcoma seen in areas of Pagetic bone or fibrous dysplasia, or sites of previous radiotherapy (if >20Gy exposure, especially if received alkylating chemotherapy). Also seen in de-differentiated chondrosarcoma.

Treatment requires a multidisciplinary approach, with neoadjuvant chemotherapy often used. Surgical treatment is to achieve local disease control. 60–70% survive long term (95% if parosteal surface osteosarcoma).

Adult tumours—cartilage forming

Benign

Enchondroma

Proliferation of hyaline cartilage in metaphysis/diaphysis, common in hands and feet. May present with pain, fracture or as an incidental finding. Solitary lesions have ~1% risk of malignant transformation to chondrosarcama, higher if multiple—Ollier's disease (30%) or Maffucci's syndrome (associated haemangiomata—up to 100% risk). Asymptomatic lesions may be observed. Symptomatic or suspicious lesions require marginal excision (curettage) ± grafting or PMMA.

Osteochondroma (exostosis)

Cartilage-capped lesion from the physis, with a narrow (pedunculated) or broad-based (sessile) stalk. Most grow away from the joint, except in Trevor's disease (growth towards the epiphysis). Growth after skeletal maturity suggests malignant transformation (1%); assess the cartilage cap depth with MRI or US. Multiple lesions present in osteochondromatosis (hereditary multiple exostoses (HME); 30% sporadic mutations), with associated short stature, bowing deformities and a 20% malignant transformation risk. Symptomatic benign lesions should be excised, with a 5% recurrence risk (higher if sessile). Others may be observed.

Chondroblastoma

Benign lesion with low metastatic potential; childhood equivalent of giant cell tumour. Lytic lesion in epiphyseal location that can cross the physis. Treat by intralesional/marginal excision ± graft.

Chondromyxoid fibroma

Rare cartilage-forming tumour with fibrous and myxoid elements. Present with pain; characteristically found around the knee in eccentric metaphyseal location. Treatment is en bloc excision.

Malignant

Chondrosarcoma

Primary or secondary to malignant transformation of chondroid lesion. Present with pain, mass, mechanical symptoms or pathological fracture. May de-differentiate to high grade (especially central lesions). Excise with wide margin; girdle lesions make limb salvage difficult. Adjuvant therapies reserved for high grade tumours as most are relatively resistant. 5yr survival 80% if low grade, 20% if high grade.

Adult tumours—giant cell tumour of bone

Definition
Primary benign tumour of unknown origin with locally aggressive features.

Epidemiology
- Peak presentation 20–40yrs; female predominance
- Despite 'benign' nature, ~1% metastatic potential to lung
- 10% chance of transformation to osteosarcoma.

Symptoms and signs
- Pain, referred to the joint affected
- Pathological fracture in 10%
- 50% found about the knee; 10% in sacrum/vertebrae.

Investigations
Radiographs—lytic, central lesion in long bone metaphysis that grows into the epiphysis, almost invariably reaching the subchondral plate. Cortical thinning with a permeative margin and 'soap-bubble' appearance.

Treatment
- Extended curettage (curette lesion; stain cavity; repeat curettage to remove stain) ± cryotherapy or phenol ablation. Defect packed with graft or PMMA cement
- Curettage alone carries 50% recurrence; supplementary cryotherapy or phenol ablation 17% recurrence; extended curettage and PMMA packing 3% recurrence.

Bone marrow tumours

Epidemiology
Incidence is 9 in 100 000 people in the general population rising to 70 in 100 000 in people >65yrs of age.

Divided into
- Leukaemias—primary neoplastic disorder of blood or bone marrow and characterized by an abnormal proliferation of blood cells, usually white blood cells. Acute leukaemias characterized by rapid increase in immature white blood cells and chronic leukaemia by excessive build up of mature white blood cells
- Others.

Leukaemias
Acute
- Acute lymphoblastic leukaemia (ALL)—affects young children and older adults
- Acute myelogenous leukaemia (AML)—affects mainly older adults.

Chronic
- Chronic lymphocytic leukaemia (CLL)—affects adults >60yrs (50%). Rarely affects people under 40yrs
- Chronic myelogenous leukaemia—affects adults, usually between 30 and 40yrs.

Other
- Myeloproliferative disorders
- Myelodysplastic syndrome
- Plasma cell neoplasm
- Multiple myeloma.

Myeloproliferative disorders
A group of diseases of the bone marrow in which there is abnormal, excessive and sustained proliferation of bone marrow cells. They are related to myelodysplastic syndrome and myeloid leukaemia.

Types:
- Polycythaemia rubra vera—occurs in 1 in 100 000 people after 40yrs. Males more than females. Increase in red cells and haemoglobin
- Myelofibrosis—occurs in people >50yrs. Increase of fibroblast activity. Splenomegaly and osteosclerosis develop
- Essential thrombocythaemia—very rare. Excessive defective platelet production.

Myelodysplastic syndrome
Description A very rare and diverse collection of haematological conditions characterized by production of abnormal myeloid blood cells. They are bone stem cell disorders that result in abnormal haematopoiesis. Usually diagnosed between 60 and 75yrs.

Clinical Signs and symptoms are non-specific and related to low blood counts.

Management Goals are to control symptoms and reduce risk of progression to acute myelogenous leukaemia. Blood products and erythropoietin are used along with chemotherapy and stem cell transplantation.

Plasma cell neoplasm

Description Monoclonal neoplastic proliferation of plasma cells.

Clinical Usually present with pain. Spinal involvement not uncommon.

Management Radiotherapy. Chemotherapy reserved for systemic disease. In the spine excision and spinal reconstruction may be necessary.

Multiple myeloma

Description

A malignant plasma cell tumour related to low blood counts. Incidence 3 in 100 000 people, rare below 60yrs of age.

Clinical

- Patient usually has bone pain, anaemia and may have signs of raised serum calcium or infection
- X-rays show punched out (osteolytic) lesions. Bone re-absorption occurs around the lesion due to osteoclast activity
- ESR and serum calcium elevated. Immunoelectrophoresis usually shows high levels of monoclonal immunoglobulins. (M spike) in the serum and a monoclonal light chain in the urine (Bence-Jones protein). Proteinuria. Immunoglobulins most commonly produced are IgG in 50% and IgA in 25%
- Bone scan shows up cold.

Management

Focused on disease suppression. Chemotherapy is used to control systemic disease and radiotherapy to control local disease. May need spinal decompression and fusion.

Complications include infections, renal failure, anaemia and neurological problems related to hypocalcaemia or compression of the neural elements.

Problems associated with these disorders:

- Red cells—anaemia due to failure of production
- White cells—high blast counts lead to sludging of white cells in small vessels. Leukaemia-related phenomena increased risk of pyrexia and fits. Neutropenia can lead to infection
- Platelets—thrombocytopenia leads to increased risk of bleeding
- Coagulation problems—increased bleeding time and there is increased risk of DIC.

For further reading, see Bulstrode *et al.*[1] and Levison *et al.*[2]

References

1 Bulstrode C, Buckwater J, Carr A, *et al.*, eds. *Oxford Textbook of Orthopaedics and Trauma.* Oxford: Oxford University Press, 2002.

2 Levison DA, Reid R, Burt AD, *et al.* *Muir's Textbook of Pathology*, 14th edn. Hodder Arnold, 2008.

Benign vascular tumours

Haemangiomas

Description Benign tumours of blood vessels which occur in adults. One of the most common soft tissue tumours (7% of all benign tumours). Consists of blood vessels and fibrous tissue. They commonly develop in superficial tissue:

- Capillary (port wine stain). Common in skin, also in liver, spleen and kidney, deep red or purple
- Juvenile capillary (strawberry naevus). Present at birth and regresses as child grows
- Cavernous. Consist of large sinus-like space. Common in skin and lips.

Clinical Symptomatic lesions are rare. They are usually found on X-rays (skin, spine and ribs).

Management Observation. Radiation and even surgery may be necessary for painful vertebral lesions or spinal cord compression.

Glomangioma (glomus tumour)

Description A rare tumour that arises from the glomus body and is composed of round cells and vascular spaces.

Clinical Seen in fingers (50%) and toes. It is very tender.

Management Excise.

Paraganglioma (chemodectomas)

Description Rare tumours arising from glomus cells. Glomus cells are part of the paraganglion system. They are found in the abdomen (85%), thorax (12%) and neck (3%).

Clinical Signs and symptoms that develop usually due to pressure on adjacent structures.

Management May require surgery, embolization and radiotherapy.

Multiple angiomatous syndromes

- Osler–Weber–Rendu disease: hereditary haemorrhagic telangiectasia (AD inheritance). Multiple small angiomas seen in skin, liver and spleen. Risk of haemorrhage
- Von Hippel–Lindau disease: AD condition. Cerebellar spinal and retinal angiomas. Associated with renal cell carcinoma and phaeochromocytoma
- Sturge–Weber syndrome: a developmental abnormality affecting the CNS and skin. Facial and meningeal angiomas. Associated with glaucoma, seizures and mental retardation.

Malignant vascular tumours

Haemangioendotheliomas

Description A very rare vascular tumour of intermediate malignancy characterized by vascular structures lined by plump endothelial cells. It involves mainly the axial skeleton.

Management Curettage of low grade lesions. For high grade lesions, radical surgical resection, radiotherapy and chemotherapy have been used.

Angiosarcoma

Description A very rare vascular tumour.

Clinical It has a wide range of differentiation. Seen in skin, bone (femur, tibia, and humerus), breast and liver.

Management Wide marginal resection or amputation as well as radiotherapy and chemotherapy. Prognosis is poor.

For further reading, see Bulstrode et al.[1] and Levison et al.[2].

References

1 Bulstrode C, Buckwater J, Carr A, et al., eds. *Oxford Textbook of Orthopaedics and Trauma.* Oxford: Oxford University Press, 2002.
2 Levison DA, Reid R, Burt AD, et al. *Muir's Textbook of Pathology*, 14th edn. Hodder Arnold, 2008.

Other connective tissue tumours

Langerhans cell histiocytosis (LCH)

Description LCH is a rare disease of unknown aetiology. It affects mainly skin, bone and lymph nodes, but multisystem disease can develop. Wide variety of severity varying from benign to progressively fatal disease. Usually affects children 1–15yrs old. Occurs in 1:200 000 children and 1:500 000 adults. Affects males twice as often as females.

Clinical LCH causes a non-specific inflammatory reaction that results in fever, lethargy and weight loss. Organ involvement results in more specific symptoms.
- Bone—swellings, pain from fractures
- Bone marrow—anaemia, symptoms of infection (pancytopenia)
- Skin—rash (80%)
- Lymph nodes—enlarged.

There may also be signs of liver, spleen and endocrine disease (hypothalamic pituitary axis), lung or, less frequently, GI tract or CNS involvement. The diagnosis is histological.

Management Solitary lesions may be excised and treated with radiotherapy. Systemic disease requires chemotherapy.

Lipoma

Description The most common form of soft tissue tumour. Common in 50–60yr old people but seen in all age groups. Lipomas are associated with hereditary conditions such as familial multiple lipomatosis.

Clinical Presents as a slow growing smooth, subcutaneous tumour. It is non-tender and mobile. There is a very low risk of malignant transformation.

Management Usually excised under local anaesthetic if unsightly, restricts movement or to exclude more sinister lesion such as liposarcoma.

Giant cell tumour of tendon sheath (GCTTS)

Description

Two forms:
- Localized (nodular tenosynovitis): often seen in women between 30 and 50 but can affect any age group, usually seen on the hand often adjacent to the interphalangeal joint, benign, slow growing, may erode bone under lesion, may recur if incompletely excised
- Diffuse (PVNS): rare, seen under 40yrs of age, slightly more common in women than men, usually seen in knee, ankle and foot, often painful and tender and prone to recurrence (rate close to 40%).

Clinical Pain, reduced range of movement of joints.

Management Treated with excision.

Schwannoma

Description A benign encapsulated nerve sheath tumour. They consist only of Schwann cells.

Clinical Presents between 20 and 50yrs. Mainly in the head and neck region. They are painful tumours. Less than 1% become malignant.

Management Treated with excision.

Lymphangiomas

Description These are lymphatic malformations resulting from benign proliferation of lymph vessels. They often present as a soft tissue mass in childhood. They may occur anywhere, but are most often found in the head and neck region (75%). Enlargement of affected organs due to proliferation of lymphatic tissue and small vessels, classified as simple (cutaneous and cavernous) or cystic hygromas:

- Simple: dermal in nature
- Cystic: involve neck, axilla and mediastinum.

Management

- Simple: no treatment. May choose to have excision for cosmetic reasons
- Cystic: may require excision due to pain, site and bulk. High risk of complications postexcision including haematoma, infection, hypertrophic scars and lymphatic fistulas.

Lymphangiosarcoma

Description A very rare malignant tumour which occurs in chronic lymphoedema. It develops in some patients after radical mastectomies (Stewar–Treves syndrome).

Clinical The sarcoma first appears as a purplish discoloration or tender skin nodule in an extremity. It metastasizes early.

Management Prevention and treatment of lymphoedema. Excision.

For further reading, see Bulstrode *et al.*[1] and Levison *et al.*[2].

References

1 Bulstrode C, Buckwater J, Carr A, *et al.*, eds. *Oxford Textbook of Orthopaedics and Trauma.* Oxford: Oxford University Press, 2002.
2 Levison DA, Reid R, Burt AD, *et al. Muir's Textbook of Pathology*, 14th edn. Hodder Arnold, 2008.

Metastatic bone disease

Definition
Distant spread of malignant tumour cells to bone.

Epidemiology
The most common cause for destructive bone lesions in adults. Occur less commonly in children. Affect ~20% of all patients with malignant tumours—commonly from breast, lung, prostate, kidney and thyroid.

Pathology
Deposits are usually found in the axial skeleton and in the most active marrow. Tumour cells induce osteoclastic activity (either locally through TNF or systemically via PTH-related peptide) and these cells resorb bone. Marrow is replaced with cancer cells and fibrous tissue.

Clinical
Usually a history of primary malignancy. Patients present with bone pain—that may be dull at rest, sharp on weight bearing or worse at night, decreased mobility, pathological fractures, hypercalcaemia (constipation, abdominal pains, lethargy) or weight loss.

Examination findings include swellings, bone tenderness, reduced range of movements of joints, lymphadenopathy, anaemia or neurological deficit.

Investigations
Bloods: Evaluate for anaemia and hypercalcaemia.

Radiology: X-rays—for metastasis to be seen they must be >1cm in size and have lost 50% of bone. Lytic lesions develop with breast, lung, thyroid, renal cell, melanoma and GI malignancies. Sclerotic lesions develop with
prostate, breast, lung and carcinoid malignancies.

Bone scans: Areas involved show increased uptake because of increased activity of osteoblasts, with the exception of myeloma, which is cold on bone scans, and false-negative results may be seen after recent chemotherapy. False-positive results may be obtained with degenerative disease or fractures.

CT or MRI: CT scan excellent for defining bone loss. MRI is best for establishing marrow involvement and tumour extension.

Biopsy: CT-guided or open biopsy if diagnosis is in question.

Any work-up for patients with metastatic disease should include blood tests (FBC, inflammatory markers, LFTs, bone biochemistry), imaging (plain radiographs of affected areas, CT of chest and abdomen, technetium bone scan) and biopsy (grade and type of tumour).

Differential diagnosis
- Multiple myeloma
- Lymphoma
- Bone infections
- Enchondromas

Management
Must establish the primary diagnosis.

Non-operative treatment: Control pain with analgesics, NSAIDs, steroids and/or radiotherapy and maintain patient's independence. Systemic therapy includes the use of bisphosphonates, radioisotopes and external beam radiation.

Operative options: Stabilization of long bones or the spine is important in preventing fractures or compression of neural elements. Prophylactic fixation preferable to fixation after a fracture has occurred or the patient develops a neurological deficit. Fixation recommended with >50% of cortical bone destruction or extensive vertebral involvement. In the spine both spinal decompression and fixation are necessary. With involvement of joints, arthroplasty may be necessary.

Prognosis
The prognosis for patients with metastatic bone disease is steadily improving. Many patients survive ≥3 years. Prognosis depends on histological type and grade of tumour.

For further reading, see Bulstrode et al.[1] and Levison et al.[2]

References
1 Bulstrode C, Buckwater J, Carr A, et al., eds. *Oxford Textbook of Orthopaedics and Trauma.* Oxford: Oxford University Press, 2002.
2 Levison DA, Reid R, Burt AD, et al. *Muir's Textbook of Pathology,* 14th edn. Hodder Arnold, 2008.

Other tumours

Neurofibroma

Definition

Benign tumours of peripheral nerves, occurring as localized, diffuse or plexiform associated with neurofibromatosis (NF) type 1 lesions. The most common benign nerve tumour. Sex distribution is equal and usually affects 20–30yr age group.

Clinical

Usually present as a painless mass located within the dermis or subcutaneous tissue. Solitary neurofibromas do not undergo malignant transformation, but those associated with NF do have a low risk of transformation.

Management

Solitary lesions can be excised, but the treatment of NF is more controversial as there is a risk of malignant transformation (reported rate 2–30%) and there is a high risk of recurrence.

Desmoid tumours

Description

A benign but locally aggressive soft tissue tumour. Very rare. More common in women than men and usually affects those between 25 and 35yrs of age. Histologically resembles a low grade fibrosarcoma.

Clinical

Presents as a swelling and may be part of a genetic syndrome (familial adenomatous polyposis). MRI is the best way of evaluating the lesion.

Management

Wide local excision and radiotherapy for local control. Chemotherapy and hormonal treatments have been tried with variable success.

Elastofibroma

Description

A painless soft tissue mass fixed to the chest wall, usually at the tip of the scapula. It is unknown whether it is a benign tumour or reactive tissue formed in response to mechanical irritation. Usually seen in those <50yrs.

Clinical

Often an incidental finding—palpable mass found by the patient. Biopsy can be used if there is doubt about the diagnosis.

Management Local excision if symptomatic.

For further reading, see Bulstrode et al.[1] and Levison et al.[2].

References

1 Bulstrode C, Buckwater J, Carr A, et al., eds. *Oxford Textbook of Orthopaedics and Trauma.* Oxford: Oxford University Press, 2002.
2 Levison DA, Reid R, Burt AD, et al. *Muir's Textbook of Pathology*, 14th edn. Hodder Arnold, 2008.

Tumour-like conditions

Lesions that resemble bone neoplasms

Unicameral bone cysts

Unilocular or partially loculated fluid filled cysts. >90% found in proximal humerus. Often asymptomatic but may fracture (and then heal). Enlarge during skeletal growth then tend to resolve spontaneously. Treat conservatively unless symptomatic, then consider steroid injection, bone marrow injection or curettage and bone grafting.

Aneurysmal bone cyst

Benign but locally destructive blood-filled cysts. Most common in long bone metaphyses, proximal humerus, distal femur, proximal tibia and fibula, and ilium. Present with pain and swelling. If indicated, excision or curettage and bone grafting.

Fibrous cortical defect (non-ossifying fibroma)

Developmental proliferation of fibrous tissue and histiocytes. Most common in distal femur, proximal tibia and distal tibial metaphyses. Mostly asymptomatic often heal spontaneously.

Bone island

Nodule of mature lamellar bone within cancellous portion of the skeleton. Often asymptomatic, exclude malignancy in enlarging lesions.

Fibrous dysplasia

Developmental abnormality consisting of slow growing abnormal bone and fibrous tissue which replaces normal bone marrow. Monostotic or polyostotic forms. Common in ribs, craniofacial bones, proximal femur, tibia and humerus. Ground glass appearance on X-ray characteristic. May cause skeletal deformity and fractures, which may require surgery.

Lesions that resemble soft tissue neoplasms

Ganglion cyst

Cystic lesion, pathologically a myxomatous degeneration of fibrous tissue of the joint capsule or tendon sheath. Most commonly dorsal and volar wrist. Often asymptomatic; may fluctuate in size or resolve spontaneously. Aspiration may lead to resolution <30%. Surgical excision may be indicated but high rates of recurrence have been reported.

Intramuscular myxoma

Rare benign, painless, slow growing mass found in skeletal muscle in patients >40yrs, diagnosis greatly helped by MRI.

Nodular fasciitis

Benign proliferation of fibroblasts and myofibroblasts. Rapid growth often follows a benign self-limiting course. Found in subcutaneous fat, muscle or skin commonly in the upper extremities.

Myositis ossificans

A condition of heterotopic ossification in muscle, usually associated with trauma. There is a heritable form (myositis ossificans progressiva) which presents in childhood and is usually fatal.

Common sites
- Quadriceps
- Gluteals
- Small muscles of the hand
- Brachialis.

Common causes
- Trauma
- Burns
- Coma
- Idiopathic.

Clinical features
- 0–3 weeks: pain, swelling, stiffness
- 3–6 weeks: painless hard mass
- 3–18 months: matures, may resolve.

Investigations
- Plain X-ray—zonal calcification which matures over time
- CT/MRI—if plain radiographs not characteristic
- Biopsy if atypical features on imaging.

Histological features
- Peripherally—mature osteoid and mineralized bone
- Centrally—proliferating fibroblasts, macrophages, plasma cells.

Treatment
- Treat symptomatically
- Allow lesion to mature (up to 18 months) before considering surgery. Less than 10% require surgical excision
- Consider postoperative indomethacin and/or radiotherapy to prevent recurrence if surgical excision is performed.

Important differential diagnoses
- Calcified haemangioma
- Osteosarcoma
- Chondrosarcoma
- Synovial sarcoma
- Calcified lipoma.

Charcot arthropathy

A rapidly progressing destructive process developing in joints with autonomic and sensory neuropathy. Disease process divided into four stages:

Stage	Clinical findings	X-ray findings
0	Local oedema and warmth	Local osteoporosis
I	Oedema and warmth with progressive deformity	Osseous destruction and collapse, joint subluxation
II	Decreased oedema	Coalescence of fracture fragments
III	Minimal oedema	Consolidation and remodelling

Treatment

- Stage 0 and I—non-weight bearing in well fitting cast
- Stage II–III—gradual increase in weight bearing in moulded ankle–foot orthosis (AFO).

Surgery reserved for correction of severe deformity or fusing unstable joints once active inflammatory process resolved.

Neck pain in adults

Epidemiology Neck pain is common, occurring in 10% of the population at any time.

Aetiology

Neck pain can represent a wide array of cervical spine disorders that can be divided into traumatic and atraumatic types.

Traumatic neck pain (common after RTAs):
- Soft tissue injuries
- Subluxations or dislocations
- Herniated disc
- Fracture.

Atraumatic neck pain:
- Degenerative—cervical spondylosis, disc disease, facet degeneration
- Inflammatory—RA, AS, polymyalgia rheumatica and polymyositis
- Shoulder problems—subacromial impingement, adhesive capsulitis, tennis elbow, repetitive strain disorder and impingement syndrome
- Other problems—infection, tumours (metastatic disease, primary bone or intradural tumours), referred pain (cardiac, cholecystisis, lymph nodes, temporomandibular joint problems).

Clinical

Cervical assessment should focus on local or regional tenderness, range of movements and a neurological assessment (UMN or LMN signs). In traumatic neck pain the neck must be immobilized until it has been confirmed there is no instability and it has been documented that there is no neurological deficit.

Common presentations are:
- Axial neck pain due to degeneration, facet joint pain or ligamentous strain. Radicular pain due to disc herniation. Myelopathic symptoms develop with chronic disc degeneration and formation of osteophytes that cause cord compression (people >55yrs of age)
- Cervical disc degeneration often produces neck stiffness, headache, and referred pain to shoulder, chest and face. Atlanto-occipital and atlanto-axial pain radiate to neck, often exacerbated by neck rotation
- Radiculopathic symptoms vary. Specific nerve root involvement affects distribution of symptoms:
  - C3: pain in back of neck and mastoid area and pinna and trapezius
  - C4: pain and numbness in the back of the neck, anterior
  - C5: pain side of neck to top of shoulder, weak deltoid, no reflex change
  - C6: pain lateral arm, forearm and thumb, weak biceps and biceps reflex
  - C7: pain middle forearm and middle finger, weak triceps and triceps reflex
  - C8: pain medial forearm/little finger, intrinsic hand atrophy, normal reflexes.

In early stages paraesthesia present. Spurlings test positive and axial neck pain mainly to the side of the pain.

Myelopathic symptoms include:
- Gait disturbance
- Spasticity, decreased manual dexterity
- Paraesthesia and weakness.

Signs of myelopathy include increased tone, hyperreflexia, weakness, positive Hoffmans test (long finger DIP tapped into extension and thumb flexion occurs). L'Hermitte's sign is present in 25% of patients—neck flexion causes electrical shock-like symptoms going down the leg. Look for an up-going plantar response. Paradoxical or inverted brachial reflex (tapping the brachialis tendon causes paradoxical finger flexion to occur). This is only positive sign of C6 involvement.

Always rule out other causes of neck pain, e.g. ischaemic heart disease.

Investigations: radiology
- Cervical spine films often show non-specific changes. Degeneration is common. The spinal canal can be seen in both the AP and the lateral views. Other useful views are oblique views used to assess neural foramina. Open mouth view to assess C1 and C2 fractures and flexion/extension views to assess stability
- MRI is being used more often to look for basal skull fractures, ligament injuries and neurological problems, nerve root compression, spinal cord compression, disc herniation and foraminal stenosis. It can display both the sites of compression and intrinsic changes in the cord that represents cord oedema. Lateral disc herniations can compress the posterolateral area and the exiting nerve root
- CT is most useful for detecting bony abnormalities.

Management

Non-operative treatment Axial neck pain due to degenerative disease is managed non-operatively in the majority of cases. NSAIDs and physiotherapy useful; manual therapy may help nerve root irritation. Patients with severe, acute root pain may benefit from a root block and those with facet joint pain may benefit from facet joint injections. Cervical collars can ease pain but prolonged use should be avoided to prevent deconditioning of cervical musculature.

Operative options Reasons for operating include neurological deficit and persistent pain. Myelopathy warrants early operation to prevent deterioration. Severe root pain that has not resolved also warrants surgical treatment. Axial neck pain secondary to degeneration is generally not treated surgically, but if there are significant changes at a single segment then a fusion may be indicated. Patients should be followed-up at 4–6 week intervals until the pain or discomfort resolves. The options of anterior or posterior decompression are determined by the type of degenerative changes that are found, and surgeon's preferences.

Back pain

Epidemiology Back pain affects 8 out of 10 adults at some stage in their lives. The incidence of low back pain in developed countries is 15–20%; it is lower in developing countries. In 90% of patients with low back pain it resolves within 6 weeks.

Aetiology

- Traumatic: fracture, dislocations, disc herniations, ligamentous tears, muscle strains
- Acquired: degenerative disc or facet disease, spinal stenosis, inflammation, arthritis, spondylosis, spondylolisthesis, infections and neoplasms.

The causes of low back pain vary with age.

Young adults

- Acute fractures
- Disc disease
- Spondylolisthesis
- Scheuermann's disease
- AS
- Metabolic bone disease
- Spinal instability.

Older adults

- Degenerative facet disease
- Spinal stenosis (severe)
- Osteoporotic compression fractures
- Metastatic disease
- Infection.

Risk factors associated with low back pain are obesity, smoking, manual labour and traumatic events.

Common types of back pain

- Discogenic back pain—pain from the innervated layer of the annulus fibrosus
- Radicular back pain—pain extending to the buttock and/or leg associated. Due to nerve root compression, usually due to a disc herniation, spinal stenosis or intraspinal pathology
- Referred back pain—aortic aneurysm, visceral disease (peptic ulcer, pelvic inflammatory disease, endometriosis, gallbladder disease, pancreatic disease, renal disease and pleural disease), infection, UTI and arthritis of the hip
- Iatrogenic back pain—dural adhesions, postoperative instability, postoperative discitis, arachnoiditis
- Psychogenic back pain—organic pathology must be excluded (Waddell's inappropriate signs often present):
  - Superficial and widespread tenderness or non-anatomic tenderness
  - Stimulation tests: pain on axial loading and simulated rotation
  - Non-anatomic sensory and motor changes
  - Distracted SLR
  - Over-reaction.

If there are more than three out of the five present then there is a high probability the patient has a non-organic component to their pain. Non-organic signs in isolation should not be equated with the presence of a psychological problem.

Clinical

Symptoms include back pain, stiffness and there may be altered sensation or motor deficits. There may be paravertebral muscle spasm, reduced movements of the spine, loss of normal thoracolumbar profile and signs of a neurological deficit (reduced SLR, nerve root tension signs, weakness, loss of sensation, loss of deep tendon reflexes, clonus, positive Babinski sign).

Low back pain with leg pain occurs with nerve root entrapment due to intervertebral disc prolapses (most common cause), spinal stenosis and spondylolisthesis and spinal tumour.

A thorough history is essential to elucidate the cause of the back pain (aggravating and alleviating factors, quality of pain, radiation, cause, associated symptoms and effects of treatment).

Examine gait, posture, trunkal balance, spinal movements, sites of tenderness, provocative movements and a full neurological examination. Examine other systems from where the pain may be referred.

Serious pathology may be heralded by so-called red flags:
• <20yrs of age or >50yrs of age at onset
• Non-mechanical pain
• Nocturnal pain
• Fever, night sweats or weight loss
• Thoracic pain
• Severe or progressive neurological deficit
• Sphincter disturbances
• Immunosuppression
• History of infection or malignancy
• Significant trauma or deformity.

Patients with these signs and symptoms must be assessed as a matter of urgency.

Compression of lumbosacral nerve roots may result in a clinical disorder known as cauda equina syndrome. The clinical signs are variable but patients with the syndrome can present with low back pain, bilateral sciatica, saddle anaesthesia, weakness of the lower extremities, impaired reflexes bilaterally, and bladder and bowel dysfunction. It is a medical emergency and these patients require urgent surgery to decompress the nerve roots.

Back pain: investigations and management

Investigations

No investigations are indicated in the majority of patients. However, patients with persistent pain or those who have signs suggesting serious underlying pathology need to be investigated.

Radiology If clinically indicated and MRI is not available, plain AP and lateral radiographs of the spine may be useful. An MRI scan is indicated for persistent or chronic pain, or when there is a suspicion of inflammatory arthropathy, infection or neoplasm.

CT scans are useful for detecting bone abnormalities (fractures, osteoid osteomas) and are also used when patients cannot have an MRI scan (cardiac pacemaker, metallic vascular clips).

Bone scan Technetium bone scans are used for detecting early infection or localizing metastatic bone lesions.

Discography The painful segment can be investigated with discograms. The architecture of the disc is defined and one can see if pain is reproduced with injection of dye into a disc. A normal disc is not usually painful when injected.

Laboratory tests No specific test. If one suspects an infection or neoplasm, FBC, ESR and CRP should be requested. In patients >50yrs there is a case for doing a myeloma screen. In patients with marked stiffness or signs of connective tissue disorders, a rheumatological screen and HLA B27 testing can be requested.

Management

Non-operative treatment: avoid rest—only very short periods are acceptable during rehabilitation. NSAIDs are helpful especially for periods of 4–6 weeks. Active approaches such as the McKenzie regime may be helpful. Active patient advice and education led by the physiotherapists and all clinicians involved in the patient's care are important. Spinal manipulations may have some benefit.

Operative options: rationale for treatment: it may be assumed that back pain can be generated from abnormal movement through mechanical means and through inflammatory sources.

The mechanical source of the pain can therefore be improved by stabilization surgically. The inflammatory type of the pain can be reduced by excision of the whole disc. Mechanical instability may be due to degenerative changes, mechanical instability or spondylolisthesis. Instability symptoms include giving way, getting stuck or a ratchety feeling in the spine.

The ideal patient is one who is a non-smoker, has undergone a comprehensive programme of non-operative treatment and has an identifiable source of his or her pain.

Surgery may involve a decompression, correction of deformity or malalignment and fusion, which could be with or without instrumentation. Lumbar disc replacements are being used for low back pain, but their use remains controversial.

Failure of surgery can be due to inappropriate patient selection, wrong level surgery, unrealistic patient expectations, problems related to surgery and secondary pathology contributing to low back pain.

For further reading, see Waddell et al.[1].

Reference

1 Waddell G, McCulloch JA, Kummel E, Venner RM. Nonorganic physical signs in low-back pain. *Spine* 1980;**5**:117–125.

Spondylosis

Epidemiology

Degenerative changes of the spine are present in as many as 65% of patients >50yrs. Of these, only a small number become symptomatic. It occurs more often in men than women.

A degenerative disorder affecting the vertebrae, facet joints, intervertebral discs and surrounding ligaments. It produces osteophytes, disc degeneration, narrowing of disc space, facet joint degeneration and can cause nerve root or cord compression.

Clinical features

- Spondylotic changes can result in spinal canal, lateral recess and foraminal stenosis. Spinal canal stenosis can result in myelopathy, whereas stenosis that occurs more laterally can cause radiculopathy.
- Degenerative changes sometimes result in painful and tender spine with reduced mobility.
- Root compression results in a radiculopathy and cord compression in a myelopathy.
- The changes can affect cervical, thoracic and or lumbar regions.

Pathophysiology

Dehydration and decreased elasticity of intervertebral disc occur with age, and cracks and fissures appear in intervertebral discs. Surrounding ligaments also have less elasticity and thicken. There is collapse of intervertebral discs. The annuli of these discs bulge outward, uncinate processes over-ride and hypertrophy (compromising ventrolateral portion of foramen) and facets over-ride and hypertrophy (compromising dorsolateral portion of foramen). Marginal osteophytes develop.

Cervical spondylosis

Neck pain from cervical spondylosis is common. It affects men and women equally, although onset is usually earlier in men. Incidence rises with age.

Clinical features

Radiculopathy Pain develops in arms and fingers with reduced reflexes. Dermatomal sensory loss and LMN weakness can be found.

There are 8 cervical nerve roots and only 7 cervical vertebrae. Cervical roots exit above their vertebrae. Thus, the lower nerve root at a given level is usually affected, e.g. C5/C6 pathology affects C6 nerve root. The intervertebral joints involved (in decreasing order of frequency) are C5/C6 (thumb sensation, inverted supinator reflex—fingers flex on eliciting reflex but there is no other movement, and biceps muscle), C5/C6/T1 (little finger sensation and interossei), C6/C7 (middle finger sensation, triceps, triceps reflex), C4/C5 (elbow sensation, biceps reflex and deltoid). Note rare T1 radiculopathy is sometimes caused by this disease but usually arises due to a Pancoast tumour at the lung apex.

Myelopathy Weakness (upper >lower limb), abnormal gait (typically broad based, stooped and spastic), decreased dexterity, sensory disturbance, spasticity and urinary disturbance (retention/frequency).

Other UMN signs include hyper-reflexia, Hoffmann's reflex (flicking one finger causes neighbouring digits to flex), clonus and Babinski sign (up-going plantars). L'Hermitte's sign: neck flexion/extension produces sensation of electric shock through upper and lower extremities and trunk (25% of patients with cervical spondylotic myelopathy).

In ~95% of patients with high cervical cord compression, scapulohumeral reflex can be elicited (tap tip of spine of scapula—positive if brisk scapular elevation and abduction of humerus). Lower extremity weakness indicates involvement of corticospinal tracts, a worrying sign.

In contrast to a radiculopathy, pain is not a common presenting feature of a myelopathy.

Differential diagnosis Multiple sclerosis, acute disc prolapse, neurofibroma of nerve root or subacute combined degeneration of the cord.

Thoracic spondylosis Pain often triggered by flexion (disc pain) and hyperextension (facet joint pain). Thoracic roots exit below their vertebrae (unlike in the cervical spine).

Lumbar spondylosis

Usually asymptomatic. It is present in 27–37% of the asymptomatic population. It appears to be a non-specific ageing phenomenon.

Spondylosis occurs as a result of new bone formation in areas where the annular ligament is stressed.

If symptomatic: lumbar spine carries most weight therefore pain on activity. Sitting for long periods may cause symptoms because of pressure on lumbar spine. Repetitive movements, e.g. lifting or bending, can also precipitate or aggravate the pain.

Patients with spondylosis may become symptomatic if they develop nerve root impingement, disc disease or spinal stenosis.

Lumbar nerve roots exit below their vertebrae, producing symptoms in the same level nerve root.

If osteophytes disappear check for aortic aneurysm—pressure caused by the aneurysm erodes adjacent vertebrae.

Investigations Plain X-rays including obliques, CT and MRI.

Treatment

Medical: analgesis, anti-inflammatories, muscle relaxants.

Non-operative options: immobilization or brace, soft cervical collar (only for short periods) or lumbosacral orthosis, physiotherapy, transcutaneous electrical nerve stimulation (TENS) and lifestyle changes.

Surgical: seldom required. Decompression or fusion may be considered (as for back pain) if there is objective evidence of a root lesion or myelopathy.

For further reading, see Lauerman and McCall[1].

Reference

1 Lauerman WC, McCall BR. Spine. In: Miller MD, ed. *Review of Orthopaedics*, 4th edn. London: Saunders, 2004:416–18.

Osteoporosis of the spine

OP is a reduction in the amount of bone (but normal composition) with associated microarchitectural failure and predisposition to fracture (qualitative definition).

Causes
- Primary—age-related; predominantly postmenopausal women
- Secondary—endocrine (NB: corticosteroid use; early menopause); malabsorption/anorexia; bone marrow disease; transplantation; inherited (e.g. type 1 osteogenesis imperfecta); chromosomal
- Idiopathic—not related to age or to any identifiable known cause
- Additional risk factors—inactivity; smoking; alcohol abuse.

Clinical features
- Symptoms due to associated fractures; in the spine, causes back pain, loss of height in upper segment (crown-pubis) and *de novo* deformity in sagittal and/or coronal planes (kyphosis and scoliosis, respectively)
- Features of systemic diseases which cause secondary OP (e.g. Cushing's).

Management
- Maximize peak bone mass
  - Regular load-bearing exercise
  - Calcium supplementation in youth—twin study evidence
- Diagnose OP and fractures
  - DEXA to determine bone mineral density (BMD). OP = BMD at least 2.5 SD below the peak bone mass
  - Plain radiographs of spine for fractures
  - MRI of spine to exclude metastases as cause of fractures
  - Blood investigations to exclude myeloma and causes of secondary OP
- Reduce bone loss
  - Avoid immobilization, excessive alcohol, smoking, corticosteroids
  - Regular load-bearing exercise
  - Calcium and vitamin D supplementation
  - Hormone-replacement therapy—reduces loss while on treatment
  - Bisphosphonates—trial evidence that treatment reduces vertebral fractures
- Prevent non-vertebral fracture (distal radius; femoral neck)
  - Falls avoidance—optimize vision and balance; treat causes of syncope
- Exclude malignant disease (metastases; multiple myeloma)
- Look for modifiable risk factors and causes of secondary OP
- Treat symptomatic vertebral fractures
  - Simple analgesia
  - Percutaneous vertebroplasty/balloon kyphoplasty with augmentation of body with PMMA cement. Balloon kyphoplasty also restores height.

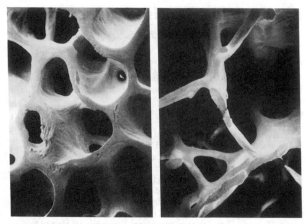

Fig. 8.3 Scanning electron microscope appearance of normal and osteoporotic bone.

Reproduced from Bulstrode et al., *Oxford Textbook of Orthopaedics and Trauma*, with permission from Oxford University Press.

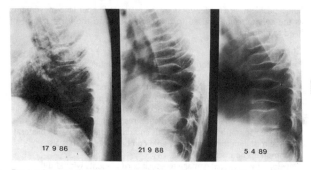

Fig. 8.4 Radiographic changes in idiopathic juvenile osteoporosis: the development and spontaneous improvement in vertebral osteoporosis in a boy aged 11.

Reproduced from Bulstrode et al., *Oxford Textbook of Orthopaedics and Trauma*, with permission from Oxford University Press.

Rheumatoid arthritis of the spine

RA can affect any part of the spine but the cervical spine is most commonly affected.

Pathology

Synovium is present at the atlantoaxial articulation and the facet joints. Destruction of the surrounding tissues leads to a number of instability patterns:

- Basilar settling—occurs in 40% of patients with RA of the cervical spine. The space between the odontoid and foramen magnum decreases steadily and pressure can be placed on the spinal cord and brainstem
- Atlantoaxial instability—occurs in 50–80% of patients with RA of the cervical spine. The transverse and apical ligaments which prevent displacement of C1 on C2 vertebral bodies are destroyed by pannus. The space available for the cord behind the dens is insufficient and pressure is placed on the cord. Radiographs show an increased space between the arch of the atlas and front of the dens (<3mm normal)
- Subaxial instability—occurs in 20% of patients with RA of the cervical spine. Excessive intervertebral movement becomes possible and the cord or nerve roots can be compressed.

Patients requiring general anaesthetic should have a preoperative cervical spine series including flexion–extension views, as many cases are asymptomatic.

Spinal problems are made worse by the restricted upper limb movements as the cervical spine is used to bring the mouth to the hand instead of hand to mouth.

Clinical

Patients may have symptoms and signs from a number of sources:

- Localized pain or deformity—from the spine itself
- Radiculitis—nerve root irritation leads to referred pain in that dermatome. Occipital headache may in fact be upper cervical root irritation referred to auricular or occipital dermatomes
- Radiculopathy—nerve root dysfunction results in LMN signs and decreased sensation. Both radiculitis and radiculopathy may be bilateral and be mistaken for peripheral nerve compression which is also common in rheumatoid disease
- Myelopathy—gradual damage to spinal cord presents with LMN signs at level of compression and upper motor signs below this level. Sensory symptoms may be confusing but may have a level above which sensation is normal. Also ask about weakness, paraesthesia, stumbling, altered gait (from loss of power, sensation or proprioception) and sphincter problems.

Look for evidence of myelopathy at every possible opportunity as missing it can result in serious harm.

Investigations

Radiology Plain radiographs of the cervical spine AP, lateral and odontoid peg views. Flexion and extension laterals are important. These should be 'patient-controlled' active rather than passive movement, to prevent harm.

MRI scans Examine the soft tissues, including the cord. Increased cord signal on T2-weighted images is suggestive of oedema, and a myelopathy may develop. A fluid-filled defect (syrinx) may develop in the cord.

Management

Non-operative treatment

- Analgesia and NSAIDs
- Medical treatment of underlying condition
- Optimize upper limb function to reduce demands on cervical spine
- Soft collar or firmer orthosis may relieve some symptoms.

Operative options

Surgical intervention may be required for pain or neurological compromise.

Myelopathy has been graded by Ranawat *et al.*[1]:

- Grade I—no neurological deficit.
- Grade II—subjective motor symptoms (weakness).
- Grade IIIA—objective motor signs but ambulatory.
- Grade IIIB—objective motor signs and non-ambulatory.

Surgery is possibly indicated in patients with grades II and IIIA disease. Patients with grade IIIB do not do as well following surgery. Surgery consists of procedures to decompress the cord and stabilize the involved unstable segment of the spine.

Other spinal problems

- Patients with RA are more prone to the usual spectrum of degenerative spinal disease
- With steroid use and generalized OP they are at high risk for vertebral collapse fractures.

Reference

1 Ranawat CS, O'Leary P, Pellicci P, *et al.* Cervical fusion in rheumatoid arthritis. *J Bone Joint Surg Am* 1979;**61A**:1003–10.

Ankylosing spondylitis

Pathology (see 📖 p. 184).

Spinal involvement in AS

Although AS affects any joint, it has profound effects on the vertebral column. The other seronegative arthropathies (enteropathic, psoriatic) may have similar manifestations in the spine.

- SIJs are affected early on in the disease process
- Syndesmophytes, ossification around the intervertebral discs, result in the formation of a solid column of bone
- Loss of the normal lumbar lordosis and increased thoracic kyphosis results in marked sagittal imbalance
- Forward gaze is affected—initially it can be achieved by hyperlordosis of the cervical spine but with increasing deformity even this becomes difficult
- Flexion deformities of the hips exacerbates the postural problems.

Clinical

Males are affected more commonly than females. Initially mild lower back pain develops which may be relieved with activity. The stiffness and typical signs may not be apparent until the disease is quite advanced. Rarely, neurological compromise of cord or roots may occur and specific symptoms should be enquired about.

In advanced cases inspection from the side reveals the 'question-mark' deformity due to the kyphosis and hip flexion deformities. Chest expansion is affected—normal is >7cm.

Assessing the severity of the deformity:
- Gaze length—as deformity increases the patient struggles to see in front of themselves. Measuring how far they can see provides a useful measure for disease progression
- Wall–tragus distance (WTD)—patients should be able to stand with heels, buttocks, shoulders and occiput flat against a wall. This may not be possible in AS. The measurement is from the wall to the tragus of the ear.

Investigations

Plain radiographs: pelvic radiograph may show abnormal SIJs. Spinal radiographs may show the syndesmophytes. When extensive disease this gives the appearance of a 'bamboo spine'.

MRI scan: if AS is suspected an MRI of the SIJs will show inflammation and is one of the earliest positive investigations. It is also useful in assessing neurological elements of the spine.

Management

Non-operative treatment: early physiotherapy can be beneficial in helping maintain the movement of the spine and hips. As the deformity becomes rigid, non-operative interventions are less beneficial. Even seating may be problematic and standard wheelchairs may not provide adequate support.

Operative options: if hip arthritis and flexion deformities are a significant factor, total hip arthroplasty combined with soft tissue releases may be beneficial. The surgery may improve the trunkal balance so that spinal surgery is not required. To gain the most benefit, bilateral simultaneous total hip arthroplasty may be required. There is an increased risk of heterotopic ossification in patients with AS.

A closing wedge osteotomy of the spine combined with an instrumented posterior fusion may be required for severe deformities. This is major surgery with high risks. Non-union is a problem in AS because of the stiffness of the adjacent joints.

Vertebral and intervertebral fractures are seen in AS (Anderson lesions). Due to the high risk of non-union and potentially fatal neurological sequelae, these injuries require surgical stabilization. Any patient with vertebral pain following trauma (even relatively low energy injuries) should be presumed to have a fracture until proven otherwise. Confirming the diagnosis may be difficult and require CT or MRI scan.

Chiari malformation

A collection of malformations of the cranio-cervical junction named after Hans Chiari who described them in the 1890s[1]. His initial reports were in children, but it is now recognized that the type I malformation predominantly occurs in adults. Type I is common and often asymptomatic. Types II–IV are rare and are associated with other major abnormalities of the cranio-vertebral axis. MRI is the most useful investigation to make the diagnosis.

Chiari I

The cerebellar tonsils (± medulla oblongata) prolapse through the foramen magnum. It is a demonstrable radiological abnormality in as many as 0.5–1% of the adult population. The clinical features do not always correlate with radiological severity and therefore attempts to assign measurable criteria to the degree of herniation are not useful.

Presenting symptoms

Are variable but may include
- Headache
- Neck pain
- Scoliosis
- Sensory disturbance
- Dysphagia
- Incoordination.

Associated abnormalities

- Syrinx
- Scoliosis
- Hydrocephalus
- Basilar impression.

Causes

- Developmentally small posterior fossa
- Acquired reduction in calvarial volume—craniosynostosis, rickets, achondroplasia, Paget's disease, acromegaly.

Chiari II (Arnold–Chiari malformation)

A more significant herniation of the hindbrain including the medulla, 4th ventricle, pons and cerebellum, into spinal canal. Almost always associated with (myelomeningocele) spina bifida and hydrocephalus. A low termination of the spinal cord (tethered cord) is also a common association.

Chiari III and IV

Type III involves a spina bifida of the cervical spine ± occiput with cerebellar herniation through the foramen magnum. Type IV is cerebellar hypoplasia without herniation.

Treatment options

- None or observation only
- Closure of spina bifida defects
- CSF shunting to relieve hydrocephalus
- Surgical decompression—relieves pressure on the neural elements and restores CSF flow which can reverse hydrocephalus and syringomyelia
  - Anterior (transoral)
  - Posterior (suboccipital craniectomy)
- Drainage of syrinx by direct aspiration or surgical myelotomy.

Reference

1 Koehler PJ. Chiari's description of cerebellar ectopy (1891). *J Neurosurg* 1991;**75**:823–6.

Spina bifida

A congenital spinal dysraphism due to incomplete closure of the embryonic neural tube. Typically affects the lumbosacral spine and is classified into 3 categories of severity.

- Spina bifida occulta—isolated vertebral defect with normal overlying soft tissue, usually asymptomatic
- Meningocele—there is a cystic herniation comprising the meninges and CSF (but no neural elements) through a bony and musculocutaneous defect
- Myelomeningocele—the most severe form where the herniation contains the meningeal sac and nerve roots or spinal cord. There is neurological dysfunction distal to the defect.

Incidence

Defects of spina bifida occulta seen in ~5–10% of lumbar X-rays. Incidence of open spina bifida (meningocele/myelomeningocele) is ~1 per 1000 live births.

Causes

Multifactorial. Genetic, nutritional and metabolic influences.

Diagnosis

Open spina bifida commonly a prenatal diagnosis on maternal USS. Serum α-fetoprotein (AFP) and amniotic fluid AFP (at amniocentesis) raised in spina bifida fetuses but not specific to this disorder.

Clinical features

If not diagnosed prenatally, open spina bifida will manifest itself at birth with a saccular lesion overlying the lumbosacral spine. Spina bifida occulta may show midline skin dimpling or a hairy patch, but often is only identifiable on radiographic examination.

Complications/associated defects

- meningitis—particularly if there is direct exposure of meninges or neural tissue
- faecal and urinary incontinence—neurogenic bladder can lead to recurrent urinary sepsis
- sensory loss predisposes to development of pressure sores
- motor loss—weakness and spasticity can lead to scoliosis, hip dislocation, lower limb contractures, foot deformities
- future walking ability depends on level of lesion. Thoracic and high lumbar lesions never walk, mid lumbar may do initially but as the child gets older many revert to chair use, low lumbar lesions are usually functional walkers
- neurosurgical problems—Chiari II malformation, syrinx formation and hydrocephalus, tethered cord
- psychological problems—mild mental retardation, depression.

Investigations (postnatal)
- MRI to image spinal cord
- Plain radiographs to assess for scoliosis and hip dysplasia/dislocation
- CT to assess hydrocephalus.

Management
- Neurosurgical closure of open defect within first 48h to minimize risk of infection
- Insertion of shunt for management of hydrocephalus
- Subsequent multidisciplinary input including physiotherapists, paediatricians, neurosurgeons, urologists
- Orthopaedic input—aim to improve/preserve function—reduce deformity, release contractures and balance muscle forces.

Prevention
Current recommendations are 400µg folic acid daily 1 month preconception and for first trimester. Increased to 5mg daily if maternal or family history of spina bifida.

Kyphosis in adults

Definition Kyphosis is excessive curvature of the spine in the sagittal plane. With normal sagittal balance, a plumb line from C7 should fall through S1, allowing wide variation in cervical and lumbar lordosis and thoracic kyphosis to achieve balance. Normal range for thoracic kyphosis is 10–40° and for lumbar lordosis is 30–80°, varying with age and gender.

Epidemiology The incidence of kyphosis varies according to the underlying pathology—occurs in 15% of Caucasian females with osteoporosis ('dowager's hump') and 5% of patients with spinal TB.

Risk factors These include family history of kyphosis, OP, spinal fracture, infection and malignancy.

Aetiology

- Congenital
- Developmental: Scheuermann's disease, developmental roundback and spondylolisthesis
- Acquired: inflammatory (AS), metabolic (OP), chondrodystrophic, neoplastic, post-traumatic and iatrogenic (postlaminectomy, postinstrumentation).

Clinical

Kyphotic deformities presenting in adults may develop from disorders of childhood. History must include family history of kyphosis, progression of the deformity and other congenital abnormalities. It is important to ask about constitutional symptoms, e.g. weight loss, fevers and night sweats, as well as neurological symptoms. Previous medical history must include medication (steroids) and history of trauma or previous surgery. Examine with the patient standing in a neutral position and bending forward. Assess coronal and sagittal alignment with range of movements of the spine and other joints. The flexibility of the kyphosis can be assessed in the erect patient by extension and with the patient lying down by prone hyperextension. Complete neurological examination is necessary.

Investigations Aimed at establishing the aetiology and evaluating the alignment of the spine to allow planning for surgery.

Radiology:

- Plain radiographs—AP and lateral views of the whole spine including the pelvis (pelvic parameters influence the thoracic and lumbar alignment). The patient must be standing with knees fully extended
- CT scan—helpful in defining bony structures
- MRI scan—shows soft tissues and neural elements and their relationships to bony structures.

Management All patients without significant neurological deficit should be managed non-operatively. Surgery is indicated when non-operative measures fail, or the patient develops intractable pain, worsening kyphosis or deteriorating neurology.

Non-operative treatment—analgesia, NSAIDs, physical therapy and regular exercise. Bracing is not normally effective.

Operative options—anterior or posterior procedures, or a combination of these. Segmental vertebral fixation improves chances of successful correction. To correct the deformity a number of osteotomies may be needed—multiple facet osteotomies, closing wedge osteotomy, pedicle subtraction osteotomy or vertebral column resection. Complications include excessive bleeding, infection, nerve root injury, paralysis, failure of fixation, persistent pain, and cardiac and respiratory complications. Large deformities, especially those with short, sharp angular malalignments, are particularly hazardous.

Ankylosing spondylitis (📖 see p. 184)
Clinical
AS involves the spine, SIJs and to a lesser extent, the peripheral joints. In the spine, there is loss of lumbar lordosis with limited back motion and hip flexion contractures. Patients may have fixed cervical, thoracic or lumbar hyperkyphosis, and this may cause marked functional limitations due to inability to face forward. Patients develop a posture described as the question mark posture. They may have diminished chest expansion.

Patients with AS have a higher incidence of spinal fracture with minimal trauma. These fractures are associated with a significant risk of spinal cord injury and permanent neurologic deficit.

Investigations
Radiology: symmetric, bilateral subchondral erosions of the SIJs and subchondral sclerosis, first on the iliac side, then on both sides of these joints. The disease affects the lumbar spine first then the thoracic spine. Vertebrae appear squared off on the lateral radiographs. Longitudinal ligaments and annulus ossify, creating marginal syndesmophytes and a so-called 'bamboo spine' appearance from the sacrum to the occiput. Facet joints are also obliterated.

Management
The aim is to balance the head over the sacrum successfully. The kyphotic spine may be corrected by osteotomies and fusion. The surgery usually involves an extension osteotomy and fusion of the spine with instrumentation. Complications of osteotomies include non-union, loss of correction, and neurological and vascular (aortic) injury.

Post-traumatic kyphosis
Kyphosis following burst fractures is common, especially following thoracolumbar burst fractures. Surgery to stabilize and correct these deformities is associated with high complication rates. Kyphosis from osteoporotic fractures is also common and is usually treated non-operatively.

Scoliosis in adults

Definition
Abnormal curvature of the spine in the coronal plane of >10° (Fig. 8.5).

Epidemiology
Incidence of adult scoliosis is between 3 and 5%. The thoracic or lumbar region may be involved.

Aetiology
The most common causes in adults are:
- Progressive congenital, idiopathic or neuromuscular curves
- Degenerative disease, often with OP
- Post-traumatic changes
- Postoperative changes.

Risk factors for progression
These include:
- Adolescent curves that are 50–75° at maturity
- OP.

Clinical
Small curves are usually asymptomatic, but as the deformity increases pain or neurological problems may occur. Worsening pain and disability are common presenting symptoms in adults. Other symptoms are asymmetrical waistline, poorly fitting clothing and prominence of one side of the chest. With scoliosis there may be trunkal asymmetry, a rib hump, loss of spinal movements, shoulder or pelvic imbalance and signs of neurological deficits due to cord or nerve root compression.

Investigations
Radiology
Scoliosis views—AP and lateral views of whole spine and pelvis. These are used to establish the cause of the scoliosis, type of curve and effects of the deformity on pelvic balance. The size of the curve is measured by determining the Cobb angle.

Lateral bending views—AP views with bending to each side to determine flexibility. Used in surgical planning (levels of fusion).

CT scan—used to assess bony structures and spinal canal. It is better than an MRI scan in showing details of the vertebrae.

MRI scan—used to image the spinal column and neural elements. It is better than CT scan in assessing soft tissues.

Bone densitometry—depending on the age of the patient, bone densitometry may be necessary to check for osteopenia.

Management

In adults, the most important consideration in deciding on the type of treatment is the severity of the patient's symptoms, rather than the size of the deformity. Treatment options include:
- Expectant management (observation)
- Orthosis
- Surgery.

Non-operative treatment

Includes analgesics, NSAIDs, physical therapy and use of orthoses.

Operative options

Indications for surgery are intractable pain, progressive deformity and neurological compromise. Anterior, posterior and a combination of anterior and posterior instrumented fusions are used. Thoracoplasty can improve the cosmesis of thoracic curves. Complications of surgery include failure of instrumentation, pseudoarthrosis, infection, excessive bleeding, visceral, vascular and neurological injuries. Persistent pain or deformity above or below fusion levels are late complications.

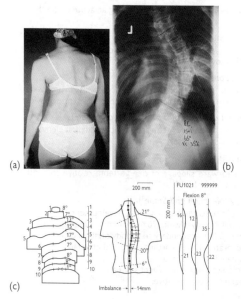

Fig. 8.5 (a) Patient with adolescent idiopathic scoliosis. (b) Radiograph of the patient. (c) Surface topography.

Reproduced from Bulstrode et al., Oxford Textbook of Orthopaedics and Trauma, with permission from Oxford University Press.

Spondylolysis and spondylolisthesis in adults

Spondylolysis
A fatigue fracture develops leading to a defect in the pars interarticularis region of the neural arch.

Epidemiology
More common in females than males. L5 level is the most common.

Risks factors
- Hereditary—AR, thin vertebral bone
- Overuse—hyperextension mechanism (gymnasts).

Clinical
Asymptomatic in most, low back pain and stiffness.

Investigations
Radiology—oblique views of the spine detect 95% of lesions (Scottie dog sign of La Chapelle).

Bone scan—increased uptake indicating an acute lesion that will probably heal.

Management
Rest from precipitating activity and analgesia. Lumbar brace and physiotherapy can be helpful.

Complications
Non-union, progression to spondylolisthesis (from widening of the fracture gap) and nerve compression secondary to spondylolisthesis.

Differential diagnosis of back pain in young adults
Scheuermann's disease, neoplasm, infection, neural elements, retroperitoneum and disc prolapse.

Spondylolisthesis
There is forward slippage of one vertebra relative to another. It usually occurs at L4/5 or L5/S1.

Aetiology (Newman and Stone[1])
Spondylolisthesis can be congenital, developmental or acquired:
- Congenital or dysplastic (20%)—often marked slippage
- Isthmic (50%)—secondary to spondylolysis (fatigue fracture)
- Degenerative (25%)—arthritis of the lumbar facet joints
- Trauma—bilateral fractures
- Pathological—tumours, Paget's disease
- Iatrogenic—postoperative.

Clinical
May be asymptomatic. Usually have insidious onset of low back pain and muscle spasm in the 2nd to 3rd decade. Flattening of the back with a spinous process step-off on palpation. Symptoms of claudication (leg pain and weakness) may signal lateral recess stenosis.

Investigation: radiology

- Confirmed with standing lateral X-ray and oblique X-rays
- CT scan provides detail of bony anatomy and is used in surgical planning.

Classification

Myerding classification: percentage of slip of the AP diameter of the vertebrae:

Grade	I	II	III	IV	V
% slip	<25	25–50	50–75	75–100	>100

Spondyloptosis—slippage >100%.

Slip angle (Boxall et al.[2]): the degree of tilting forward of the L5 body on the sacrum. Good correlation with clinical deformity and rate of progression. On a lateral X-ray the angle is normally >0°.

Risk factors for slip progression:

Young age at presentation, female, slip angle >10°, high-grade slip, dome-shaped sacrum and inclined sacrum (>30° beyond vertical).

Management

Non-operative treatment:—reduce sports and other high impact activities, brace and arrange physiotherapy. Serial X-rays are used to monitor the deformity.

Operative options—surgery is indicated if the slip is >50%, tilt angle >30° or if there is progression, failure of non-operative treatment, or development of significant neurology.

Surgery: grade I or II—*in situ* fusion with decompression. Repair of the pars defects with lag screws for slips <25%. Grade III or IV—extended *in situ* fusion and decompression. Decompression without fusion can be considered for elderly degenerative spondylolisthesis. A failed posterior fusion may require anterior interbody fusion.

For further reading, see Sengupta and Herkowitz[3] and Beutler et al.[4].

References

1 Newman PH, Stone KH. The etiology of spondylolisthesis. *J Bone Joint Surg Br* 1963;**45**:39–59.
2 Boxall D, Bradford DS, Winter RB, et al. Management of severe spondylolisthesis in children and adolescents. *J Bone Joint Surg Am* 1979;**61**:479–95.
3 Sengupta DK, Herkowitz HN. Degenerative spondylolisthesis: review of current trends and controversies. *Spine* 2005;**6S**:S71–81.
4 Beutler WJ, Fredrickson BE, Murtland A, et al. The natural history of spondylolysis and spondylolisthesis: 45-year follow-up evaluation. *Spine* 2003;**28**:1027–35.

Infections of the spine: pyogenic infections and tuberculosis

Pyogenic infections
Pyogenic infections of the vertebral body is relatively uncommon and frequently missed or diagnosed late. Requires a high index of suspicion.

Site
Lumbar spine is most common. Thoracic and cervical infections have a higher incidence of paralysis.

Risk factors
Elderly, IV drug abuse, infection elsewhere, bacterial endocarditis, immunocompromised, and use of steroids.

Spread
Haematogenous (Batson's complex—posturological procedures). The infection leads to thrombosis, infarction and abscess formation.

Organisms
Staphylococcal aureus is the most common, others include β-haemolytic streptococcus, Gram-negative organisms, *Salmonella* (in SCD), *Pasteurella*, TB and fungal infections.

Complications
Paravertebral and/or epidural abscess, vertebral collapse and neurological sequelae.

Clinical
Onset of symptoms is often insidious. Back pain (night) is the most common presentation. Look for the triad: fever, back pain and tenderness. Up to 40% incidence of neurological compromise in patients with spinal disease.

Differential diagnosis
Tumours (disc destruction is atypical) and degenerative spinal disease.

Investigations
Radiology: X-rays—may be normal for several weeks with progressive disc space narrowing, erosions, sclerosis, new bone formation and intervertebral fusion by 6–12 months.

MRI scan: early diagnosis as possible and the modality is sensitive and specific.

Blood tests: FBC ESR, CRP, blood cultures, antistreptolysin O titre and tuberculin test.

Others: urine culture and sensitivity and technetium bone scan (high sensitivity after 48h).

Management
Identify organism (blood, urine, biopsy).

Non-operative treatment: IV antibiotics (microbiology advice)—at least 2 weeks with oral for 3 months. Use ESR to follow disease. Favourable course expected in patients <60yrs with normal immune status and decreasing ESR.

Operative options: Need open biopsy to find the causative organism. Surgery indicated with worsening neurology, spinal instability, abscess formation and failure of medical treatment. The aim of surgery is to debride, decompress and stabilize the spine.

Approaches

- Anterior approach—good exposure for abscess drainage, especially psoas—decompression and fusion
- Posterior approach—to drain epidural or disc space infections and if long instrumented fusion is necessary.

Tuberculosis

Spine involved in 50% of patients with bone and joint TB. Commonly in children and young adults. Usually involves two adjacent vertebrae.

Pathology

There is osteolytic infarction with pus formation and collection of necrotic debris. Erosion of bone and intervertebral disc leads to collapse and instability. TB spondylitis may occur by haematogenous spread or secondary to direct extension from infected viscera.

Clinical

Patients present with insidious onset of back pain with fever, night chills, weight loss and loss of appetite. Neurological symptoms may develop. In advanced disease there may be a spinal deformity (gibbous deformity).

Investigations

Microbiology—blood, sputum cultures and tissue samples are obtained—needle or open (detection of acid-fast bacilli on Ziehl–Nielson staining).

Radiology—spine X-rays demonstrate disc space narrowing, vertebral collapse, spondylolisthesis; soft tissue thickening may be found. MRI can show extent of infection and compression of spinal cord or nerve roots.

Management

Chemotherapy. The spine may need to be debrided of necrotic tissue and stabilized. Anterior, posterior and combined approaches to the spine are used depending on the extent of the infection, compression of the neural elements and stability of the spine.

Complications include

- Abscess tracking (cervical—retrophalangeal abscess, thoracic—pleural cavity, lumbar—femoral triangle)
- Formation of mycotic aortic aneurysm
- Respiratory or renal problems with disseminated disease.

Infections of the spine: discitis

Non-specific inflammation of the intervertebral disc and endplates in the skeletally immature. Lower thoracic/lumbar.

Presentation

Generalized malaise, history of upper respiratory tract infection, backache, stiffness, postural abnormality, fever, reduced mobility, abdominal pain.

Aetiology

May be unclear, includes—trauma, apophysitis, infection.

Diagnosis

History, inflammatory markers, urine/blood cultures, X-ray—disc space narrowing, endplate erosions. Increased uptake on bone scan. MRI is the gold standard. Disc aspiration.

Treatment

Rest, spinal brace, IV antibiotics if toxic signs.

Spontaneous interbody fusion is rare. In most, gradual restoration of disc height occurs.

For further reading, see Weinberg and Silber[1], Hsieh et al.[2] and Quinones-Hinojosa et al.[3].

References

1 Weinberg J, Silber JS. Infections of the spine: what the orthopaedist needs to know. *Clin Neurosurg* 1978;**25**:296–304.
2 Hsieh PC, Wienecke RJ, O'Shaughnessy BA, *et al.* Surgical strategies for vertebral osteomyelitis and epidural abscess. *Neurosurg Focus* 2004;**17**:E4.
3 Quinones-Hinojosa A, Jun P, Jacobs R, *et al.* General principles in the medical and surgical management of spinal infections: a multidisciplinary approach. *Neurosurg Focus* 2004;**17**:E1.

Disc lesions: overview and herniated disc

Anatomy

Intervertebral discs—make up a quarter of the spinal column's length. There are no discs between C1 and 2 and within the coccyx. They are avascular and rely on diffusion across the endplates for nutrition. Discs are fibrocartilaginous structures serving as shock-absorbing system to protect the spine. The movement at each disc is very small. They allow extension, flexion and limited rotation.

Intervertebral discs are composed of an outer annulus fibrosus (AF) which is a strong radial-like structure made up of type II collagen orientated at various angles. It contains water and a proteoglycan (PG) matrix containing chondrocytes. The nucleus pulposus (NP) contains more water and PGs in a hydrated gel-like matrix that resists compression. Vascular and neural elements are found only within the outer layer of the AF.

Pathology

Age-related changes occur within the disc. PG synthesis falls and less water is retained. Collagen levels increase. The discs become stiffer and the AF transmits more load.

The discs are able to withstand large forces (10 000N). With excessive loads, the first structure to fail is normally the bony vertebral endplate.

Herniated disc

Aetiology

The cause of disc herniation is related primarily to normal degenerative processes that occur with ageing. Endplate fractures cause disruption of the nuclear homeostasis and trigger autoimmune processes. Repetitive stresses across the discs may accelerate the process. Disc degradation leads to the resorption or herniation.

(a) Thoracic disc

Epidemiology

Thoracic disc herniation is rare, occurring in only 0.5% of all prolapsed discs. Peak in the 4th decade. Approximately 75% occur below T8 and largely at the T11/T12 level. They present with thoracic back pain and there may be upper motor neuron signs involving the lower limbs. Thoracic disc herniation may produce chest, abdominal or even groin pain, mimicking cardiac, GI or urogenital problems.

Investigations

Diagnosis is confirmed with an MRI scan.

Management

Treatment is non-operative—rest and use of NSAIDs and physiotherapy. If pain persists despite non-operative treatment surgery may be indicated. Costotransversectomy or transthoracic approach is used to minimize cord compression, and a fusion may be added.

(b) Lumbar disc

Clinical

Patients present with radiating lower limb pain (radiculopathy). The distribution of the pain is related to the level and position of disc prolapse as this determines which nerve root is involved. Most disc prolapses that result in compression of neural elements occur in the posterolateral position. Far lateral disc prolapses comprise 6–10% of disc prolapses.

Epidemiology

Lumbar disc prolapse occurs commonly in patients 30–50yrs old. The lumbar spine is the spine region most commonly affected, and L4, L5 disc that which herniates most often, followed by the L5, S1 disc.

Lumbar disc herniations are a major cause of acute and chronic back and lower limb symptoms.

Classifications

By morphology:
- Protruded—localized bulge with annulus and posterior longitudinal ligament (PLL) intact
- Extruded—protrudes through the annulus but is in continuity with the disc space
- Sequestrated—protrudes through the annulus and there is a free fragment of disc in the epidural space.

By location:
- Central—often associated with back pain only
- Posterolateral—most common. Usually affects the ipsilateral nerve root of the lower lumbar vertebrae
- Far lateral—usually affects the ipsilateral nerve root of the upper lumbar vertebrae.

A thorough history should include the onset, nature and course of the pain, changes in bladder or bowel function, previous medical history, history of trauma, risk factors and constitutional symptoms. The neurological examination for patients with suspected nerve root compression should include a careful assessment of motor and sensory functions, and nerve root tension signs must be elicited if present.

Disc lesions: disc prolapse and discogenic pain

Disc prolapses and nerve roots affected:

- L2/3 posterolateral—L3 nerve root; L2/3 far lateral—L2 nerve root
- L3/4 posterolateral—L4 nerve root; L3/4 far lateral—L3 nerve root
- L4/5 posterolateral—L5 nerve root; L4/5 far lateral—L4 nerve root

The patient's gait must be assessed and back examined to assess function and exclude other pathologies.

'Rules of Three' (Apley):

- Three guidelines. (i) Young and very old seldom have acute disc prolapse. (ii) Look for infection, benign tumours and spondylolisthesis in adolescents. (iii) Look for vertebral compression fracture and malignancy in the elderly
- Three warnings. (i) Sciatica is referred pain which can also come from facet joints, SIJs or infection. (ii) Disc prolapse at most occurs at two levels; with multiple levels suspect a neurological cause. (iii) In severe, unrelenting pain, suspect tumour or infection
- Three major disorders to exclude. (i) Infection and inflammatory. (ii) Vertebral tumours. (iii) Nerve tumours.

Natural history

About 90% of patients improve in 6 weeks.

Investigation

MRI is the investigation of choice.

Management

Non-operative treatment—the majority can be treated with modification of activities, a short period of rest, analgesics and NSAIDs, physiotherapy. Epidural or nerve root injections are used.

Operative options—surgery is indicated for unrelenting leg pain, motor deficits or cauda equina syndrome. Surgical approaches include posterior midline or paramedial approaches. A large central disc may compress the cauda equina causing loss of perianal sensation, saddle anaesthesia, bilateral LMN signs in the legs, sphincteric disturbance with inability to sense bladder filling, painless retention or urinary incontinence, loss of anal tone and faecal incontinence. This is a surgical emergency requiring an emergency MRI and spinal decompression within 24h of onset of symptoms.

Discogenic pain

Discogenic pain can defined as back pain without a radicular component with no evidence of neural compression or segmental instability.

Aetiology

Discs have sensory nerve endings in the outer third of the annulus. Pressure within the disc can produce back pain by stimulating nocioceptors in the PLL.

Clinical

The diagnosis is one of exclusions. Patients usually have a long history of back pain, often with radiation to buttocks and posterior thighs. There is usually significant paravertebral spasm. There are no focal neurological signs.

Investigations

Radiology—plain X-rays are normal or show degenerative changes. MRI scan is used to establish there is degenerative disc disease—loss of signal on T2-weighted images, annular tears, loss of disc height and associated endplate changes.

Discography—altered disc architecture and a positive provocative test (pain reproduced with injection of contrast under pressure) constitute a positive response. A positive test should also include a normal level as a reference.

Causes

Infection (discitis), torsional injury (circumferential tear of the annulus) and internal disc disruption.

Classification

- Grade 0: no disruption
- Grade 1: disruption to inner third
- Grade 2: middle third
- Grade 3: outer third.

Management

Non-operative treatment—physiotherapy and epidural injection of local anaesthetic and steroid.

Operative options—fusion (anterior or posterior) usually with instrumentation or disc replacement for persistent, severe pain.

For further reading see Guyer and Ohnmeiss[1] and Thompson et al.[2].

References

1 Guyer RD, Ohnmeiss DD. Intervertebral disc prostheses. *Spine* 2003;**15**:15–23.

2 Thompson RE, Pearcy MJ, Downing KJ, et al. Disc lesions and the mechanics of the intervertebral joint complex. *Spine* 2000;**23**:3026–30.

Spinal stenosis

Epidemiology
The incidence is 2–8%. Symptoms usually develop in the 5th and 6th decades.

Pathology
Disc dehydration leads to loss of disc height and this increases loading of the facets. The facets hypertrophy and this, together with a bulging annulus and thickening of ligamentum flavum, lead to stenosis. Spinal stenosis is narrowing of the spinal canal or neural foramina producing root ischaemia and neurogenic claudication.

Types of stenosis
- Central—causes: medial encroachment, congenitally narrow canal ('trefoil' shape), spondylolisthesis; central disc herniation and trauma or surgery
- Lateral—causes: compression of the nerve root by lateral disc herniation, thickening of the ligamentum flavum and hypertrophy of the superior articular process. Lateral recess stenosis often affects the traversing nerve root
- Foraminal—causes: loss of disc height, disc herniation and osteophyte formation. The exiting nerve root compressed in foramen.

Clinical
Patients, who are usually ≥60yrs of age, present with unilateral or bilateral leg pain with or without back pain on walking upright (increases the spinal stenosis). It is often preceded by longstanding low back pain. The walking distance that precipitates the pain is unpredictable and is relieved by sitting or leaning forwards (leaning on a shopping trolley). Phalen provocation test—leg pain brought on by extension of the spine.

It is important to differentiate between neurogenic and vascular claudication. Neurogenic claudication (spinal stenosis) causes pain, tightness and numbness and subjective weakness in the lower limbs.

Table 8.2 A comparison of vascular and neurogenic claudication

	Vascular	Neurogenic
Walking distance to onset of pain	Constant	Variable
Pain	Calf	Prox–mid thigh
Relieved	Standing	Sitting, bending
Lying flat	Relieves	May worsen
Uphill walking	Symptoms soon	Symptoms late

On examination there is often loss of lumbar lordosis, decreased lumbar movements and occasionally there may be nerve root tension signs or evidence of a motor or sensory deficit.

Natural history

Symptoms remain unchanged in 60–70%, worse in 15–20% and improve in 15–20% of patients.

Investigation: radiology

- X-rays: degenerative changes are seen but poorly defined
- CT scan: look for lateral and central stenosis. Cross-sectional dural area of <100mm^2 denotes stenosis. Dural sac with anteroposterior diameter of <10mm consistent with lumbar stenosis.
- MRI: gold standard. Allows visualization of the vertebral discs, neural elements, ligamentum flavum and thecal sac.

Management

Patient selection is the key to successful treatment.

Non-operative treatment—analgesia, physiotherapy, epidural or nerve root injections, flexion brace, treatment in the setting of a rehabilitation programme or pain clinic.

Operative options—indications: cauda equina compression, progressive or severe neurological deficit, intractable back or leg pain, failed non-operative treatment and worsening deformity. Procedures include posterior approach with laminotomy or laminectomy and decompression of the nerve roots. Resection of a facet joint is sometimes necessary to ensure nerve root decompression.

Fusion with autogenous or synthetic bone added to decompression if spinal instability or spondylolisthesis demonstrated.

Problems with surgery—selecting the correct level (pre- and intra-operative), persistent pain (insufficient decompression, preoperative neuropraxia), recurrent pain (scar tissue), postoperative instability, non-union of fusion, degenerative changes can develop at other levels.

For further reading, see Pratt et al.[1], Jolles et al.[2] and Amundsen et al.[3].

References

1 Pratt RK, Fairbank JC, Virr A. The reliability of the shuttle walking test, the Swiss spinal stenosis questionnaire, the Oxford spinal stenosis score and the Oswestry disability index in the assessment of patients with lumbar spinal stenosis. Spine 2002;**27**:84–91.

2 Jolles BM, Porchet F, Theumann N. Surgical treatment of lumbar spinal stenosis: five year follow up. J Bone Joint Surg Br 2001;**83**:949–53.

3 Amunsden T, Weber H, Nordal H, et al. Lumbar spinal stenosis: conservative or surgical management? A prospective 10 year study. Spine 2000;**25**:1424–36.

Coccydynia

The coccyx is the most inferior part of the axial skeleton and represents a vestigial tail consisting of four or more bones fused together. It articulates with the sacrum through a vestigial disc and ligaments.

Epidemiology

More common in females—coccyx rotated and facing backwards which makes it more susceptible to trauma. The female broader pelvis places sitting pressure on the coccyx in addition to the ischial tuberosities.

Pathology

It is not clearly understood where the pain arises but it probably arises from the ligaments or the disc. A soft tissue or bone tumour is rarely the cause of this pain.

Aetiology

Local trauma and childbirth (baby's head rides over the coccyx) are the most common causes. Tumours, especially those involving the sacrum, can mimic coccydynia.

Clinical

Pressure on the coccyx aggravates the pain. History is aimed at identifying potential causes. Examination should include pelvic and rectal palpation to feel for a mass or tumour and local tenderness. Coccygeal tenderness is strongly suggestive of coccydynia. If negative look for referred causes of pain (disc herniation or degenerative disc disease).

Investigations: radiology

- Radiographs of the sacrum and coccyx—to rule out a fracture or a large tumour
- MRI scan to look for infection or tumour
- Bone scan and CT add little.

In most patients with coccydynia all investigations are negative.

Management

Non-operative treatment—analgesia, NSAIDs. A doughnut-shaped pillow may ease pressure on the coccyx. The patient must understand that improvement is often not rapid. If no improvement a local anaesthetic injection in and around the sacrococcygeal joint may be helpful. Manipulations and stretching of the ligaments can be tried for persisting pain. Physiotherapy may be helpful. If pain persists, significant pathology (sacral or pelvic tumour, infection) needs to be excluded.

Operative options—surgical indications include failure of conservative treatment or diagnosis of a tumour. Coccygectomy is rarely performed. A small incision directly over the coccyx, periosteum is elevated and soft tissues mobilized from the distal sacrum. The coccyx is then excised. The patient may have discomfort for some time and recovery may take up to

12 months. Outcome is dependent on patient selection. Complications occur if the plane of dissection is not strictly subperiosteal, the rectum is at risk. Rectal perforation may lead to a serious infection, and a diverting colostomy may be required. Wound healing and superficial infection occurs. The most common postoperative problem is ongoing or worsening coccygeal pain.

For further reading, see Wray et al.[1] and Wray and Templeton[2].

References

1 Wray C, Easom S, Hoskinson J. Coccydynia. Aetiology and treatment. *J Bone Joint Surg Br* 1991;**73**:335–8.

2 Wray A, Templeton J. Coccygectomy. A review of thirty-seven cases. *Ulster Med J* 1982;**51**:121–4.

Thoracic outlet syndrome

Thoracic outlet syndrome is a condition that causes chronic neck, shoulder and arm pain. Neurological and/or vascular symptoms and/or signs may develop in the upper limbs during certain activities or in certain provocative positions of the head or upper limb.

Aetiology

- The brachial plexus runs between scalenus anterior and scalenus medius along with the subclavian artery. The subclavian vein runs in front of scalenus anterior
- Any abnormality in this region, classically a cervical rib, may cause compression of neurovascular structures in certain arm positions. Other causes include fibromuscular bands or muscle hypertrophy
- Less common causes include an aneurysm of the subclavian artery and repeated trauma.

Differential diagnoses

Thoracic outlet syndrome must be differentiated from cervical spine disease, in particular a cervical radiculopathy. Other causes include:

- Musculoskeletal pain
- Subclavian vascular steal syndrome
- Peripheral nerve entrapment
- Raynaud's disease.

History

Patients usually present with pain, weakness and paraesthesia, and may have had investigations or even surgery for other diagnoses but have failed to respond to treatment.

Symptoms include:

- Vague upper limb pain not fitting a particular dermatome or peripheral nerve distribution
- Vascular phenomenon due to arterial spasm including colour changes
- Cramping sensation in muscles with certain activities
- One must ask about position of the neck and limbs when symptoms occur and a history of previous trauma to the clavicle or first rib.

Examination

- A full peripheral neurological and vascular examination is required in any atypical arm pain presentation
- Examine the cervical spine for evidence of nerve root compression
- Subclavian bruit
- Asymmetrical upper limb pulses
- Special tests aim to reproduce the provocative position. Arm abduction and neck rotation are typical positions used to provoke symptoms. With involvement of upper nerve roots (C5, C6 and C7) symptoms are reproduced by turning head to opposite side, tilting head and lifting and straining, whereas with lower nerve root involvement (C8, T1) elevating the arm, reaching and lifting reproduces symptoms.

Investigations

- These will be indicated by history and examination
- Plain radiographs of cervical spine. Look for cervical rib or elongated C7 transverse process
- MRI of cervical spine and posterior triangle of neck
- Angiography
- Electrophysiological studies can exclude a more peripheral cause of symptoms or cervical root problem
- Infiltration of the anterior or middle scalene muscle with local anaesthetic can be used as a confirmatory test.

Management

- Non-operative measures such as postural and muscle strengthening exercises may control or alleviate symptoms. If related to muscle hypertrophy (e.g. body builders), resting the muscles involved may ease symptoms
- Persistent symptoms may be treated surgically. Operations that may be required include:
  - Cervical rib excision
  - Repair of subclavian aneurysm
  - Fibrous band/muscle release
  - With a transaxillary approach for first rib resection 80–90% of patients report a satisfactory result. Despite surgical intervention, symptoms recur in 15–20% of patents and usually in those who have involvement of the upper cervical nerve roots.

For further reading, see Parziale et al.[1] and Edwards et al.[2]

References

1 Parziale JR, Akelman E, Weiss AP. Thoracic outlet syndrome. *Am J Orthop* 2000;**29**:353–60.
2 Edwards DP, Mulkern E, Raja AN. Trans-axillary first rib excision for thoracic outlet syndrome. *J R Coll Surg Edinb* 1999;**44**:362–5.

Osteoarthritis of the upper limb: shoulder and elbow

Primary OA of the upper limb is not as common as in the lower limb.

When OA of the upper limb is present there may be an underlying cause such as trauma, crystal arthropathy or abnormal joint biomechanics.

Epidemiology

Older patients and more common in males.

Shoulder girdle

Sites: OA may affect the GHJ or, more commonly, the ACJ. Acromioclavicular arthritis may be painful directly or may cause irritation of the underlying rotator cuff muscles and present with impingement (see ▭ p. 284). Glenohumeral OA may follow rotator cuff tear where the centralizing effect of the cuff muscles is lost. This is termed 'cuff arthropathy'.

Acromioclavicular joint

Clinical: patients with joint arthritis have pain and tenderness localized to the ACJ. Pain aggravated by adduction. It often develops after trauma (distal clavicle fractures, ACJ dislocations).

Investigations:
• Radiographs—degenerative changes of the ACJ
• Local anaesthetic—injection of lignocaine into the joint can be used to confirm diagnosis.

Management:
Non-operative treatment—most patients with ACJ arthritis respond to non-operative treatment: modification of activities, NSAIDs and corticosteroid injections.

Operative options—resection of 1.5–2.0cm of distal clavicle, either as an open procedure or arthroscopically.

Glenohumeral joint

Clinical

Glenohumeral OA pain is felt deep within the shoulder and lateral aspect of the arm. Stiffness may be confused with a frozen shoulder. Osteophytes may act as blocks to range of motion. Characteristics on examination include the sensation of crepitus with movements and pain throughout the range of movement.

Investigations

Diagnostic injections of local anaesthetic into suspected sites. Radiographs show the typical features of OA (see ▭ p. 193) and may show a high riding humeral head suggesting dysfunction of the rotator cuff muscles. (see ▭ p. 284).

Management

Non-operative treatment—includes analgesia and anti-inflammatory medications. Physiotherapy and hydrotherapy can be beneficial in retaining range of movement (ROM) and strength.

Operative options—surgical options are limited but arthroplasty has good results and the, often large, osteophytes can be removed. Options include resurfacing arthroplasty or stemmed designs which can be cemented or uncemented. The decision to replace the glenoid surface depends on the distribution of the disease, remaining bone stock and expertise of the surgeon. Pain relief and function are improved with total joint arthroplasty in some series, but loosening of the glenoid component is common and problematic.

Elbow

Clinical

Pain around the elbow may be a presenting feature, but often the patient notices the elbow stiffness and loss of full extension. Symptoms suggestive of ulnar neuropathy at the elbow may be present if there is a pronounced flexion contracture or osteophytes around the elbow. Loose bodies may cause intermittent locking of the joint. Extension may be blocked by osteophytes in the olecranon fossa and anterior capsule contractions. Further passive extension causes pain due to impingement. Flexion can also be blocked by anterior osteophytes at the tip of the coranoid process or fossa. Pronation and supination may be affected by radiocapitellar involvement.

Investigations

Plain radiographs are usually sufficient to demonstrate the arthritis and any bony loose bodies, though occasionally high definition CT may be helpful.

Management:

Non-operative treatment—similar to those used in the shoulder joint.

Operative options
- Ulnar neuropathy in the presence of a flexion deformity may benefit from anterior transposition of the ulnar nerve
- Symptomatic loose bodies can be excised by an open procedure or arthroscopically. In the olecranon fossa this can be performed directly from the back. Anterior loose bodies can be removed arthroscopically or through a window made in the base of the olecranon fossa from posteriorly
- Joint replacement—may be indicated in selected patients for relief of pain. Long-term results are not excellent and longevity is reduced in all but low activity individuals. Results are not as good as when performed for RA.

Osteoarthritis of the upper limb: wrist and hand

Wrist

Clinical OA of the wrist usually follows trauma, e.g. scaphoid fracture non-union or osteonecrosis, scapholunate ligament disruption, other instability pattern or Kienbock's disease of the lunate. Pain and stiffness are usual complaints. In manual workers this may interfere with tasks and threaten employment. Grip strength is reduced. Pronation and supination may be preserved if the distal radioulnar joint (DRUJ) is preserved, but other movements are reduced.

Investigations radiographs show arthritic changes which may initially be localized to one articulation.

Management *Non-operative treatment*—depends on precise location of degenerative change and the demands of the patient. Splintage is therapeutic in some cases and simulates wrist fusion if this is considered an option.

Operative options:
- Fusion—partial fusions retain some movement but complete transcarpal fusion has a more predictable outcome. The position is chosen after a careful assessment of the patient's needs
- Radial styloidectomy
- Proximal row carpectomy
- Wrist denervation.

Hand

Clinical Most commonly affected joints of the hand are the DIPJs of the fingers and carpometacarpal joint (CMCJ) of the thumb. The IPJs of the fingers may be involved, presenting with pain, deformity (osteophytes of the called Heberden's nodes) or mucous cysts (a ganglion-like cyst arising from a degenerate joint). The first ray CMCJ and trapezial articulations may be arthritic.

Investigations Radiographs of the hand—AP and lateral views.

Management
Non-operative treatment—splintage and hand therapy may be beneficial.

Operative options—surgical treatment options for interphalangeal OA include debridement, arthroplasty and arthrodesis. For OA involving the trapeziometacarpal joint, arthroplasty (excision, interposition or replacement) may be indicated for advanced disease. Fusion is an option for young patients with high demands.

Rheumatoid arthritis of the upper limb

The most visible effects of rheumatoid disease can be seen in the upper limb, especially in the hands. Arthritis of the lower limbs may increase demands on the upper limbs during mobilization, and this should be taken into consideration when deciding on management.

Upper limb functions

- ADL—feeding, washing and dressing
- Communication
- Mobility—sticks and wheelchairs
- Sensory organs—through touch.

Clinical

Patients with RA involving the upper limbs present with pain, loss of function and deformity. In addition to the disease, patients can present with problems related to treatment, e.g. steroid use resulting in osteonecrosis. Thorough assessment of the cervical spine must be performed to rule out instability or compression of neural structures. As patients with RA have numerous problems it is important to take a history focused on the currently most disabling ones. However, it is important to consider joint involvement in the context of local and syndrome problems and overall goals and treatment plans. To achieve this, each patient should have a team looking after them that includes a rheumatologist, surgeon, physiotherapist and occupational hand therapist.

Presenting symptoms are:

- **Pain:** multiple possible sources including cervical spine, joints, nerve entrapment and soft tissue problems
- **Deformity:** sudden onset may indicate tendon ruptures. A swelling may be due to synovitis, rheumatoid nodules or prominence of bones due to joint subluxations
- **Loss of function:** the summation of the deformities, pain, stiffness and neurological impairments result in progressive disability
- **Previous treatments:** medical, surgical and therapist modalities. Modification of home and use of modified utensils.

Investigations Haematological and biochemical investigations to monitor the disease. Radiology—includes plain radiographs, CT scan, MRI scan and US.

Management

Non-operative treatment—May include NSAIDs, immunosuppressive agents, disease-modifying agents and corticosteroids. Physiotherapy and occupational therapy to maintain movements. Splintage can be helpful.

Operative options—Surgical treatment options can be classified as preventative (synovectomy), corrective (tendon transfers, soft tissue reconstruction, synovectomy, nerve decompression) and salvage (total joint arthroplasty and arthrodesis).

Rheumatoid arthritis of the upper limb: clinical problems

Shoulder

Clinical

Patients are younger and tend to be female. They typically have multiple joint involvement, synovitis, joint erosion and rotator cuff dysfunction. Marked muscle atrophy may be present. High incidence of rotator cuff abnormalities.

Management

Non-operative treatment—medical management of systemic disease. Analgesia and physiotherapy.

Operative options—number of surgical options related to joint or rotator cuff. Aim is to provide pain-free movements.

Elbow

Clinical

Some patients develop stiff elbows (decreased range of movement) whilst others become very mobile (unstable). Function may be very good despite dramatic appearances on radiographs. Examination must include assessment of soft tissues around the joint and radial and ulnar nerves.

Management

Non-operative treatment—may include NSAIDs, immunosuppressive agents, remitive agents and corticosteroids. Physiotherapy and occupational therapy to maintain movements. Splintage can be helpful.

Operative options—surgery indicated for intractable pain and progressive deformity. Surgical options include synovectomy (contraindicated in severe instability and stiffness), capsular release, radial head excision and arthroplasty (interposition or replacement).

Wrist

Clinical

The effects of the disease on the joint and volar ligaments result in dissociation of the DRUJ and distal subluxation of the ulnar head. Reduction of this may be painful ('piano key' sign). The radiocarpal joint becomes eroded and subluxes volarly and ulnar wards, and rotates into radial deviation.

Management

Non-operative treatment—medication and physiotherapy.

Operative options—distal radioulnar resection at the distal ulna (Darrach procedure), hemiresection interposition technique or fusion of the DRUJ and creation of pseudarthrosis in distal ulna (Sauve–Kapandji procedure). Radiocarpal reconstruction: tendon transfers, partial or total wrist arthrodesis or wrist arthroplasty.

Hand

Clinical problems that develop include:

- MCPJ subluxation occurs due to synovitis destroying the capsule and the abnormal pull of tendons
- Swan neck deformities (hyperextension of the PIPJ and flexion of the DIPJ) occurs due to laxity of volar structures at the PIPJ (volar plate, FDG) or dorsal structures at the DIPJ (mallet finger)
- Boutonnière deformity (flexion of PIPJ with hyperextension of DIPJ) occurs because of damage to the central slip over the PIPJ allowing subluxation of the lateral bands of the extensor mechanism which hyperextend the DIPJ
- The thumb can develop either swan neck or Boutonnière deformity or become unstable at the CMCJ or MCPJ.

Management

Non-operative treatment—medication to relieve/suppress inflammation. Physiotherapy and occupational hand therapy. Injection therapy and splinting is important.

Operative options—soft tissue reconstruction provided some cartilage is preserved (synovectomy, tendon transfers, tendon relocation, capsular reefing). Arthroplasty or arthrodesis used in more advanced disease.

Patients with RA that require joint reconstruction or salvage procedures should be treated in a specialized hand unit.

Tendons

Clinical

Tendon ruptures occur due to attrition over bony prominences or ischaemia in a fibro-osseous tunnel exacerbated by synovitis.

- Vaughan–Jackson syndrome—rupture of the ulnar digital extensor tendons over the DRUJ
- Mannerfelt lesion—rupture of the FPL tendon at the distal radius or scaphoid tubercle.

Nerves

Peripheral neuropathies are common.

Upper limb nerve entrapment 1

A peripheral nerve consists of the axons of sensory, motor and autonomic nerves supported by Schwann cells producing myelin sheaths and connective tissue with rich vascular supply. Various substances travel along the axons from the cell body in the dorsal root ganglion (sensory) or anterior horns of the spinal cord (motor). Anything disrupting this transport or the vascular supply of the nerve results in dysfunction.

Entrapment syndromes occur when compression of the nerve is present in one of the fibrous, muscular or osseous tunnels through which the nerve passes. The nerve may be surrounded by fibrosis.

Although most upper limb nerve entrapments are idiopathic, there are a number of conditions which can predispose to developing neuropathy or cause swelling in the tissues surrounding the nerve.
• Predisposing conditions to exclude—diabetes mellitus, alcoholism
• Causes of nerve compression—synovitis due to rheumatoid disease or other causes, pregnancy, myxoedema.

Treatment of these conditions usually relieves the compression, and symptoms associated with pregnancy usually resolve with childbirth.

The differential diagnosis includes viral neuritis and radiation neuritis.

Clinical

The presenting features of nerve root entrapment include:
• Pain—often poorly localized to the area of compression or the course of the nerve
• Paraesthesia—the exact site of 'pins-and-needles' can be crucial in the diagnosis as the distribution reflects the sensory innervation distal to the site of compression
• Numbness—decrease or loss of sensation in the innervated region. Can be quantified with threshold testing using filaments of various thickness
• Weakness of innervated motor units—a late sign or symptom as other motor units hypertrophy to compensate
• Others—swelling, soft tissue wasting (pulp of digits), altered temperature or hydration, stiffness, loss of dexterity.

Provocative tests—these are positive if they reproduce the symptoms with which the patient presents. Tapping over the nerve produces an electric shock-like pain in the distribution of that nerve, suggesting irritability. Compression of the nerve with digital pressure or a joint position which reduces the size of the fibro-osseous canal may also reproduce the symptoms.

Investigations

- Plain radiographs—with abnormal presentations may reveal bony protuberances which may compress the nerve
- MRI scans—may reveal fibrous bands causing compression
- Neurophysiology tests—may show slowing of the conduction across the region of compression (normal in upper limb is >50m/s) suggesting demyelination. Reduced amplitude implies loss of the total number of axons available (see 📖 p. 38). EMG may reveal denervation fibrillation potentials. Normal physiology tests do not exclude compression, and vice versa.

Management

Non-operative treatment—once the site of compression has been identified the entrapment can be addressed.

- Physiotherapy—aimed at stretching tight muscles or bands. Nerve gliding exercises are specific for particular nerves and may promote improved perfusion of the nerve
- Splintage—especially night splintage. Prevents patient adopting provocative postures such as wrist flexion compressing median nerve or elbow flexion compressing ulnar nerve. Splints may be off-the-shelf or custom moulded for the patient
- Steroid injection—around the nerve. Can reduce inflammation. Useful if there is evidence of synovitis.

Operative options

- Surgical decompression or transposition. Common syndromes usually respond to decompression at the site of compression. Less common syndromes may have multiple possible sites of compression and require more extensive decompression
- Surgery usually results in rapid relief of paraesthetic symptoms. Sensory and motor losses take longer to recover and may do so only incompletely. It is important to warn patients of this
- Longstanding motor deficits may not recover and tendon transfers may be required to restore function.

Upper limb nerve entrapment 2

Specific nerve entrapments can occur at almost any point along the course of a nerve, so it is vital to know the normal anatomy and common variants of the peripheral nervous system.

Median nerve

Proximal compression: may involve the whole nerve or just the AIN which has no cutaneous sensory distribution.

Anterior interosseous syndrome: testing the AIN involves getting the patient to form an 'O' with their index finger and thumb (the 'OK' sign) and pinch hard. Hyperextension of the IPJ of the thumb and DIPJ of the index finger occurs due to weakness of the FPL and FDP to the index finger. Pronator quadratus (PQ) is also supplied by the AIN and its strength can be assessed with resistance to pronation of the forearm with the elbow in flexion.

Treat non-operatively for 3 months and if symptoms do not resolve surgical exploration of the nerve is indicated.

Pronator syndrome: compression of the median nerve occurs where it passes between the two heads of the pronator muscle. Forearm pain is usually caused or worsened by resisted flexion of the elbow with the forearm pronated. The syndrome requires surgery if muscle weakness persists despite non-operative care. May need to explore area between heads of pronator muscle, lacertus fibrosis and arch of the FDS.

Other sites of compression
- Supracondylar, ligament of Struthers and proximal edge of the FDS
- Carpal tunnel syndrome (see 📖 p. 308).

Distal compression: ulnar nerve—cubital tunnel syndrome
The ulnar nerve is compressed between the two heads of the FCU muscle.

Clinical: patient complains of pain or paraesthesia in the ulnar one and a half digits on the palmar aspect of the hand but also more proximally including the dorsal ulnar border of the hand supplied by the dorsal branch of the ulnar nerve. Symptoms worse with elbow flexion. Patients may be woken from sleep with symptoms. Wasting of the intrinsic muscles of the hand (excluding those supplied by the median nerve) can be seen in the space between the metacarpals ('guttering') especially in the first web space. Froment's test examines this specifically and is positive if thumb adduction is replaced by flexion at the IPJ by FPL. Claw hand leads to hyperextension of the MCPJs and flexion of the PIPJs of the ulnar two digits due to the unopposed action of FDS and ED tendons.

Management: Prolonged elbow flexion should be avoided. If splintage and physiotherapy fail to relieve symptoms the nerve can be decompressed behind the epicondyle where it passes between the two heads of FCU. It can also be transposed to lie subcutaneously anterior to the epicondyle. Medial epicondylectomy is also an option. Occasionally the ulnar nerve subluxes over the epicondyle with elbow flexion causing symptoms. This must be excluded before operations are performed around the elbow.

Guyon's canal—ulnar entrapment syndrome

Clinical: entrapment at this site may produce motor signs, sensory signs or both due to branching of the nerve in the canal—altered sensation, pain or weakness. Hyperaesthesia in ulnar two digits, muscle atrophy and reduced filling of ulnar artery may occur.

Management: rest and immobilization and avoidance of repetitive trauma. Surgical decompression if symptoms persist.

Ulnar entrapment may occur at arcade of Struthers, at the distal end of the humerus, proximal to the epicondyles or in the olecranon groove.

Ulnar paradox—distal entrapment of the ulnar nerve produces a greater claw hand deformity as the FDP is unaffected and so its action is unopposed.

Radial nerve

The radial nerve and its main branches, the PIN—a motor nerve—and the SRN—a sensory nerve, are less commonly involved in entrapment syndromes.

Radial nerve: posterior interosseous nerve syndrome

Clinical: the PIN may be compressed at the proximal edge of supinator (arcade of Frohse). This may produce a motor syndrome with weakness of ED or ECRB, or a sensory syndrome with pain in the forearm (PINs have sensory fibres from the wrist joint) but no sensory loss. The so-called 'Saturday night' palsy may develop from prolonged pressure on the PIN. The sensory syndrome must be differentiated from tennis elbow (see 📖 p. 293).

Management: may resolve spontaneously. Surgical decompression if symptoms persist.

Suprascapular nerve entrapment

Entrapment of the nerve occurs as it passes under the transverse scapular ligament.

Clinical: rare condition. Patients present with deep pain in the paravertebral area of the shoulder and wasting of the supraspinatus and infraspinatus muscles. Occurs as the nerve passes under the transverse scapular ligament.

Peripheral nerve injuries

Description
Nerves may be injured by laceration (knife, glass, sharp bone edge, scalpel), pressure (hard surface, tourniquet), traction or ischaemia (tourniquet, arterial injury, burn eschar, compartment syndrome).

Classification
Seddon:
- Neurapraxia—a temporary conduction block. Nerve intact. No Wallerian degeneration distally. No distal muscle denervation. Diagnosis of exclusion. Recovery within 6 weeks usual
- Axonotmesis—discontinuity of the axon but the supporting connective tissue tube is intact and the nerve recovers slowly (1mm/day) as the axon regrows. Distal Wallerian degeneration and muscle denervation
- Neurotmesis—the nerve is completely divided and chances of recovery are slight without repair or nerve grafting.

Sunderland:
- Neurapraxia
- Loss of endoneurium
- Loss of endoneurium and perineurium
- Loss of endoneurium, perineurium and epineurium
- Neurotmesis.

Clinical Nerve injuries are often associated with other injuries including vascular.

History should include:
- Mechanism of injury
- Development of neurological symptoms—onset and severity (immediately after injury, later or after an intervention)
- Cause—any improvement (more proximally innervated muscles recover first)
- Past medical history—if surgery has been performed get a copy of the operation note.

On examination look for:
- Specific distribution of sensory loss
- Loss of autonomic function, e.g. loss of sweating. This is useful in those who cannot explain sensory loss, particularly in children
- Pattern of muscle involvement—what muscles are not working and what muscles are still working (could be used for transfers)
- Advancing Tinnel sign—tapping on a peripheral nerve from distal to proximal, pain felt at point where regeneration has reached.

Investigations
- Radiology: plain radiographs—to establish if there is an associated fracture and to look for radio-opaque foreign bodies
- Neurophysiology tests (see 📖 p. 38)—NCS and EMG can assess grade of nerve injury after 3–6 weeks
- Angiography—can be useful if a concomitant vascular injury is suspected.

Management

Indications for exploring a nerve injury include:
- Penetrating injuries
- Open fractures
- When nerve injury follows an intervention such as surgery
- When no recovery has occurred—the timing for this is controversial. It should be noted that motor endplates are unlikely to recover if not reinnervated within 18 months. This includes the time to nerve repair or grafting as well as time for recovery at ~1mm/day.

Which injuries can be left?

If there is a motor deficit the joints affected should be passively mobilized and splinted in a safe position to prevent contractures whilst awaiting recovery. Sensory deficits should be protected from injury such as burns.
- Closed or incomplete injuries
- Patients with paraesthesia associated with closed crush injury or low energy fracture patterns and no evidence of compartment syndrome.

Principles of repair

- Repair must not be under tension—transposition of nerve may reduce tension, e.g. ulnar nerve injuries. Graft can span defect to reduce tension
- Oppose fascicles anatomically, motor to motor, sensory to sensory. Surface blood vessels aid orientation
- Use least traumatic method for repair—small sutures (8/0 to 10/0) and microinstruments
- Place repair in healthy vascularized bed of tissue.

Sources for nerve grafts

Nerve graft material can be taken from any source where there will not be a functional deficit. Patients should be warned of areas of anaesthesia though these should not include areas where protective sensation is vital such as the sole of the foot. In major, multiple nerve lesions, some of the damaged nerves may be considered beyond possibility of repair and can thus be used for graft.
- PIN from dorsum of wrist (supplies wrist joint only)
- Sural nerve
- Medial cutaneous nerve of the arm
- Vein or artery interposition—provides a tube for nerve regeneration
- Synthetic tubes.

Postoperative care

As for injuries awaiting recovery (see above). Tension can be reduced temporarily by splinting in an advantageous position, e.g. slight wrist flexion with wrist median nerve injuries.

Shoulder dislocations

The shoulder joint has the greatest range of movement of all the joints in the body, and instability may develop.

Shoulder instability can be described in a number of ways:
- Directional—majority of cases are anterior instability with some posterior and others multidirectional
- Temporal—acute dislocation present for <3 weeks, chronic >3 weeks
- Aetiological—traumatic or atraumatic
- Patient influenced—recurrent, habitual (able to be done voluntarily) or obligatory (occurs with limb in particular position).

The shoulder is the most commonly dislocated joint—45% of all dislocations.

Acute anterior dislocation

Clinical

Usually follows a traumatic event such as contact whilst playing sport or a fall from height.

Patient presents with pain and inability to move the arm. Deformity may be present due to the humeral head bulging anteriorly, but may be absent in large individuals.

It is important to assess neurological and vascular function of upper limb (including axillary nerve sensation over lateral arm and deltoid muscle function) prior to any intervention.

Investigations

Plain radiographs—AP and lateral views of shoulder to confirm diagnosis and exclude a fracture dislocation.

Management

Prompt reduction of the dislocation is required. This should not require excessive force. Ideal conditions would be with patient fully anaesthetized with a muscle relaxant administered.

Awake sedation with analgesia is an option but should only be carried out by experienced clinicians. Full monitoring and resuscitation facilities should be available. Infiltration of the joint with local anaesthetic may be sufficient to allow reduction in patients who do not have well developed shoulder girdle muscles.

Always consent patient for an open reduction before attempting a closed reduction. Open reduction is rarely required in simple dislocation.

Technique of closed reduction: Patient placed in supine position. Image intensifier must be available to confirm reduction. Assistant can provide countertraction. Most important component is longitudinal traction. Gentle external rotation helps disimpact the head from the glenoid. Thumb pressure anteriorly helps move the humeral head over the glenoid rim. Blocks to reduction include long head of biceps or fracture fragments.

Confirm reduction and exclude iatrogenic fracture, with check radiographs. Recheck distal neurovascular function.

Postreduction management: Prolonged immobilization does not reduce the risk of recurrence. Aim for early, active mobilization, as comfort allows, and strengthening exercises to improve rotator cuff function. Immobilization in external rotation may reduce the risk of recurrence.

Acute posterior dislocation

Clinical
This injury occurs in the elderly, epileptics during seizures or electric shock victims. The profile of the shoulder girdle can be deceptively normal, especially in bilateral cases. External rotation is usually limited and may be mistaken for a frozen shoulder.

Investigations
Plain radiographs. The AP view may show the humeral head in oblique profile ('light-bulb' sign) or look almost normal. A lateral (axillary preferably) is mandatory to exclude dislocation.

Impaction fracture of the posterior glenoid lip or anterior humeral head may be present and require further evaluation with a CT scan.

Management
Closed reduction using longitudinal traction. The humeral head can be disimpacted with internal rotation of the humerus. If open reduction is required an anterior approach is the preferred option.

Acute inferior dislocation

Clinical A rare injury presenting with an inability to adduct the arm (luxatio errecta).

Management Closed reduction with longitudinal traction is indicated.

Inferior subluxation

Clinical Following shoulder trauma or surgery, a joint effusion combined with weakness of the rotator cuff muscles allows the humeral head to drift inferiorly with the effect of gravity on the upper limb.

Management No specific treatment for this is required but it should not be confused with true dislocation.

Missed dislocation

An old (>3 weeks) missed dislocation will probably require an open reduction and reconstruction, and is not an emergency.

Occasionally, in elderly low demand patients, function is maintained despite the dislocation and the risks of open reduction outweigh the benefits. These patients are more suitably managed with a physiotherapy rehabilitation programme provided pain is not a major problem.

Shoulder instability

Recurrent shoulder instability

Description

Subluxation or dislocation may occur recurrently when any of the stabilizing structures of the shoulder are lost. The pathology varies depending on whether the initial dislocation was traumatic or relatively atraumatic.

Traumatic: instability is most commonly anterior.
- Bankart lesion—avulsion of the glenoid labrum from the glenoid
- Glenohumeral ligament avulsion or tear from the glenoid or humerus (HAGL—humeral avulsion of inferior glenohumeral ligament)
- Hill–Sachs lesion—impaction fracture of posterior humeral head in anterior dislocations (reversed in posterior dislocations) which reduces the contact area of the humeral head.

Atraumatic: instability is more likely to be multidirectional.
- Generalized ligamentous laxity—may be familial or inherited as part of a recognized syndrome such as Ehlers–Danlos syndrome. Other joint laxity may be evident such as the knees, elbows and hands. Patients are usually young
- Rarely the glenoid may be hypoplastic or abnormally orientated.

Clinical
Note:
- Age of the patient. Under 25 years—high risk (up to 90%) of recurrence following traumatic dislocation. Over 40 years—lower risk of recurrent dislocation
- Wilful dislocation and relocation—if this is the patient's party trick or method of gaining attention it is less likely to respond to surgical interventions. This is termed habitual dislocation
- Symptoms may be non-specific in young patients who compensate well with dynamic stabilizers. Pain, arm paraesthesia and apprehension may be present. If these follow a traumatic episode subtle instability should be suspected.

On examination, the following are found:
- Signs of laxity: these include generalized laxity
  - Sulcus sign—pulling arms inferiorly produces an increased subacromial space evident as a visible and palpable skin sulcus
  - Load-shift sign—holding the scapular neck firmly with one hand and humeral head with the other, the humerus can be displaced in an anterior or posterior direction more on the affected side
- Signs of instability:
  - Apprehension/relocation—for anterior instability. The abducted arm is externally rotated and the patient resists the movement. When repeated, with anterior pressure over the humeral head the patient is more comfortable
  - Posterior apprehension—posterior force on a flexed arm reproduced patient symptoms.

Investigations
- Radiology:
  - Plain radiographs—looking for fractures or Hill–Sachs lesions
  - CT arthrogram—can show disruption to the labrum or capsular structures as well as bony architecture
  - MRI or MR arthrogram—has excellent soft tissue definition. In anterior instability the inferior capsule may also be loose
- Examination under anaesthesia (EUA): negates the effects of dynamic muscular stabilizers
- Arthroscopy: may be required in less obvious cases to decide on the exact pathology.

Management
Anterior instability—in patients younger than 25, recurrence is so common in this group that early intervention aimed at correcting the pathology is often indicated. Sporting individuals are more at risk for recurrence.

Once the initial trauma has settled the shoulder can be investigated as above or a EUA and arthroscopy performed with the patient consented for reconstruction at the same operation.

Surgical options include repair of the labrum to the glenoid and tightening of the inferior glenohumeral ligament, subscapularis advancement and bony operations such as transfer of the tip of the coracoid to the anterior aspect of the glenoid.

Specific risks of such interventions include axillary nerve damage, loss of external rotation and late arthritic changes.

Anterior instability—older patients
With increasing age the risk of recurrence decreases and the risk of stiffness increases. A structured physiotherapy programme following 1 or 2 weeks of immobilization is appropriate. Less commonly stabilization procedures are required. Physiotherapy is aimed at cuff muscle strengthening exercises and maintaining range of motion.

Multidirectional instability
Surgical intervention is possible with capsular shift procedures. They have a high failure rate and it is vital to ensure all conservative options are exhausted before embarking on surgery and that any psychological problems are addressed. Majority of patients grow out of the problem.

Management summary (after Matsen)
- TUBS—Traumatic aetiology, Unidirectional instability, Bankart lesion present and Surgical management
- AMBRI—Atraumatic, Multidirectional instability, Bilateral involvement, Rehabilitation vital and Inferior capsular shift is surgical option.

Calcific tendonitis

Calcific tendinitis of the shoulder is characterized by the presence of macroscopic deposits of hydroxyapatite (a crystalline calcium phosphate) in any tendon of the rotator cuff, usually the supraspinatus tendon.

Aetiology

- The increase in calcium deposits is due to degenerative calcification
- The hypovascular critical zone of Codman undergoes fibrocartilaginous metaplasia
- Calcium hydroxyapatite is deposited in this area
- Trauma or other event stimulates an intensely painful response to the calcification.

History and examination

Calcific tendinitis may present in 3 ways:
- Chronic pain with intermittent flares, usually when the condition is in the formative phase
- Mechanical symptoms due to a large calcific deposit that may block elevation of the shoulder
- More severe pain due to inflammation, usually in the resorptive phase.

Pain commonly radiates from the point of the shoulder to the deltoid insertion and aggravated by elevation of the arm above shoulder level or by lying on the shoulder. Stiffness, catching or weakness of the shoulder are other presenting symptoms. On examination there is loss of range of motion with a painful arc of motion from 70 to 110° of shoulder flexion. There may be crepitus or impingement signs.

Investigations

The calcific deposit can be characterized by its location (i.e. which tendon is affected) and its size. The appearance may change rapidly over days.
- Plain radiographs of the shoulder show an area of calcification; in supraspinatus tendonitis this is just proximal to the greater tubercle. This should not be mistaken for an avulsion fracture
- Ultrasonography demonstrates well the presence of calcification within the affected tendon. In experienced hands, ultrasonography is more sensitive than plain X-rays.

Differential diagnoses

- Neuralgic amyotrophy or brachial neuralgia—a postviral condition associated with intense shoulder girdle pain
- Rotator cuff syndrome—chronic calcific depositions may be present on imaging but are not the source of pain. Impingement pain is the principal finding.

Management

- Acute phase
  - Rest
  - NSAIDs
  - Subacromial injection with steroid preparation and local anaesthetic
- Persistent symptoms
  - Decompression of tendon by penetrating calcium deposits with a hypodermic needle. US guidance can make localization more accurate
  - Surgical decompression can be performed as an open procedure or arthroscopically. Either technique can be combined with a subacromial decompression.

Natural history

This condition is self-limiting in all cases. Intervention should only be considered where pain relief is not achieved with simple measures.

For further reading, see Uhthoff and Loehr[1].

Reference

1 Uhthoff HK, Loehr JW. Calcific tendinopathy of the rotator cuff: pathogenesis, diagnosis, and management. *J Am Acad Orthop Surg* 1997;**5**:183–91.

Rotator cuff syndrome

The rotator cuff is the group of muscles which maintain the position of the humeral head in the glenoid concavity when the power muscles are acting on the shoulder. Damage to the tendons of these muscles (most commonly supraspinatus) results in pain either directly or due to the imbalance of the other muscles acting on the shoulder girdle.

Aetiology

The pathogenesis of rotator cuff disease is multifactorial with intrinsic and extrinsic factors.
- Intrinsic pathology—the tendon of supraspinatus has an area of poor vascularity just proximal to its insertion point. This area may become inflamed due to an increased propensity to trauma
- Extrinsic pathology—impingement of the supraspinatus between the greater tubercle and the overlying coracoacromial arch results in tendon damage and inflammation. The tight subacromial space may be made worse by osteophytes on the undersurface of the acromion and ACJ or by local inflammation.

Stages

Neer[1] identified three stages of subacromial impingement (Table 8.3).

Table 8.3 Stages of subacromial impingement syndrome

Stage	Age (years)	Pathology	Course	Treatment
I	<25	Oedema and haemorrhage	Reversible	Conservative
II	25–40	Fibrosis and tendonitis	Activity-related pain	Conservative and/or acromioplasty
III	>40	Spur formation and cuff tear	Progressive disability	Acromioplasty and/or repair

History

The typical patient is aged between 40 and 60yrs. A short-lived tendonitis may affect a younger age group after intense activity. Presenting symptoms are often:
- Pain—typically occurs as the shoulder is abducted or flexed and felt over the lateral aspect of the arm. There may be a 'painful arc', a range of movement associated with pain where pain is less with movements below or above this range
- Sleep disturbances—pain worse when lying on the affected shoulder.
- Difficulty with overhead activities.

Examination

- Thorough examination of the neck and both upper limbs and a neurological assessment is essential. Local wasting, swellings, instability and tenderness are important signs, and both active and passive range of movement of both shoulders must be measured
- Pain may be experienced through the painful arc though further passive movement may be possible and sustainable once achieved
- At the point of impingement pain external rotation may relieve the pain and internal rotation worsens the pain
- An injection of local anaesthetic into the subacromial space may relieve the impingement pain within minutes, allowing an increased range of active movement while the patient is still in clinic
- Although painful, the cuff muscle power should be intact.

Differential diagnoses

- Humeral head pathology—tumours or infection
- Calcific tendonitis
- Referred pain from neck or cervical radiculitis.

Investigations

- Plain radiographs—three views should be taken at 90°. Typical signs of rotator cuff disease include sclerosis on the undersurface of the acromion ('sourcil' sign), cyst formation in the greater tuberosity, osteophytes of the ACJ and, with a cuff tear, narrowing of the subacromial space. A lateral view may show a 'hooked' acromion or an os acromiale
- Arthrography—useful in detecting rotator cuff tears
- Ultrasonography—allows comparison of shoulders and is particularly useful in assessing patients who have had a rotator cuff repair
- MRI—demonstrates bony structures and soft tissues, particularly identifying partial tears. MR arthrography is the investigation of choice for assessing the labrum and glenohumeral ligaments.

Management

Most rotator cuff disease can be managed non-operatively with:
- Changes in activity
- Analgesics and NSAIDs
- Injection—subacromial local anaesthetic and steroid injection
- Physiotherapy and exercise programme—aimed at improving rotator cuff muscle strength and ensuring the humeral head is centred in the glenoid.

Surgical management is reserved for failed conservative treatment.
- Surgical options—arthroscopic subacromial decompression and ACJ excision (excision of the lateral 1cm of clavicle). Open surgical repair is recommended when there is a full thickness rotator cuff tear.

For further reading, see Matsen[2].

References

1 Neer CS II. Impingement lesions. *Clin Orthop* 1983;**73**:70.
2 Matsen FA III. Rotator cuff. In: Rockwood CA Jr, Matsen FA III, eds. *The Shoulder*, 3rd edn. Philadelphia: WB Saunders Co., 1998:755.

Rupture of the rotator cuff

This is a condition closely associated with rotator cuff or impingement syndrome. Supraspinatus is most commonly affected, though large tears may involve infraspinatus, teres minor or subscapularis. Tears can be classed as partial thickness or full thickness.

History
Patients aged usually >50yrs old. They may present with:
- Pain or loss of function following a low energy traumatic event
- A history of shoulder problems suggestive of impingement
- Difficulty with activities requiring the arm to be held above shoulder height
- In young, athletic patients the rotator cuff may be torn as a result of high energy trauma.

Examination
- Findings will depend on which tendon is torn and the extent of the tear
- Inspection may reveal wasting or asymmetry
- Tenderness, which may be minimal
- Active abduction may be limited to ~30° and associated with a 'shrug' as the whole scapula is raised. Compensatory movements of the whole body are common and may mask the severity of active motion loss
- Passive movements may be nearly normal and can be sustained by deltoid
- Biceps long head tendon ruptures may also be evident.

Investigations
- Plain radiographs—the humeral head may be noted to migrate superiorly due to the unopposed pull of deltoid. In longstanding tears, there may be secondary arthritic changes ('cuff arthropathy')
- USS—in experienced hands partial- or full-thickness tears can be detected. The size of tear can be assessed
- MRI—the tear can be identified. The muscle belly of supraspinatus can also be assessed for fatty degeneration which indicates a longstanding tear and makes it less likely that the patient will do well with a repair.

Classification of full-thickness tears
Tears are classified by the size of tear (amount of retraction of the tendon).
- Small: <1cm
- Medium: 1–2cm
- Large: 2–5cm
- Massive: >5cm.

Management

Rotator cuff tears may be asymptomatic and initial conservative management is indicated. Partial thickness tears are commonly more painful but will usually respond to analgesia and anti-inflammatory medication. Physiotherapy is beneficial in strengthening the remaining cuff muscles and maintaining passive range of movement whilst awaiting recovery.

Surgery is indicated in active individuals who are working and who fail to respond to conservative measures. The aims of treatment are pain relief, removal of the cause for the tear, which is often impingement on the coracoacromial arch, and restoration of function. In planning treatment it must be remembered that the cuff tendons are degenerate. The surgical options are:

- Open or arthroscopic subacromial decompression (SAD)—in all patients with partial-thickness tears and in less active individuals with large tears
- Open or arthroscopic reattachment of cuff to greater tubercle followed by a structured rehabilitation programme—in patients with small to large full-thickness tears. They may require a subacromial decompression
- Tendon transfers or advancement procedures may be required—in massive cuff tears that are not amenable to reattachment, especially if the muscle is contracted
- GHJ arthroplasty may be indicated in patients with a cuff arthropathy. A reverse geometry prosthesis (convex glenoid component, concave humeral component) may be beneficial. In the presence of a degenerate GHJ, cuff repair alone is not indicated.

For further reading, see Matsen[1].

Reference

1 Matsen FA III. Rotator cuff. In: Rockwood CA Jr, Matsen FA III, eds. *The Shoulder*, 3rd edn. Philadelphia: WB Saunders Co., 1998:755.

Adhesive capsulitis (frozen shoulder)

An idiopathic condition associated with initial pain followed by decreased range of movement with a gradual, often incomplete, recovery over months to years ('freezing, frozen and thawing'). The criterion for diagnosing adhesive capsulitis is a painful shoulder with restricted active and passive glenohumeral and scapulothoracic motion for at least 1 month duration and has either reached a plateau or worsened.

Patients with primary frozen shoulder have no significant findings on the history, clinical examination or radiographic imaging to explain the loss of motion and pain, whereas patients with secondary frozen shoulder have a history that preceded shoulder symptoms, such as trauma or surgery to the affected upper extremity. Systemic disorders such as diabetes mellitus, hypothyroidism, hyperthyroidism and hypoadrenalism are associated with frozen shoulder.

Pathology
- Aetiology is unclear but autoimmune responses, biochemical changes, neurological dysfunction, trauma and psychological problems have been implicated
- Histological changes in the capsule are consistent with chronic inflammation and resemble the changes seen in Dupuytren's disease
- The capsule is avascular and tense and adherent to the humeral head, resulting in reduced joint volume. The coracohumeral ligament is often tightly contracted.

History and examination
- Initially the shoulder is very painful but later there is gradual loss of movement
- Symptoms are often worse at night
- There is typically a global reduction in active and passive movements
- There may be a preceding, sometimes minor, traumatic event
- Examination of the cervical spine, both shoulders and the trunk must be performed to exclude other pathology
- The range of motion of both shoulders must be accurately documented.

Investigations
- Plain radiographs are usually normal but are important in ruling out other causes of a stiff shoulder
- Arthrography is not useful due to the difficulty of performing the examination—the contrast medium cannot easily be injected into the constricted joint space.

Differential diagnoses
The diagnosis of frozen shoulder should only be made once other diagnoses have been excluded:
- Rotator cuff disorders
- Dislocation—may be missed especially in a confused or multiply traumatized patient

- Arthritis—osteophytes or articular damage may result in painful stiffness
- Any painful condition of the shoulder—tumour or infection are vital to exclude.

Management

Freezing stage

During the early painful stage, analgesia and gentle, active assisted ROM exercises are helpful.

Frozen stage

Pain is less of a problem but the limited ROM can limit function. ROM may improve with physiotherapy. If the patient is unable to cope with waiting for natural recovery further options are available that include:

- Manipulation under anaesthesia—with the patient under general anaesthesia the capsular adhesions are torn by manual force. Short lever arms should be used (one hand stabilizing the scapula, the other holding the humerus as close to the shoulder as possible). The humerus is gently forced into abduction, flexion, external rotation and internal rotation until the adhesions give with a tearing sensation. Repeating each movement once there has been some release with other movements is beneficial. The GHJ is then injected with steroid and local anaesthetic. Postoperatively the patient should start physiotherapy early. Risks include fracture of the humerus or dislocation
- Open or arthroscopic release—the procedure aims to divide the contracted tissues such as the coracohumeral ligament. Surgical release reserved for patients with osteopenia, rotator cuff thinning and failed manipulation or arthroscopic release. The benefit of these procedures compared with simple manipulation is unclear.

For further reading, see Harryman et al.[1]

Reference

1 Harryman DT II, Lazarus MD, Rozencwaig R. The stiff shoulder. In: Rockwood CA Jr, Matsen FA III, eds. *The Shoulder*, vol 2, 2nd edn. Philadelphia: WB Saunders Co.,1998:1064.

Acromioclavicular joint disruption

The ACJ is usually disrupted by a direct blow to the top of the shoulder. Initially the capsule and ligaments of the ACJ are damaged but with increasing energy the supporting coracoclavicular (CC) ligaments and the adjacent supporting muscles may be disrupted.

History and examination

There is a history of trauma resulting in pain and swelling over the ACJ. The injury usually occurs in young athletes playing contact sports.

Open dislocations are rare. Localized tenderness may be the only sign in ACJ sprains. With ligament disruption the lateral end of the clavicle becomes more prominent. In late presentations examine the contralateral side to compare ACJ mobility. In high energy injuries cervical spine neurovascular injuries must be excluded.

Investigations

- Plain X-ray: routine shoulder trauma series should be obtained. An AP view of the clavicle is important; can be improved with 10° cephalic tilt
- Stress views—weights of 2–5kg are suspended from each arm and AP radiographs are taken. The images help evaluate the integrity of the CC ligaments. Useful with delayed presentation.

Classification[1]

Displacement is based on depth of ACJ on AP radiographs.

- Type I—no clavicle displacement on plain radiographs. A sprain
- Type II—slight superior displacement of clavicle
- Type III—125–200% displacement of the clavicle
- Type IV—posteriorly displaced clavicle buttonholes through trapezius
- Type V—more than 200% displacement of the clavicle
- Type VI—clavicle displaced inferiorly under the coracoid process.

Management

In general, types I–III should be managed non-operatively and types IV–VI should be reduced and stabilized.

- Types I and II: 1 week of rest in broad arm sling followed by active full range of motion
- Type III: non-surgical treatment as for types I and II usually sufficient despite prominence of the clavicle. In some patients, especially if more active, open reduction and ligamentous reconstruction with temporary CC fixation may be advisable
- Types IV–VI: a good outcome is unlikely unless treated by open reduction and reconstruction of the ligaments
- Reconstruction of CC ligament—includes transfer of the CC ligament (Weaver–Dunn technique[2]) or screw fixation from the clavicle to the coracoid (Bosworth technique) to augment repair. The lateral 1cm of clavicle can be excised as part of the procedure. These procedures can be done in the acute phase or for late pain from an ACJ injury.

References

1 Rockwood CA Jr, Williams GR, Young DC. Injuries to the acromioclavicular joint. In: Rockwood CA, Green DP, Bucholz RW, *et al.*, eds. *Fractures in Adults*, vol 2, 4th edn. Philadelphia: Lippincott-Raven, 1996:1341.
2 Weaver JK, Dunn HK. Treatment of acromioclavicular injuries, especially complete acromioclavicular separation. *J Bone Joint Surg Am* 1972;**54**:1187.

Sternoclavicular joint dislocation

Sternoclavicular joint (SCJ) dislocation is much rarer than ACJ disruption, but important to recognize. There can be anterior or posterior dislocation. Posterior SCJ dislocation is associated with major vascular injuries and airway compromise. The injury is often caused by RTAs or direct trauma.

Sternoclavicular joint injuries can be imaged best with a CT scan.

For acute anterior sternoclavicular dislocations, non-operative treatment is indicated. Closed reduction is not indicated in this highly unstable injury because the reduction cannot be maintained. A sling may be worn for comfort. For posterior sternoclavicular dislocation closed or even open reduction is indicated.

For further reading, see Bicos and Nicholson[1].

Reference

1 Bicos J, Nicholson GP. Treatment and results of sternoclavicular joint injuries. *Clin Sports Med* 2003;**22**:359.

Tendinopathies around the elbow

Tendinopathies around the elbow are made up of two main conditions, lateral epicondylitis (tennis elbow), and medial epicondylitis (golfer's elbow).

Epidemiology

Not exclusive to sports persons, these conditions affect 1–3% of the population, are most common in the 40–50yr old age group, and occur in men more than women (2:1).

Anatomy and pathology

- Tennis elbow: common extensor origin predominantly ECRB
- Golfer's elbow: common flexor origin, pronator teres and FCR
- Pathology: degenerative angiofibroblastic hyperplasia within the tendon origin, not an inflammation of the epicondyle as the name suggests.

Clinical evaluation

- Activity-related pain around medial or lateral epicondyle
- Local tenderness at epicondyle
- Pain on resisted wrist or finger extension (tennis elbow) or wrist flexion (golfer's elbow).

Investigation

- Generally not necessary
- X-ray is often normal (may show calcification in lateral epicondylitis)
- USS or MRI may be useful if diagnostic doubt.

Treatment

- Non-operative: rest, activity modification, counterforce brace, physiotherapy, NSAIDs. Steroid injections (into tendon not epicondyle). 90% will resolve with non-operative management in 2yrs
- Operative: surgical release of common extensor or flexor origin. Tennis elbow approach: Kocher's incision and approach between ECRL and anconeus; release common extensor origin and remove any abnormal ECRB tendon.

Elbow instability

Instability of the elbow may be acute, chronic or recurrent. An acute traumatic dislocation is common and may lead to chronic instability.

Anatomy and pathology

The elbow is a complex hinge joint consisting of 3 articulations within a common joint capsule:
- ulnotrochlear joint
- radiocapitellar joint
- proximal radioulnar joint.

Stability is provided by the bones, the joint capsule, muscular action and the ligamentous restraints. The important ligaments are the medial collateral ligament and the lateral ligament (which consists of the lateral ulnar collateral, the annular and the radial collateral ligaments). A dislocation is named according to the direction the radius and ulna move relative to the humerus, most commonly posterior or posterolateral after a fall onto the outstretched hand. Occasionally the ulna and radius are separated by the injury (divergent dislocation).

Acute dislocation

Types of injury
- Open or closed
- Simple—no associated fracture
- Complex—associated with fracture, commonly coronoid, radial head or neck, capitellum or epicondyles
- Terrible triad—dislocation with radial head and coronoid fractures. This has a bad reputation, with a predisposition to recurrent instability and poor prognosis.

Clinical evaluation
- History—mechanism of injury
- Neurovascular status
- X-ray—AP and lateral views.

Treatment
- Closed reduction—by traction on forearm/countertraction on arm
- Make an assessment of postreduction stability
- Repeat radiographs to ensure concentric reduction
- Splint elbow in 90° of flexion.

Postreduction management
- Simple—if stable after reduction, mobilize early (7–10 days in splint). If unstable keep in splint for longer (up to 3 weeks)
- Complex—fractures may require internal fixation; radial head/neck fractures require replacement if not reconstructable. If instability persists after ORIF (open reduction internal fixation) consider ligament reconstruction or hinged external fixation. Specialist referral may be required.

Chronic instability

This is an uncommon condition which can be secondary to:
- Repetitive trauma in the throwing athlete—usually to the medial collateral ligament complex producing valgus instability
- A previous elbow dislocation
- RA.

Posterolateral rotatory instability

Is a consequence of insufficiency of the ulnar lateral collateral ligament. Symptoms may be of pain, clicking or clunking in the elbow. Examination of the elbow may reveal no abnormality, but the lateral pivot-shift test may reveal the instability.

Treatment of chronic instability

- Activity modification
- Bracing for provocative activities
- Ligament reconstruction or repair.

Radioulnar synostosis

Bony union of the radius and ulna limiting forearm rotation is a rare condition seen most commonly after high energy comminuted forearm fractures but also occurs as a congenital abnormality.

Congenital radioulnar synostosis

Due to *in utero* failure of longitudinal segmentation of radius and ulna (4–7 weeks). Usually affects proximal forearm; may not present until late childhood or adolescence with lack of forearm rotation. 60% are bilateral. Usually sporadic. 1/3 associated with other skeletal abnormalities.

Anatomy and pathology

Range of synostosis from proximal fibrous union to total synostosis of radius and ulna. Limits forearm rotation; most common clinical presentation is a fixed pronation deformity.

Investigation

AP and lateral radiographs. CT if uncertainty whether fibrous or bony union.

Treatment

Often none is required as patients compensate well with shoulder movement. Surgery is considered in severe cases most often when fixed in marked pronation. Surgical excision of synostosis with soft tissue interposition often fails due to re-fusion. Rotational osteotomy to more functional position (20–30° supination) may yield better results.

Post-traumatic radioulnar synostosis

Occurs in ~2% of forearm fractures. Seen most commonly in association with the following factors.
• High energy injury/polytrauma
• Head injury
• Open fractures
• Delayed fixation
• ORIF of both bones through single incision.

Treatment

Often amenable to surgical excision after 1–2 yrs and interposition of, for example, fat, muscle or silicone to prevent recurrence. Consider NSAIDs as prophylaxis in head injury cases where heterotopic bone formation is likely.

Avascular necrosis of the carpal bones

AVN of the lunate (Kienbock's disease)

Kienbock's disease (pronounced Keenbock's), or lunatomalacia, is an uncommon but important differential diagnosis of wrist pain.

Anatomy and pathology

The lunate is the keystone of the carpus, transmitting 50% of the compressive load across the wrist joint (normally, 80% of any load is transmitted via the radius, 20% via the ulna). Mostly covered by articular (hyaline) cartilage, the blood supply is usually by vessels entering the dorsal and volar poles. There is a rich anastomotic network within the bone (intraosseous supply). Compromise of this supply causes AVN. Aetiological theories include trauma, repetitive microtrauma and there is an association with a relatively short ulna (negative ulnar variance).

Clinical evaluation

Insidious onset of wrist pain, stiffness and weakness often in the young adult. Localized dorsal lunate tenderness.

Investigations

- AP and lateral X-ray
- MRI (low signal change on T1).

Treatment

Dependent on symptoms and radiographic stage.

Classification of radiographic stages

- Stage I No X-ray changes visible, changes seen on MRI only. Non-operative treatment
- Stage II Sclerosis of lunate increased density. Consider radial shortening
- Stage III Sclerosis and fragmentation of lunate. Consider radial shortening, proximal row carpectomy
- Stage IV Degenerative arthritis in adjacent joints. Wrist fusion

AVN of the scaphoid

AVN of the scaphoid is most commonly seen postfracture (see 📖 p. 408). Idiopathic AVN of the scaphoid or Preiser's disease (pronounced prizers) is a rare condition. Average age of onset 40yrs, may respond to immobilization. End-stage arthritis may require salvage procedures.

Very rare sporadic cases of AVN affecting other carpal bones have been reported.

Carpal instability

Carpal instability is a dysfunction of the carpus, and should be considered after any wrist trauma, and in any case of chronic wrist pain.

Anatomy

The carpus comprises a proximal row (scaphoid, lunate, triquetrum) and distal row (trapezium, trapezoid, capitate, hamate). The pisiform lies separately in the tendon of FCU. The proximal row acts as an intercalated segment between the tightly bound distal row and the radiocarpal joint.

Intrinsic ligaments bind bones within the same carpal row. The important proximal row ligaments are scapholunate and lunotriquetral ligaments. Extrinsic ligaments span more than two bones or the radiocarpal joint.

Kinematics

Flexion/extension can occur at both the radiocarpal and midcarpal joints.

During radial deviation the proximal row flexes; during ulnar deviation the proximal row extends.

Classification of carpal instability

May be categorized by chronicity, severity (static or dynamic), aetiology, location (e.g. radiocarpal, midcarpal, intercarpal), direction or pattern[1].

Direction of instability (see Fig. 8.6)

- DISI: dorsal intercalated segment instability, lunate is angled dorsally, scapholunate angle >70°. Causes: scapholunate dissociation, scaphoid
- VISI: volar intercalated segment instability, lunate is angled volarly, scapholunate angle <30°. Causes: lunotriquetral ligament disruption.

Patterns of instability

- CID: carpal instability dissociative: within a row
- CIND: carpal instability non-dissociative: between rows
- CIC: carpal instability combined: both within and between rows
- CIA: carpal instability adaptive: secondary to pathology outside the carpus, e.g. malunion of a distal radius fracture.

Mayfield classification[2]

A classification of progressive perilunate instability (a CIC type). Ranges from stage 1 (scapholunate ligament tear) to 4 (lunate dislocation).

Clinical assessment

- History of an acute fall onto an outstretched hand, or failure of a 'wrist sprain' to resolve
- Examination requires a detailed palpation of wrist landmarks and assessment of neurovascular status
- Be alert to median nerve compression in acute injuries
- Special tests, e.g. Watson's test for scapholunate instability (see wrist examination, 📖 p. 15), Reagan's shuck test (shears the lunotriquetral joint)
- AP and lateral wrist X-ray—normal features: scapholunate angle = 30–60°. Smooth arc of carpal rows and Gilula's lines (Fig. 8.7). Scapholunate interval ≤3mm (widening of this interval = the Terry Thomas sign)
- MR arthrogram/wrist arthroscopy may help in occult diagnosis.

Treatment

- Acute lunate/perilunate dislocation—reduction and pinning. Median nerve decompression as clinically indicated
- Acute ligament ruptures—open repair and/or pinning
- Chronic ligament disruptions—options include capsulodesis, excision of part of the carpus, intercarpal fusions or formal wrist fusion
- Radial malunion—radial osteotomy.

Complications

- Degenerative changes may occur in the intercarpal and radiocarpal joints, e.g. scapholunate advanced collapse (SLAC) in chronic scapholunate dissociation.

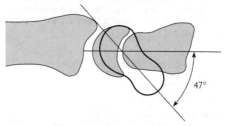

47°

Fig. 8.6 Lateral scaphulonate is measured by the angle subtended by the axes of the scaphoid and the linate. The normal value is 47° with a range of 30–60°.

Reproduced from Bulstrode et al., *Oxford Textbook of Orthopaedics and Trauma*, with permission from Oxford University Press.

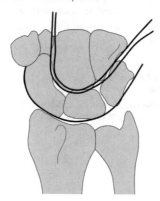

Fig. 8.7 Gilula's lines.

Reproduced from Bulstrode et al., *Oxford Textbook of Orthopaedics and Trauma*, with permission from Oxford University Press.

References

1 Larsen CF, Amadio PC, Gilula LA, Hodge JC. Analysis of carpal instability: 1. Description of the scheme. *J Hand Surg Am* 1995;**20**:757–64.
2 Mayfield JK. Mechanism of carpal injuries. *Clin Orthop* 1980;**149**:45–54.

The paralytic hand

Paralysis of any of the muscles of the hand leads to compromise of this vital functional unit. Assessment and treatment should occur within a specialist unit.

Anatomy and pathology

Causes of paralysis of the hand muscles are related to pathology of the CNS (e.g. CP), brachial plexus, peripheral nerves, or muscles or tendons. The most common aetiology is traumatic.

Clinical evaluation

A careful history and examination must be performed to identify the cause and muscles affected by the paralysis. Most importantly the functional difficulties that the patient experiences in their ADL and employment must be carefully evaluated.

Treatment

Treatment must be directed towards clearly identified goals.
- Prevent contractures
- Preserve existing ROM and power
- Maximize use of functioning units.

Non-operative: occupational, hand and physiotherapy. Splints may often facilitate certain functions, e.g. splinting a wrist drop in extension aids grip strength.

Operative (for CP see 📖 p. 304):

Consider **tendon transfers**. Aim is to replace the function of a paralysed muscle unit and/or return balance to a paralysed hand.

Tissue equilibrium must be achieved before consideration of tendon transfer.

Key questions to ask are
- What function is missing?
- What is available for transfer?
- How are these best combined?

Criteria for a transferable tendon: expendable, with adequate amplitude strength, length, excursion, glide, and correct line of pull on a mobile joint.

Table 8.4 Common tendon transfers

Pathology	Functional loss	Tendon transfer
Ruptured EPL (e.g. distal radius)	Thumb extension	EIP transfer
EDM, EDC rupture (e.g. rheumatoid synovitis)	Finger extension	EIP transfer
Radial nerve palsy	Wrist extension	Pronator teres to ECRB
	Finger extension	FCU/FCR to EDC
	Thumb extension	Palmaris longus to EPL

EPL = extensor pollicis longus, EIP = extensor indicis proprius, EDM = extensor digiti minimi, EDC = extensor digitorum communis, ECRB = extensor carpi radialis brevis, FCU/FCR = flexor carpi ulnaris/radialis.

Volkmann's contracture

Contracture and paralysis of the upper limb originally described in 1881 by Richard von Volkmann. It is due to muscle necrosis and fibrosis secondary to an untreated ischaemic insult.

Anatomy and pathology

Venous stasis, and/or disruption to arterial flow leads to tissue ischaemia. Subsequent tissue oedema and swelling further compromise tissue blood supply, leading to further ischaemic muscle damage. The muscles most severely affected are FDP and FPL, followed by FDS and pronator teres.

Ischaemic nerve damage occurs, leading to irreversible sensory changes and motor paralysis.

Causes
• Vascular injury
• Direct trauma
• Compartment syndrome.

Management

The key to management of this condition is prevention. Volkmann's contracture is most frequently seen as the sequelae to compartment syndrome. High vigilance and prompt intervention is vital in patients at risk of compartment syndrome to avoid the irreversible changes of Volkmann's ischaemic contracture.

Injury phase

In the early stages of ischaemia, emergency steps should be taken to restore vascularity to the upper limb and if necessary perform fasciotomies to alleviate compartment syndrome.

Established contracture

Careful functional evaluation must be performed of this difficult condition by a specialist with an interest in this field. In the majority of cases, non-operative management is indicated.

Cerebral palsy hand

Cerebral palsy (CP) is an evolving disorder of movement, posture and motor function due to a non-progressive abnormality in the immature brain. Upper limb involvement is present in all types of CP patients and the hand is affected to a varying degree.

General evaluation

A multidisciplinary team is required to manage CP patients—carers, occupational and physiotherapists, social workers, paediatricians and surgeons should all be involved in their assessment. This will be an ongoing process over several visits and a significant period of time for most patients.

Hand function is affected by the condition of the rest of the upper limb and by the general neurological state. Surgery is therefore individualized and should be designed to meet very specific goals. Only a small proportion of patients with hand involvement can be helped by surgery.

Evaluation of the hand

Important elements of the examination include:
- Sensation—stereognosis, sensory thresholds (using Semmes–Weinstein monofilaments), proprioception, temperature perception. A hand that is ignored may be insensate, and surgery is unlikely to restore function
- Muscle examination—strength, degree of spasticity, coordination for each major muscle. Also assess proximal control of the upper limb (i.e. shoulder and elbow function—for hand placement)
- Joints—determine if deformities are static (fixed joint contracture) or dynamic (correctable by overcoming spasticity or by changing position of adjacent joints)
- Note resting position of the hand and ability to grip and release.

Non-operative management

Daytime splinting usually impedes function and spasticity is abolished in sleep. Splints and therapy are therefore most commonly used postoperatively.

Goals of surgery

- Improve hand function—allow grasp and release
- Correct deformities that hinder hygiene, dressing or transport
- Cosmetic improvement.

Principles of surgery

- Spastic deformities respond best to soft tissue surgery. Surgery is less helpful in other forms of CP unless arthrodesis is required for joint stability
- Abnormal joints should be restored to a functional position
- The muscular forces on that joint should be rebalanced to prevent recurrent deformities.

Surgical options

- Lengthenings or releases—of tendon, musculotendinous junction, fractional lengthening of the muscle or release from its origin
- Tendon transfer
- Tenodesis
- Joint procedures—joint excision, arthrodesis, or capsular release.

Common situations

- Wrist flexion deformity—dynamic deformities can be treated by flexor releases/lengthening and a tendon transfer. There are many motors that can be transferred to ECRB (e.g. FCU, FCR, ECU). Release of the flexor–pronator origin has been used for more severe deformities. Wrist fusion reserved for severe contractures
- Thumb-in-palm deformity—in the most common type, release of the adductor pollicis ± Z plasty of the webspace is required. With flexion deformites of the thumb, release of FPB ± FPL is needed. Stabilization of the MCPJ may be necessary if it is in hyperextension. Thumb abduction may require augmentation by tendon transfer
- Finger flexion deformities—requires lengthening of the flexors and augmentation of finger extension (by FDS, FCR or FCU). If using FDS this can also power the wrist
- Swan neck deformity of fingers—treated by central slip tenotomy or FDS tenodesis.

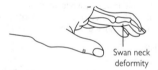

Swan neck
deformity

Fig. 8.8 Swan neck deformity.

Reproduced from Davies, R, and Everitt, H, *Musculoskeletal Problems*, 2006, ISBN 978-0-19-857058-5, with permission from Oxford University Press.

For further reading, see Saeed[1].

Reference

1 Saeed, WR. Cerebral palsy of the upper extremity: the surgical perspective. *Curr Orthopaed* 2003;**17**:105–16.

Dupuytren's disease

A proliferative thickening and subsequent contracture of the palmar fascia of the hand. It is highly prevalent in the Scandinavian population (30% of men in Norway >60yrs), and is common in the UK (15% of men in England >60yrs). It can be present without the resultant contracture, which most commonly affects the ring and little fingers.

Risk factors

Family history, male sex, age, smoking, alcohol, diabetes, epilepsy (or antiepileptic drugs).

Anatomy and pathology

Dupuytren's disease affects palmar and digital fascia of the hand. Bands of fascia are referred to as cords when affected by Dupuytren's disease.

- Pretendinous cords run longitudinally from proximal palm to base of the digit
- The spiral cords are made up of the diseased pretendinous band, spiral band, lateral band and Grayson's ligament. They pull the neurovascular bundle towards the midline, proximally and superficially
- Histology—normal fascia is replaced by a proliferating fibroblast and myofibroblast population producing cords of thicker and, in the case of contracture, shorter, bands of fascia with a higher ratio of type III to type I collagen than normal
- Dupuytren's diathesis is an aggressive form of the disease affecting younger individuals, also characterized by fibromatosis in the plantar fascia (Lederhosen's disease) and the penis (Peyronie's disease).

Clinical evaluation

- Ask about risk factors
- Look and feel for cords, skin nodules and pits in both hands
- Assess symptoms, cosmesis and function (face washing, ability to put hand in pocket or glove). Pain is usually absent
- Measure MCPJ and PIPJ contracture. A quick method to establish significant contracture is the ability to put the hand flat on the table (Hueston's table-top test)
- Digital Allen's test to assess arterial supply to the fingers.

Treatment

Conservative management with splintage has no proven benefit. Steroid injection may help with pain, but does not affect contracture. There are many options for surgery. Incisions, skin, fascia and joints all need to be dealt with.

- Incision—Bruner zig-zag or straight incision and then Z-plasties
- Fascia—fasciotomy (needle or knife) good for isolated pretendinous cord with MCPJ contracture. Alternative is fasciectomy (removal of fascia) which formally dissects the neurovascular bundle proximally and traces distally, removing fascia causing contracture
- Skin—can be left open in the palm if necessary to heal by secondary intent. In the fingers, extra length can be gained by Z-plasties. Skin grafts are sometimes required for coverage. In dermofasciectomy, the aim is to remove both skin and fascia to try and prevent recurrence, especially in Dupuytren's diathesis or recurrent disease

- Joints—almost any degree of MCPJ contracture is correctable. PIPJ contracture is more difficult to deal with. It may correct with passive manipulation, otherwise release of palmar plate and accessory collateral ligaments may be required.

Indications for surgery

Symptomatic significant or progressive contracture. Recurrence is common (>50% at 10yrs) but may not require further surgery. *Salvage procedures*—PIPJ fusion, amputation.

Complications of surgery

- Delayed wound healing
- Digital nerve or artery injury
- Recurrence
- Persistent or incomplete PIPJ correction
- Loss of flexion, i.e. stiff straight finger which may be more disabling than the original contracture
- Infection.

For further reading, see Smith[1].

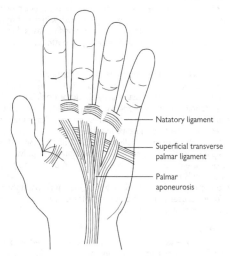

Fig. 8.9 Anatomy of the palmar fascia.

Reproduced from Hand Clinics, 7, Strickland and Leibovic, Abatiny and Pathogenesis of the digital cords and nodules, see 📖 pp. 645–57, Copyright Elsevier 1991.

Reference

1 Smith, P. Dupuytren's disease. In: *Lister's The Hand*, 4th edn. London: Churchill Livingstone, Harcourt Publishers, 2002.

Carpal tunnel syndrome

Carpal tunnel syndrome is a collection of clinical features due to compression of the median nerve as it passes beneath the transverse carpal ligament in the wrist.

Anatomy

The carpal tunnel is made up of a floor of carpal bones and a roof of the transverse carpal ligament running from the pisiform and hook of hamate medially to the scaphoid tubercle and trapezium laterally. It transmits the median nerve, FDP, FDS, FPL and FCR tendons.

Incidence

~1:1000 per year, middle age, the most common peripheral nerve entrapment.

History

- Typically nocturnal dysaesthesia that wakes the patient and is relieved by shaking the hand or hanging it over the side of the bed
- Pain or paraesthesia when gripping, e.g. holding a steering wheel, telephone or book
- The paraesthesia should be in the distribution of the median nerve; thumb, index, middle fingers. There may be wrist pain ± proximal radiation, and patients have difficulty performing fine tasks due to numbness (e.g. picking up a needle or doing up buttons).

Examination

- Blunting of sensation in the median nerve distribution
- Weakness, even wasting, in the muscles supplied by the median nerve distal to the carpal tunnel (most reliably abductor pollicis brevis)
- Tinel's test: tapping over the median nerve in or just proximal to the carpal tunnel produces tingling in the median nerve distribution or reproduces the patient's symptoms in a positive test
- Phalen's test: hold both wrists fully flexed for 1min; a positive test provokes paraesthesia in a median nerve distribution. Applying direct pressure over the median nerve with the wrist in the flexed position may reinforce this test
- Exclude other causes of wrist pain, e.g. de Quervain's, basal thumb OA, and other causes of neurological symptoms, e.g. thoracic outlet compression syndrome, cervical root impingement.

Investigations

- Electrophysiology—nerve conduction velocity is reduced across the carpal tunnel with increased latency and reduced amplitude. Normal velocity = 30–40m/s.

Causes of carpal tunnel syndrome
Idiopathic (the majority), Colles fracture, Cushing's disease, rheumatoid, acromegaly, amyloidosis, mass lesion, diabetes, myxoedema, pregnancy, sarcoid, SLE.

Treatment
Non-operative
- Nocturnal neutral position wrist splints may help with night symptoms, and may be worn for daytime provocative activities
- Steroid injections into the tunnel (**not into the nerve**) may provide relief in the early stages (<6 months from onset).

Operative
- Open decompression—longitudinal release of the transverse carpal ligament in line with radial border of the ring finger. Soft tissue dissection superficial to the ligament should be performed with care to avoid damage to the palmar cutaneous branch of the median nerve
- Complications: infection, pain, wound problems, weakness, nerve damage, CRPS (chronic regional pain syndrome), recurrence (~10%).

Prognosis
Duration of symptoms may not influence final functional outcome after surgery. Preoperative severity does seem to indicate a worse final outcome, but surgery is still beneficial.

For further reading, see Burke et al.[1]

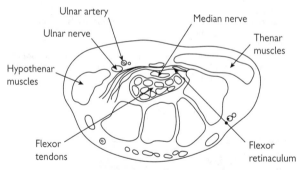

Fig. 8.10 Cross-section of the carpal tunnel.

Reference
1 Burke FD, Wilgis EF, Dubin NH, et al. Relationship between the duration and severity of symptoms and the outcome of carpal tunnel surgery. *J Hand Surg Am* 2006;**31**:1478–82.

de Quervain's syndrome

This is a painful disorder of the first dorsal compartment of the wrist. The cause is unknown, overactivity is not causal but is often aggravates the condition. It is more common in females and may arise during or just after pregnancy.

Anatomy and pathology

The disorder affects the APL and EPB in the first dorsal compartment of the wrist (Fig. 8.11). There may be fibrillation or delamination of the tendon surface with collagen fibril thickening, and fibrocartilage metaplasia. No evidence of inflammation has been discovered.

Clinical evaluation

- Pain over the first dorsal compartment during use of the thumb
- Swelling and tenderness over the compartment
- Pain on resisted thumb extension
- Finkelstein's test[1]—production of pain on ulnar deviation of the wrist with thumb in palm
- Exclude other causes of pain in this area, e.g. basal thumb arthritis, scaphoid injury/non-union.

Management

- Non-operative
  - Rest
  - Analgesia
  - Splintage with thumb immobilization
  - Steroid injection (avoid subcutaneous injection, leads to skin atrophy and depigmentation)
- Operative
  - Transverse skin incision over compartment, avoid superficial branch of radial nerve (damage may result in neuroma), longitudinal dorsal release of compartment and any subcompartments.

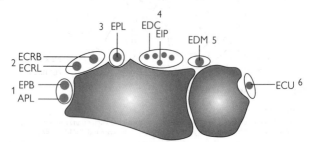

Fig. 8.11 The six extensor compartments of the wrist shown diagrammatically. Courtesy of Dr E. McNally.

Reference

1 Finkelstein, H. Stenosing tendovaginitis at the radial styloid process. *J Bone Joint Surg Am* 1930;**12**:509–40.

Trigger finger

Trigger finger or stenosing tenosynovitis is a common cause of pain and disability in the hand.

Anatomy and pathology

Trigger finger in the adult is due to a nodular thickening on the flexor tendon, accompanied by stenosis of the first annular pulley (A1) at the level of the MCPJ. It is most common in middle-aged females and usually affects the ring, middle finger and thumb. It is mostly idiopathic, but is seen in rheumatoid, diabetic and renal dialysis patients (amyloid deposition).

Clinical evaluation

Patients present with clicking or locking of the finger in flexion/extension. Often the finger is found locked in the palm on waking and needs to be straightened by the opposite hand (often painful). Although the patient often points to the IPJ as the problem, tenderness and palpable clicking are felt over the site of pathology at the A1 pulley.

Management

Non-operative
• May resolve spontaneously
• Night splintage in extension
• Steroid injection of tendon sheath (60–70% success).

Operative
• Indicated after failure of conservative management
• Local anaesthesia, surgical release of the A1 pulley
• Transverse or longitudinal skin incision over A1 pulley at MCPJ
• Protect neurovascular bundle then perform longitudinal release of A1 pulley
• Consider regional anaesthesia in rheumatoid patients to allow for synovectomy.

Trigger thumb

Trigger thumb is more common in young children and often presents with a painless flexion deformity of the IPJ. Initial treatment is with night splintage; failure of resolution is treated with surgery.

Infection in the hand

Paronychia
Infection (usually *S. aureus*) of the eponychial fold. Treatment involves release of pus under pressure by probing nail fold or formal incision and drainage under digital nerve block. Symptoms usually settle quickly. Oral antibiotics may hasten resolution.

Felon
Pulp space infection. Often exquisitely painful due to increased compartment pressure between unyielding fibrous septa of pulp. Treat with incision and drainage through mid lateral incision releasing septae from bone (approach from ulnar side of digit except thumb and little finger).

Bite injuries
Human bites: often follow punch injury over knuckle ('fight bite'). MCPJ frequently violated, mandates formal exploration and irrigation. X-ray to exclude fracture or tooth fragment in MC head. Organisms include α-haemolytic *Streptococcus*, *S. aureus* and *Eikenella corrodens*. All puncture wounds should receive antibiotics, e.g. augmentin (amoxycillin/clavulanic acid) even if joint/tendon sheath not apparently involved.

Animal bites: organisms include α-haemolytic *Streptococcus*, *Pasteurella multocida*, *S. aureus* and anaerobes. Treatment similar to human bites; special care with cat bites as sharp canines often puncture joint or tendon sheath mandating surgical drainage.

Tendon sheath infection
Kanavel's cardinal signs:
• Fusiform (sausage) swelling
• Flexed posture
• Tenderness along tendon sheath
• Pain on passive extension.

Early diagnosis and prompt treatment with elevation/IV antibiotics essential. Open drainage and washout is required in all confirmed cases of tendon sheath infection. Delayed treatment can lead to fibrosis, joint contracture or extension of infection to deep palmar spaces: index and thumb to thenar space; middle, ring and little finger to mid palmar space.

Deep space infections
Web space abscess: form either side of transverse metacarpal ligament leading to swelling on palm and dorsum of hand and abduction of the adjacent fingers. Drain through dorsal and volar incisions to avoid scars in the web space which heal with contracture.

Deep palmar infections: thenar, midpalmar and hypothenar spaces. Present as tender, boggy volar swellings with pain on movement of tendons passing through the space. Treatment involves open drainage (palmar approach) followed by elevation and IV antibiotics. Splintage should be in the Edinburgh position (MCPJ flexed, IPJ extended) to avoid contracture of collateral ligaments and permanent stiffness.

Ganglia

Fluid-filled cysts which originate from a joint and usually present as subcutaneous lumps, which may fluctuate in size. They are most commonly found in the hand and account for 50% of all hand swellings.

Presentation

- Dorsal wrist ganglia are the most common and originate from the dorsal wrist capsule in the scapholunate interval. They are usually only a cosmetic nuisance, but can cause discomfort with wrist extension
- Palmar wrist ganglia are usually found on the radial side of the wrist and originate from the scapholunate or scaphotrapezial joint
- Flexor tendon sheath ganglia are usually small, hard, tender lumps found over the proximal digital crease. May cause pain on gripping
- Digital mucous cysts are a form of ganglia originating from an arthritic DIPJ. Present as swellings to the side of the midline at the base of the nail. The growth of the nail may be affected (grooved)
- Intraosseous ganglia are rare.

Examination

The smooth hard cyst transilluminates when sufficiently large. They are usually non-tender and may be mobile, especially if they are attached to the joint by a long pedicle.

Investigation

- Usually none required
- Radiographs may be useful in dorsal digital ganglia to show arthritic change in joints, or to rule out other causes of pain
- USS or MRI for occult ganglia
- The simplest test to confirm diagnosis is to aspirate the ganglion. The fluid is viscous and clear.

Management

- Reassurance—most ganglia are best left alone. Many will resolve spontaneously
- Historically, rupture of ganglia was performed by a blow from the family Bible!
- Aspiration of the ganglion cyst contents can be reassuring for patients, but recurrence is common. Aspiration then steroid injection probably does not reduce the incidence of recurrence
- For flexor sheath ganglia aspiration is usually not possible but needle puncture will often disperse the cyst and surgery can often be avoided
- For the recurrent symptomatic wrist ganglion, surgical excision of the sac with excision of the pedicle back to the joint of origin has a lower incidence of recurrence
- Digital mucous cysts can be excised, the skin defect may need a local skin flap for coverage.

For further reading, see Dias et al.[1]

Reference

1 Dias JJ, Dhukaram V, Kumar P. The natural history of untreated dorsal wrist ganglia and patient reported outcome 6 years after intervention. *J Hand Surg Eur Vol* 2007;**32**:502–8.

Tumours of the hand

History

- Age—primary bone tumours occur in younger age groups. Metastatic tumours in older age groups
- Pain
  - Night pain—associated with neoplasia
  - Throbbing—associated with infection
- Trauma—possible fracture callus or malunion
- Constitutional symptoms—night sweats, malaise, fatigue, weight loss
- Family history—multiple exostoses (HME), NF
- Past medical history—malignancy, gout, RA?

Examination

Examine for site, size, shape, etc. as you would for any lump. Of particular relevance to the hand:

- large ganglia may transilluminate
- check for mobility/tethering to adjacent structures
- Always examine regional lymph nodes.

Investigations

- Blood tests—Ca^{2+}, ALP, uric acid, inflammatory markers
- Blood cultures if patient pyrexial
- Imaging
  - X-ray—to look for any bony involvement
  - MRI—gives excellent definition to the tumour; the gold standard
  - US—to ascertain whether the tumour is cystic
- Biopsy—often excisional which may be the only treatment required.

Tumour classification

Non-neoplastic lesions

- Ganglion cyst—the most common hand swelling (palmar or dorsal wrist ganglia, digital mucous cyst, ganglion of tendon sheath)
- Others—e.g. dermoid cyst.

Tumours of bone

- Benign—exostosis (may be multiple, think of HME), osteoid osteoma (occasionally occurs in phalanges/metacarpals)
- Malignant—osteosarcoma, Ewing's—extremely rare.

Tumours of cartilage

- Benign—enchondroma (quite common, may be an incidental finding, if multiple = Ollier's disease)
- Malignant—chondrosarcoma.

Tumours of vascular apparatus

- Benign:
  - Glomus tumour—usually under nail bed, exquisitely tender, gives bluish tinge)

- Arteriovenous malformations—capillary haemangiomas (strawberry naevi/port wine stain) or more substantial arterial/venous abnormalities
- Malignant—haemangiosarcoma.

Tumours of nerves
- Benign—Schwannoma/neurilemmoma
- Malignant.

Tumours from other cell origin
- Benign—GCTTS (common, localized form of PVNS—treatment is excision)
- Malignant—synovial sarcoma, epithelioid sarcoma.

Tumours of skin cells
- Basal cell carcinoma
- Squamous cell carcinoma
- Melanoma.

Metastases
- Rarely present in the hand.

Entrapment syndromes of the lower limb

Structures causing entrapment
- Congenital osseous/fibrous bands
- Benign tumours, e.g. exostosis, ganglion
- Iatrogenic, e.g. scar tissue, surgical implants.

Types of entrapment
- Nerve—most common
- Vascular
- Tendon.

Spinal nerve root entrapment
- From intervertebral disc prolapse, or degenerative lateral recess stenosis.

Meralgia paraesthetica
- An entrapment syndrome of the lateral femoral cutaneous nerve—results in pain and paraesthesia in a variable area of the lateral thigh
- May be compressed as it enters the thigh from the abdomen, or as it courses superficially below and medial to the anterior superior iliac spine.

Tarsal tunnel syndrome
- Entrapment of the tibial nerve or its branches (medial and lateral plantar nerves, calcaneal branch) by the flexor retinaculum as it courses around the medial malleolus
- Symptoms may include pain, paraesthesia and numbness
- Isolated pain may be confused with plantar fasciitis.

Morton's neuroma
- Due to compression of a common digital nerve between the metatarsal heads as it passes deep to the intermetatarsal ligament to enter the webspace. The 3rd webspace is usually affected
- Symptoms range from a dull ache to symptoms very similar to metatarsalgia
- The Mulder's click test (squeezing the metatarsal heads together while applying AP compression with the other examining hand) helps to clinically diagnose the condition.

Piriformis syndrome
- Compression of the sciatic nerve or its contributing parts by piriformis in the gluteal region
- Causes pain on sitting
- Symptoms may be confused with spinal nerve root entrapment.

Popliteal artery entrapment
- Variant anatomy may cause extrinsic compression of the artery
- Leads to pain, claudication in young patients.

Peripheral nerve injuries in the lower limb

Peripheral nerve injuries in the lower limb are less common than their counterparts in the upper limb.

Causes of peripheral nerve injuries

- Trauma
- Iatrogenic.

Anatomical classification of peripheral nerve injuries[1]

(see Peripheral nerve injuries, 📖 p. 276)

- Neurapraxia
- Axonotmesis
- Neurotmesis.

Specific lower limb injuries and peripheral nerves at risk

- *Posterior hip dislocation.* The sciatic nerve lies posterior to the proximal femur and may undergo a traction injury as the hip dislocates or a compression injury as the hip is relocated. This highlights the importance of assessing neurological status on initial assessment of an injured limb and again following an intervention
- *Pavlik harness.* Complications of Pavlik harness in the management of developmental dysplasia of the hip include compression of the femoral nerve by prolonged and excessive hip flexion
- *Iliac crest bone harvesting.* The lateral femoral cutaneous nerve usually exits the pelvis inferior and medial to the anterior superior iliac spine, but its course is variable and is therefore prone to iatrogenic damage when harvesting bone graft
- *Below knee casting.* The fibular head, as well as other bony prominences, should be padded prior to applying the cast, in order to prevent pressure sores and direct compression of the common peroneal nerve nerve as it courses around the fibular neck
- *Saphenous vein cannulation.* The saphenous nerve lies adjacent to the vein at the ankle and is easily damaged, resulting in sensory loss to the medial border of the foot
- *Compartment syndrome.* This surgical emergency occurs when the intracompartmental pressure rises to within 30mmHg of the systemic diastolic BP. This results in loss of tissue perfusion to the affected compartment, with the contents becoming increasingly ischaemic. Peripheral nerves are poorly tolerant of ischaemic damage.
- *Total hip replacement.* During THR, injury to the femoral, sciatic or superior gluteal nerves can occur with excessive retraction. The nerves usually recover over several weeks but a few persist
- *Achilles tendon repair.* The surgical approach should be on the medial border of the Achilles tendon, to avoid damaging the sural nerve, which runs near the lateral border of the tendon.

Reference

1 Seddon HJ. Three types of nerve injury. Brain1943;**66**:237–88.

Osteoarthritis of the hip

A non-inflammatory degenerative disease of the hip joint involving hyaline cartilage, fibrocartilage, bone and synovium. Primary or idiopathic OA is diagnosed when no known cause is identified. OA can be secondary to AVN, infection, trauma, paediatric hip disease (DDH, Perthes, slipped upper femoral epiphysis (SUFE)).

Incidence

~1% in <55 yrs, 4–6% in >65yrs with a modest male predominance.

Risk factors
- General—age, family history
- Local—any of the diseases causing secondary OA (see above)
- Increased body weight does not increase the risk for developing hip OA (in contrast to knee OA).

History
- Insidious groin, thigh or buttock pain frequently referring to anterior, medial or lateral thigh and occasionally to the knee. Pain is aggravated with activity, on weight bearing and at night
- Stiffness with characteristic difficulty in hip flexion (e.g. putting on socks, cutting toenails)
- Restriction in mobility with reduction of walking distance.

Clinical features
- Antalgic or Trendelenburg gait
- FFD as revealed by Thomas' test
- Reduced ROM, commonly a loss of internal rotation
- Trendelenburg sign (pelvic tilt on single leg stance)
- Leg length measurements may show some discrepancy (especially if, for example, DDH or shortening after fracture)
- Patrick's test (figure-of-four) is useful in differentiating hip pain from sacroiliac joint pain
- The apprehension test (extension and external rotation) is useful in dysplasia and labral pathology, and the impingement test (flexion, adduction and internal rotation) is useful in assessing for anterior labral pathology and impingement.

American College of Rheumatology diagnostic criteria for hip OA[1]

Hip pain and at least 2 of the following 3
- ESR <20mm/h
- Radiographic femoral or acetabular osteophytes
- Radiographic joint space narrowing.

Investigations

- Radiographs: AP pelvis and lateral hip X-ray. Typical features: narrowing of joint space, subchondral sclerosis, cyst and osteophyte formation. Shenton's line is a reliable method to assess for subluxation of the joint. In cases of hip dysplasia, the acetabulum may be more vertically oriented with increased sourcil angle and reduced Wiberg angle. False profile views can be very useful as they may demonstrate reduced anterior coverage of the femoral head
- CT scanning and a 3-D reconstruction may be useful in the preoperative planning especially in cases of DDH
- MR arthrography may be useful if labral pathology is suspected
- FBC, ESR, CRP.

Treatment

- Conservative—activity modification, self-help arthritis programmes, physiotherapy (ROM, strengthening exercises, aquatic exercise programmes), occupational therapy (joint protection, assistive devices), non-opioid analgesics, NSAIDs, opioid analgesics, self-help programmes
- Operative
  - Preserving the joint: femoral or acetabular osteotomy is indicated in cases where cartilage is at least partly preserved and joint congruity is present, in younger patients with underlying structural cause for early degeneration (e.g. acetabular dysplasia)
  - Replacing the joint: THR or hip resurfacing arthroplasty
  - Excising the joint: Girdlestone's procedure—historic first-line treatment, now used only for salvage, e.g. infected joint replacement
  - Fusing the joint: arthrodesis rarely used in young patients.

Complications of surgery

- Infection, thrombosis, dislocation of replaced hip, leg length discrepancy, periprosthetic fracture, nerve and vessel injuries, prosthetic loosening, osteolysis, heterotopic ossification
- Primary THR early complication rate is 1–2% with implant survival at 10yrs of ≥90%
- Osteotomies can be complicated by non-union, malunion, undercorrection or over-correction.

Reference

1 Altman R, Alarcon G, Appelrouth D, et al. The American College of Rheumatology criteria for the classification and reporting of osteoarthritis of the hip. Arthritis Rheum 1991;34:505–14.

Rheumatoid arthritis of the hip

Incidence
The hip may be affected in 15–28% of all patients with RA. The prevalence of progressive hip joint involvement requiring joint arthroplasty was 15% after disease duration of 6yrs. Patients with RA also have an increased risk of fracture of the proximal femur possibly due to generalized OP and periarticular osteopenia.

History
- Younger presentation compared with hip OA
- Bilateral involvement is frequent
- Morning stiffness
- Severe disability.

Clinical features
- Early manifestations of hip RA are often not apparent as the hip may present with synovitis that does not produce characteristic symptoms
- There may be significant contractures around the hip and/or the ipsilateral knee
- Concomitant problems usually encountered in these patients are dermatitis, vasculitis, fragile skin, osteopenia and muscle wasting.

Investigations
- RhF: found in the serum of 85% of patients with RA and ~5% of healthy individuals
- FBC, ESR, CRP
- Plain radiographs. Classic signs are uniform joint space loss, periarticular osteopenia and marginal erosion. Later typical degenerative findings may be superimposed on the classic signs. Protrusio acetabuli is common in patients with hip RA
- Bone scan may be useful in documenting multiple joint involvement
- A team approach of these patients with the rheumatologist involved in the orthopaedic treatment plan is mandatory.

Treatment
- Treatment can be difficult and controversial. Goals of treatment are pain relief, prevention of cartilage destruction and joint function improvement
- General measures of education, adequate rest, and physical and occupational therapy and the use of aids are important
- NSAIDs, corticosteroids and disease-modifying antirheumatic drugs (DMARDs) may be helpful
- Osteotomies have not yielded good results in hip RA

- When significant degeneration occurs, THR has yielded satisfactory results. The complication rate is higher in RA patients after THR than in patients with OA, with infection rates reaching ~4% and also aseptic loosening having a higher prevalence. DMARDs need to be stopped perioperatively. Periprosthetic fractures during surgery are also more common. If both the ipsilateral hip and knee are involved, THR precedes knee surgery. In bilateral hip involvement, single-stage bilateral THRs may be performed. Cemented THRs has yielded good results, although loosening of the acetabulum component can reach 26%. Severe osteopenia often makes cementless fixation difficult and intraoperative femoral fracture is a danger. Despite this, successful use of cementless femoral and acetabular components has been shown in several series.

Avascular necrosis of the hip

Definition
Osteonecrosis, producing sclerosis, lucency, flattening of the femoral head.

Epidemiology
Occurs most often in men in the fourth or fifth decade.

Risk factors
AVN can be primary (~30%) or secondary. Recognized risk factors are: trauma, alcohol abuse, systemic steroid use, gout, Caisson disease, Gaucher's disease, renal osteodystrophy, haemoglobinopathies (such as SCD), vasculitis (as in SLE), diabetes, hyperlipidaemias.

Features
Regardless of cause, the histological picture of AVN of the femoral head is the presence of empty lacunae in the trabecular bone.

Symptoms and signs
- Insidious groin pain exacerbated with ambulation and activity
- Stiffness
- Patients with early disease can be asymptomatic
- Pain can be severe for a few weeks and then subside
- Pain is usually present before radiographic appearances present.

Differential diagnosis
- Transient OP (use MRI to delineate)
- Hip OA
- Hip infections.

Classification
Various systems have been proposed, such as Ficat and Arlet, Steinberg and ARCO.

Correlation of symptoms with imaging and pathology:
- Stage 0 (preclinical): no symptoms, normal X-ray, MRI ischaemic marrow changes noted, bone scan decreased uptake?
- Stage 1 (preradiological): none or mild symptoms, normal X-ray, cold spot on bone scan, infarction of weight-bearing part of head, abundant dead marrow cells, osteoblasts, osteogenic cells
- Stage 2: mild symptoms, density changes in femoral head on X-ray, increased uptake on bone scan, spontaneous repair of infarcted area and new bone deposited between necrotic trabeculae.
  - Stage 2A: sclerosis or cysts on X-ray. Normal joint space, normal head contour
  - Stage 2B: flattening (crescent sign)
- Stage 3: mild to moderate symptoms, loss of sphericity and collapse of femoral head, increased uptake on bone scan, subchondral fracture, collapse, compaction and fragmentation of necrotic segment, dead bone trabeculae and marrow cells on both sides of fracture line

- Stage 4: moderate to severe symptoms, joint space narrowing with acetabular changes, increased uptake on bone scan, osteoarthritic changes with degeneration of acetabular cartilage.

Investigations

- Plain radiographs. They show changes later than MRI and bone scan
- MRI. Decreased signal from ischaemic marrow on T1 images. Double line sign on T2 images. 100% sensitivity, 98% specificity
- Bone scan. 75–80% sensitivity for stages 1 and 2. Increased uptake on both sides of joint may suggest OA
- SPECT (single photon emission CT). 3-D isotope scanning technique. Useful in the mapping of osteonecrosis and treatment follow-up.

Treatment

Depends on stage of the disease at the time of diagnosis.

Conservative treatment

- Protective weight bearing, withdrawal from exposure to risk factors.

Operative treatment

- Core decompression—suitable for stages 1 and 2
- Trapdoor procedure—indicated for precollapse stages
- Non-vascularized/vascularized fibula graft—suitable for stages 2 and 3
- Intertrochanteric osteotomy of the proximal femur—suitable for stages 2 and 3 with partial AVN of the femoral head
- Arthrodesis is considered in young adults
- THR is considered in stage 4—results vary depending on pre-existing risk factors.

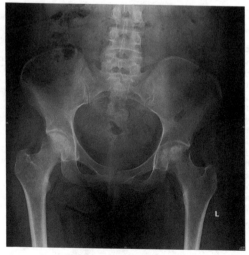

Fig. 8.12 X-ray showing avascular necrosis of the hip.

Knee osteoarthritis

Causes

- Primary OA
- Secondary—to trauma (NB: menisectomy increases risk of OA×10), OCD, osteonecrosis.

Risk factors

- Obesity
- Previous menisectomy
- Instability, e.g. ACL insufficiency
- Angular malalignment of limb.

History and examination

- Confirm that the knee is the source of pain—examine hip, ankle and spine to exclude referred pain
- Establish the level of disability—functional restrictions, rest pain
- Determine effectiveness of other treatments tried (and those possible)—activity modifications; weight loss; analgesics; intra-articular therapies (hyaluronidase; corticosteroid; arthroscopic therapies)
- Decide on likely site of pain—patello-femoral; meniscal; tibio-femoral.
- If surgery is considered, is the patient suitable?—general medical condition; neurovascular status of limb; state of local soft tissues. NB: skin, ligaments, quadriceps mechanism; past history of local infection.

Investigations

- Weight-bearing AP and lateral views
- Flexion views show (early) antero-medial arthritis
- Patellar skyline views sometimes indicated
- General investigations as medical condition dictates.

Treatment options

- Non-operative—weight loss and lifestyle modifications; physiotherapy to strengthen quadriceps mechanism; analgesics/short-term NSAIDs
- Intra-articular corticosteroid or hyaluronidase (limited efficacy)
- Arthroscopic debridement of degenerate meniscal tears or chondral flaps/tears
- Osteotomy—distal femur if valgus, proximal tibial if varus. Subsequent arthroplasty shown to be less successful
- Arthroplasty—unicompartmental if isolated disease prostheses for the patello-femoral and both medial and lateral tibio-femoral compartments exist. Good long-term survivorship reported for medial unicompartmental replacement with correct patient selection
- Total knee arthroplasty—fixed or mobile bearing surface replacements, or linked (hinge) replacements for unstable knees
- Arthrodesis—now rarely used as a primary treatment but may be an option, e.g. as salvage for an infected knee or infected TKR.

Meniscal tears

Meniscal injuries are the most common reason for knee arthroscopy.

The medial meniscus (and especially the posterior horn) is more frequently torn than the lateral. After the age of 50 meniscus tears are degenerative. Almost 60% of people >50 have a degenerative tear. Most of these are asymptomatic.

Classification
- Longitudinal
- Radial
- Horizontal cleavage
- Bucket handle
- Flap and inverted flap tears
- Complex tears.

Clinical
- Usual mechanism is a twisting strain while weight bearing
- Joint line pain, catching, popping and locking, giving way
- Tenderness along the joint line and effusion. When the tear is only in the avascular more central part of the meniscus (white zone) then effusion may slowly develop and haemarthrosis does not occur
- (+)ve McMurray's test: clicking or pain along the joint line with forced knee flexion and rotation
- Deep squats and duck-walking are painful
- When the meniscus is completely displaced the knee undergoes painful locking, unable to extend fully. It is more frequent for the torn meniscus to cause pain, intermittent catching and occasionally locking as it flips into and out of the area of contact between the femur and the tibia.

Imaging
- MRI is the gold standard in diagnosing meniscal injuries, with a sensitivity of >93% for the medial meniscus. Sensitivity is lower with the lateral meniscus. MRI is useful in excluding patients from unnecessary arthroscopy.

Treatment and prognosis
- Conservative: limitation of activity
- Manipulation to unlock the knee and reduce the meniscus
- Arthroscopic partial meniscectomy—excise unstable flaps back to stable rim
- Meniscal repair can be considered for peripheral tears in younger patients in a stable knee. This can be performed either open or arthroscopically—there are various suture techniques or fixation devices available
- When ACL is torn then it must also be reconstructed, especially when the meniscus has been repaired.

Ligamentous disorders around the knee

Introduction
Ligament injuries can occur in both contact and non-contact activities. It is frequently the case that more than one structure is injured as all ligaments and menisci function together.

Classification
- Grade I: stretching of the ligament with no detectable instability
- Grade II: further stretching of the ligament with detectable instability, but with fibres in continuity
- Grade III: complete disruption of the ligament.

Medial collateral ligament
- Two layers: superficial is the main restraint against valgus stress at 25° of knee flexion. Deep layer is attached to the medial meniscus and adds further stability to valgus stress. Injury to MCL is the most common injury to the knee ligaments
- Clinical: isolated MCL injuries present with pain along the ligament, localized swelling, pain and instability with valgus and Slocum, test and **no** haemarthrosis
- Instability should be checked with the knee at 30° as in full extension the posterior capsule may contribute to false impression of stability
- As cruciate ligament injuries may co-exist they must be checked carefully
- Treatment: in isolated injuries early functional motion with protective weight bearing and crutches helps with a valgus-stabilizing brace. Surgical treatment is rarely necessary.

Lateral collateral ligament
- LCL injuries are less common than MCL injuries. They are usually more extensive, involving the cruciates and/or the posterolateral corner of the knee. These injuries may represent a reduced knee dislocation, and careful neurovascular assessment is necessary
- Clinical: varus stress should be tried with the knee at 30° and at full extension. External rotation needs to be checked in comparison with the controlateral side at 30 and 90°. The peroneal nerve may sustain a stretch injury
- Treatment: can be difficult. Reconstruction of the posterolateral corner and the cruciates, when injured, should not be delayed. Stiffness or instability are frequent sequelae of these injuries.

Anterior cruciate ligament
- Most common in sports where the foot is planted solidly on the ground and the leg is twisted by the rotating body. The patient may hear a pop when the injury occurs and is unable to continue activity
- Incidence: peaks at the 3rd decade of life. In children the injury may be an ACL avulsion fracture from the tibial origin

- Acute injury presents with pain, muscle spasm, haemarthrosis, (+)ve Lachman's (either increased translation or soft end-point), (+)ve pivot-shift test (but often difficult unless patient anaesthetized). Comparison with the uninjured knee is crucial. Consider EUA and arthroscopy
- Chronic injury: ACL deficiency, knee 'giving way'. Usually obvious laxity with (+)ve pivot-shift test. Long-term instability produces OA
- Acute treatment needs to be individualized. The outcome of conservative treatment depends on the degree of instability, other knee injuries, age, job demand and general health
- Early reconstruction indicated for world-class athletes
- Direct repair is not successful. Replacement with an autograft is the treatment of choice. Graft options are bone–patellar tendon–bone fixed with screws, gracilis and semi-tendinosus tendon grafting in a single or double band, allografts of patellar tendon (risk of disease transmission), synthetic substitutes (not successful)
- Chronic case: it is important to discriminate if the cardinal symptom is pain or instability. If it is instability and quadriceps and hamstrings muscles have good strength, ACL reconstruction can be considered. Even with mild OA significant improvement can be expected. If weak quadriceps and hamstrings are present then strengthening rehabilitation with a derotational brace and activity modification may help
- Prognosis: current rehabilitation protocols achieve full motion very quickly after operation. Open kinetic chain exercises are avoided initially, to prevent shear strain on the graft. About 90% of patients are reported to have a normal or near to normal life after ACL reconstruction.

Posterior cruciate ligament

- Primary restraint to posterior translation of the tibia. Twice as strong as the ACL. Runs from the lateral aspect of the medial femoral condyle to the posterior aspect of the tibia, below the joint line
- Injuries to PCL are much less common than those of the ACL. The menisci are rarely damaged. Combined injuries of the other ligaments can occur, especially in dislocation cases
- Usual mechanisms are falls or dashboard injuries
- Clinical: findings may be subtle. Misdiagnosis usual. Important to delineate permanent posterior subluxation of the tibia. This is checked with the knee at 90°
- Imaging: lateral radiographs with posterior tibial stress are useful. MRI can confirm the diagnosis
- Treatment: most can be treated conservatively. Some surgeons suggest reconstruction when PCL injury is isolated and posterior tibia translation is >15mm. Strengthening the quadriceps may help to compensate for the torn ligament. If patients are symptomatic of instability after physiotherapy then reconstruction is considered. This surgery is more difficult and less predictable than ACL reconstruction.

Instability of the knee

The shape of the condyles and menisci and dynamic action of the muscles and ligaments and joint capsule determine stability of the knee. Instability occurs when there are changes in these structures that lead to abnormal motion usually due to direct or indirect trauma. It occurs frequently after a ligamentous injury of the knee, e.g. ACL injury. Symptoms may be a sense of giving way or abnormal movement due to instability (with knee at 30 and 90° flexion).

Bony stability: shape of distal femur and proximal tibia.

Ligamentous stability: ACL, PCL, MCL and LCL.

Capsule: Posteromedial and posterolateral elements of the joint capsule.

Muscles: those involved in active movement of the joint.

Posterolateral corner instability

Definition
Rotation of the lateral tibial plateau with posterior translation in relation to the femur and opening of knee joint.

Clinical
- Need to differentiate between LCL, PCL and posterolateral corner injuries
- Varus stress test
- External rotation of tibia (dial test at 30 and 90°)
- External rotation recurvatum test
- Reversed—pivot-shift test
- Check common peroneal nerve function.

Imaging
- X-rays: segond fracture (AP view)—avulsion fracture of lateral tibia is associated with an ACL injury
- MRI: used to assess posterolateral corner, ACL, PCL and the location of the injuries.

Management
Invariably surgery is necessary. Structures that may need to be addressed are the lateral meniscus, capsule, popliteus attachments, arcuate ligament, LCL repair, biceps tendon and iliotibial band.

Patellofemoral instability

Patellofemoral joint instability may present as anterior knee pain (AKP, patellofemoral subluxation or patellofemoral dislocation. It is common in young women.

Risk factors
- Related to bone
  - Shallow femoral trochlea
  - Patella shape

- Patella alta
- Hypoplastic lateral femoral condyle
- Soft tissue
  - Ligamentous laxity
  - Strength and tone of vastus medialis muscle
  - Tight hamstrings and gastrocnemius muscles
- Malalignment
  - Increased femoral anteversion
  - Increased genu valgum
  - External tibial torsion
  - Increased Q angle.

Clinical

Must assess mechanism of injury, previous treatment and state of contro-lateral knee. Examine:

- Palpation of patellar facets
- Q angle
- Apprehension test
- ACL integrity.

Imaging

- Lateral knee X-ray (at 30° of flexion)
  - The superior pole of the patella should be beneath a line extended from the central part of the distal femoral growth plate = Blumensaat's line
  - Insall–Salvati index: length of patella to length of patella tendon is normally one. With patella alta it is <0.8
  - Blackburne–Peele index: length of patella articular surface relative to the distance of its inferior margin from the tibial plateau: normally it is 0.8–1.1
- Skyline view:
  - Trochlear signs—look for dysplastic condyles and trochlear depth (normally <8mm)
  - Sulcus angle (normally it is 126–150°)
  - Congruence angle: angle between a line bisecting the sulcus angle and a line through the lowest point of the patella articular ridge. Positive on the lateral side, negative if on medial side (normal 16°)
- AP and tunnel views are useful for osteochondral fractures
- CT or MRI.

Treatment is based on patient's lower extremity alignment, joint motion, ligamentous laxity and muscle strength. In the first instance, this should be aimed at increasing dynamic stability:

Physiotherapy: VMO (vastus medialis oblique) exercises

Surgical intervention includes

- Arthroscopy: diagnostic and lateral retinacular release
- Medial reefing with VMO transfer
- Medial hamstring transfer (Galeazzi technique) may be required to provide a tenodesis effect
- Tibial tubercle realignment.

Osteochondritis dissecans of the knee

Definition
A rare, acquired, potentially reversible disorder that affects one or more ossification centres and leads to changes to the subchondral bone that may result in separation and instability of the overlying articular cartilage.

Incidence
- 15–21 per 100 000 knees
- Usually presents at 10–20yrs of age, but may occur in any age group. Male to female ratio 2:1. Increased incidence in adolescents engaged in sport
- Involves the posterolateral aspect of the medial femoral condyle in 70%
- Medial femoral condyle affected in 80%
- Patella in 10%
- Bilateral in 15–30%.

Diagnosis
- Symptoms may be vague and poorly localized
- Joint pain, swelling, external rotation gait
- Locking may occur if loose body present
- Progressive degenerative arthritis may occur
- May find effusions, quadriceps weakness, and loss of full extension. Wilson's test: flex knee to 90° whilst internally rotating the tibia— positive if pain elicited at 30° and is relieved with external rotation
- Radiographs: AP, lateral, Merchant's and tunnel views
- MRI can depict the surrounding oedema in the subchondral bone.

Classification
Lesions are classified according to the integrity of articular cartilage and the stability of the underlying subchondral bone.
- Grade I—intact articular surfaces
- Grade II—articular cartilage breach with rim behind fragment
- Grade III—partially detached lesions. On MRI T2 sequence there is high signal behind the fragment
- Grade IV—craters with loose bodies (salvageable or unsalvageable)

Natural history
The natural history is directly dependent on age at presentation:
- In the juvenile type (children with open distal femoral physis), the prognosis is excellent if the lesion is stable
- In the adolescent with partial physeal closure, the prognosis is unknown because the lesion may behave as either the juvenile or adult type
- The adult type (closed physis) has a poorer prognosis because of limited healing potential.

Treatment

In skeletally immature patient
Conservative treatment is recommended. Stable, closed lesions usually heal. Protected crutch walking and gentle knee motion for several months

is thought to have beneficial effects on cartilage healing. Unstable lesions or lesions that have failed to respond to conservative management may require fixation with wires or screws.

In skeletally mature patient

Treatment is based on the grade and extent of the lesion:

- Removal of loose bodies
- Arthroscopic drilling or fixation of unstable fragment
- Osteochondral autograft or allograft
- Microfracture to encourage fibrocartilage cover of an osteochondral defect
- Autologous chondrocyte implantation.

In both groups analgesics and NSAIDs may be needed to control the pain.

Prognosis

In general, the prognosis of OCD is better in younger patients, but also depends on the size, grade and depth of the lesion.

Spontaneous osteonecrosis of the knee

Definition
A usually self-limiting condition that represents a subchondral bone insufficiency. Usually reported as a radiolucent area in the femoral condyle surrounded by a sclerotic halo and associated with a focally active bone scan. Can be a precursor of OA of the knee. Can present in the medial femoral condyle, lateral femoral condyle or medial tibial plateau.

Epidemiology
More common in postmenopausal females. Two separate entities exist. Spontaneous osteonecrosis of the knee usually occurs as a single focal lesion in patients >60yrs. Secondary osteonecrosis of the knee usually occurs as a multifocal lesion in patients <45yrs.

Pathophysiology
- Unknown
- Vascular theory
- Trauma theory: microfracture in the subchondral bone. This allows fluid to enter through the articular cartilage into the subchondral bone and marrow space, creating increased interosseous pressure and pain. This increased pressure in a closed space interferes with the blood supply and triggers the cycle of compromised circulation and results in osseous ischaemia. However, only 10% of patients give a history of trauma
- Insufficiency theory: insufficiency stress fracture in osteopenic bone. Association with OA
- Secondary causes: steroids, alcohol, renal transplantation, Gaucher disease, haemoglobinopathies, Caisson's disease, SLE.

Clinical manifestations
- Acute, well localized pain usually on the medial side of the knee, with nocturnal aggravation.

Radiology

X-rays
- Stage 1—normal
- Stage 2—slight flattening of the condyle
- Stage 3—area of radiolucency surrounded by subchondral sclerosis. Collapse of subchondral bone plate
- Stage 4—the radiolucency is surrounded by a definite sclerotic halo of variable thickness and density
- Stage 5—secondary arthritic changes.

Bone scans
- Increased uptake is necessary to make the diagnosis
- The osteonecrotic lesion appears as a focally intense area of uptake.

MRI
- T1—discrete low intensity signal in the femoral condyle
- T2—corresponding low signal intensity area in the central lesion, with a high intensity signal about the margin (surrounding oedema).

Differential diagnosis
- OCD
- Primary OA
- Meniscal tears
- Transient OP of the knee
- Bone marrow oedema
- Pes anserinus bursitis.

Prognosis
- Prognosis is related to the size, location and number of lesions
- Many lesions may progress to degenerative joint disease
- A large lesion (>50% of the width of the femoral condyle, or >5cm^2) has a poor prognosis in terms of joint preservation.

Treatment
- Recognizing the osteonecrosis early is difficult but may prevent unnecessary surgery and delays
- Initially, conservative treatment, especially for small lesions (protected weight bearing with crutches, analgesia, physiotherapy)
- Surgical options: arthroscopic debridement (has mixed results), proximal tibial osteotomy, drilling, with or without bone grafting, core decompression, unicompartmental or TKR, osteochondral allografts.

Jumper's knee and adolescent apophysitis

Painful conditions of the extensor mechanism of the knee due to repeated mechanical overload.

Causes

Repetitive jumping/landing on a semi-flexed knee, loading the extensor mechanism. Pain may be from the **ligamentum patellae** (tendonosis or peritendonitis) or its insertion to the **inferior patella** or tibia. The **quadriceps** insertion into the superior pole can also be affected.

In adolescents similar activities cause traction apophysitis of the inferior pole of the patella (Sinding–Larsen–Johanssen disease—SLJ) or tibial tuberosity (Osgood–Schlatter disease—OS).

Risk factors

- Frequent sport-playing with rapid acceleration/deceleration/direction change
- Possibly activities on hard floors.

Symptoms and signs

- Spectrum from pain (following activity or during activity) to tendon rupture
- Swelling with pain on kneeling with SLJ and OS
- Local tenderness at site of pain, but knee itself normal.

Investigations

- Plain radiographs—ossicle formation in tendon near bony attachments through avulsions in OS/SLJ; may persist into adult life
- US—inflammatory changes or heterogeneity
- MRI—cystic degeneration on T2; partial or complete tendon disruption.

Treatment

Adolescent apophysitis

- Maintain athletic activities as far as possible with symptomatic treatment
- Periods of rest as required—occasionally splint/plaster immobilization
- Persistently symptomatic ossicles may need excision in adult life.

Adult tendonosis

- Physiotherapy (quadriceps/hamstring stretches; local ice)
- Occasionally rest ± immobilization
- Debridement of degenerate tendon with excision of any ossicle
- Repair or reconstruction of ruptured tendons then rehabilitation.

Failure of hip and knee arthroplasty

Survival analysis, a technique borrowed from oncology trials of chemotherapy allowing data with varying lengths of follow-up meaningfully to be pooled, is popular now for studying long-term results of arthroplasty using implant failure or revision, rather than death, as the end-point. Modern joint registries produce just such data. 10yr survival rates for most THR (hip replacement) or TKR (knee replacement) now exceed 90% at 10yrs.

The classic article on modes of failure for THR was written by Charnley himself, but pertains mainly to cemented components. A number of factors may contribute to implant failure.

Infection

Can be early (<3 months postoperative) or late. May present as overt suppuration or in more indolent fashion with pain due to loosening of components. Common organisms include *S. aureus* and *S. epidermidis*; the latter has low virulence but can become pathogenic in the unique biological environment around an implant. Biofilm formation on the implant reduces antibiotic penetration to bacteria which assume a dormant state, further frustrating mechanisms of antibiotic action. Requires revision to new components after excision of all infected metalwork and soft tissue, either in a single procedure or 2 stages separated by a period with a 'spacer' implant which elutes antibiotic locally.

Instability (THR)

Three factors may lead to recurrent dislocation of a THR:
- Poor choice of implants, e.g. small head with reduced range of stable motion or insufficient head/neck offset
- Incorrect implantation; common mistake is to misjudge acetabular anteversion. Placing a retroverted socket through a posterior approach leads almost inevitably to posterior dislocation
- Neuromuscular disease, e.g. Parkinson's, CVA or otherwise poorly preserved soft tissue restraints to dislocation.

Risk is therefore higher with revision surgery.

Mechanical failure

Potential failure mechanisms depend on site (THR or TKR), type of component (cemented or uncemented), bearing surface (polyethylene, metal, ceramic or any combination of these and other surfaces) and position of the components.

Lysis around a cemented implant, previously described as 'cement disease', most likely represents resorption secondary to the inflammatory response to wear debris from the articulation (commonly metal on polyethylene historically) which has found its way into the bone/cement interface as a result of poor pressurization technique[1]. A more aggressive form of lysis has been reported with cemented titanium stems where a chemical reaction known as 'crevice corrosion' takes place.

An uncemented implant relies on initial press-fit or screw fixation with subsequent bone ongrowth (and ingrowth if implant has a biological coating) to provide long-term stability. Failure leads to painful micromotion and interposition of fibrous tissue at the bone–implant interface.

Rarely, components can fracture, leading to immediate catastrophic failure. This may be due to poor design, a faulty batch of materials or poor component alignment.

Stress shielding

A highly rigid canal-filling (typically uncemented) femoral component in THR can unload the proximal femur, transmitting all load directly to the shaft and bypassing the metaphysis, which can lead to disuse osteopenia. This may predispose to fracture and complicate a revision.

Periprosthetic fracture

May occur around a well-fixed implant, commonly at tip where the modulus of elasticity mismatch (high for bone, low for implant) causes a 'stress riser'. Alternatively bone loss around the implant, from a variety of causes, creates a zone of weakness allowing pathological fracture with minimal trauma. Revision requires either an implant which bypasses the deficient zone or a procedure to restore bone stock around the new implant.

Investigation of a painful arthroplasty

- Plain radiographs for component geometry and gross radiographic signs of loosening and/or infection (bone lysis at implant/bone interface)
- Inflammatory markers/FBC for infection
- 99mTc bone scan; increased uptake suggestive of loosening and/or infection
- Labelled white cell scan for low grade infection
- Joint aspiration for microscopy, culture and sensitivities.

Reference

1 Horowitz SM. Studies of the mechanism by which the mechanical failure of polymethylmethacrylate leads to bone resorption. *J Bone Joint Surg Am* 1993;**75**:802–13.

Osteoarthritis of the ankle and foot

Definition
Degenerative changes within the ankle or other joints of the foot.

Epidemiology
Relatively uncommon compared with OA in other joints. Most cases present in middle age.

Aetiology
- Secondary to trauma (related to angular deformity after fracture or due to minor repeated trauma)
- Ankle instability
- As part of systemic arthropathy
- Osteonecrosis
- Infection
- As a complication of bleeding disorder.

History
Pain, loss of function and past history of injury
- Pain caused by walking uphill with loss of dorsiflexion and walking across rough ground for subtalar OA
- Unable to wear high heels or pain on push off (1st MTPJ)
- Deformity
- Giving way.

Examination
Examine the patient seated and standing. Observe gait and look for:
- Swollen joints
- Decreased movement
- Palpable osteophytes
- Deformity
- Neurological deficit
- Vascular deficit.

Examine the patient's shoes for uneven wear pattern.

Investigations: radiology
Obtain a set of ankle views—AP, lateral and mortice views. Look for:
- Loss of joint space
- Sclerosis
- Cyst formation
- Osteophyte formation

A CT scan may show evidence of early arthritis.

Management

Non-operative treatment: analgesics and NSAIDs, steroid injections, weight loss activity and shoe wear modification. Orthoses—heel insoles for ankle OA, arch supports or even AFOs.

Surgical options: indicated if non-operative treatment fails after 5–6 months. Surgery includes:
- Osteotomy correcting varus deformity at the ankle (results are variable)
- Arthroscopy and debridement (improves symptoms for 3–5yrs)
- Arthrodesis: good short-term results but increases loads on other joints leading to degenerative changes, and has a nonunion rate of 5–10%
- Arthroplasty: no long-term results in ankle or 1st MTPJ.

For further reading see Bulstrode et al.[1]

Reference

1 Bulstrode C, Buckwater J, Carr A, et al., eds. *Oxford Textbook of Orthopaedics and Trauma*. Oxford: Oxford University Press, 2002.

Rheumatoid arthritis of the ankle and foot

Incidence
90% of RA patients have foot involvement, which is almost always bilateral. In 17% of RA patients the joints of the feet are the first to be affected. The forefoot is most commonly involved but the subtalar and the ankle joint is involved in 1/3 of patients.

Natural history
RA of the foot and ankle progresses through 3 stages:
- Chronic synovitis destroying the supporting structures
- Joint erosions, tendon dysfunction and instability
- Progressive deformities (dorsal subluxation and eventual dislocation of the MTPJs), loss of intrinsic–extrinsic muscle balance and claw toe deformity.

Clinical findings
Careful history taking and medication regime. Important to ascertain whether disease is currently in an active or a quiescent stage. Evaluation of vascular status of leg and condition of skin (as well as skin healing potential history).
- Hindfoot—valgus ankle joint and hindfoot (resulting in tight Achilles tendon); posterior tibial tendon dysfunction is also very common in an attempt to stabilize the medial arch
- Midfoot—flattening of the longitudinal arch, flattening and pronation of the foot. Talonavicular and naviculocuneiform articulations usually affected
- Forefoot—painful plantar callosities, present or past ulcerations, hallux valgus, swelling of MTPJs with dorsal subluxation or dislocation (due to synovitis) and large plantar bursae, interdigital neuromas, severe hammer toe and claw toe deformities, tendon ruptures, tarsal tunnel syndrome
- Also look for associated features—peripheral vascular disease/vasculitis, neurology
- Diagnostic local anaesthetic injections sometimes help to localize the source of pain.

Radiographs
AP, lateral and weight-bearing views. Bilateral involvement is usually asymmetric.

Management

- **Non-operative:** analgesia, NSAIDs, DMARDs, physiotherapy to stretch the Achilles tendon and to maintain range of motion of the hindfoot and the MTPJs, taping, foot orthosis, canes and crutches, local injections of steroids to joints or tendon sheaths (tendon rupture is a potential risk)
- **Operative:** check skin condition and blood supply first, consider stopping methotrexate and steroids 2 weeks before, consider alignment of whole lower limb. Main goal is to alleviate pain and achieve stability. If severe hip and knee deformity exists, it must be corrected before the ankle and foot deformity.

Ankle

- Initial synovitis can be treated with synovectomy (open or arthroscopic)
- If there is joint destruction but no deformity, ankle arthroplasty may be considered
- If the joint is deformed then arthrodesis is the operation of choice.

Hindfoot

- RA in the hindfoot can cause either a loose mobile joint in planovalgus which responds poorly to surgery or a stiff joint which can be fused e.g. talonavicular or triple fusion in subtalar joint subluxation. Patients should remain non-weight bearing in a short-leg cast for 6 weeks.

Midfoot

- The tarsometatarsal and intertarsal joints are less frequently involved with RA. Custom-moulded, soft orthosis used. In severe cases arthrodesis is indicated.

Forefoot

- This is the most common part of the foot affected by RA
- Arthrodesis of the 1st MTPJ. The lesser MTPJs can be corrected by releasing the extensor tendons, resection arthroplasty (excising the heads of the metatarsals and reducing the displaced fat pad)
- Hammer toes can correct by closed osteoclasis or an open procedure and Kirschner wires stabilization for 4 weeks.

Common complications of foot and ankle surgery in RA patients are: infection, delayed wound healing, neurovascular compromise, amputation, recurrence of deformity.

The unstable ankle joint

Definition

Two categories of instability:
- Functional: pain that causes the ankle to give way
- Mechanical instability: weakened static ankle restraints that lead to excessive lateral ankle subluxation and resultant pain. Ligamentous laxity syndromes and neuromuscular conditions may present with this type of instability.

Incidence

Ankle sprains are the most common sports injuries, but only 20% of patients will have residual symptoms.

Classification

Three grades exist for lateral collateral ankle ligament injuries.
- Grade I—confined to anterior tibiofibular ligament
- Grade II—injury to anterior talofibular ligament and calcaneofibular ligament with mild laxity
- Grase III—as in II with significant laxity.

Clinical findings

- Tenderness over anterior talofibular ligament and/or calcaneofibular ligament
- (+)ve anterior draw test
- (+)ve inversion test (talar tilt)
- Pain squeezing the tibia and the fibula together
- Painful external rotation of the foot
- Subtalar instability is difficult to diagnose. Clinical examination alone fails to distinguish between tibiotalar and subtalar instability (need X-ray). Abnormal tibiotalar tilt is defined as between 3 and 15° relative to the contralateral side and talar translation on the tibia >3mm.

Imaging

- AP and lateral views of the ankle and foot. AP standing view
- EUA and stress X-rays
- US of the ankle
- MRI scan (when osteochondral injuries are suspected)
- CT scan (when fractures are suspected).

Treatment

Conservative

- Ankle and hindfoot sprains are initially treated with RICE (rest, ice, compression bandage, elevation), usually in plaster of Paris for 2–3 weeks

- Most patients with ankle instability will improve with early weight bearing and rehabilitation (this includes a gradual programme of strengthening the peroneal and dorsiflexor muscles, stretching of Achilles tendon, isometric exercises with rubber bands and at a later stage proprioceptive training)
- In severe strains protect ankle with pneumatic brace or taping for sports for 3–6 months.

Operative

Should aim at anatomic reconstruction and functional stability
- Arthroscopy. Note that ~25% of patients having arthroscopy for instability symptoms have another intra-articular pathology
- If the residual lateral ligamentous tissues are amenable to repair then imbrication of the anterior talofibular ligament and/or calcaneofibular ligament with augmentation of the inferior extensor retinaculum is carried out
- Alternatively the peroneus brevis, semi-tendinosus or gracilis tendons can be used as augmentation grafts
- Bioabsorbable or metallic suture anchors have been used to achieve primary fixation
- If hindfoot varus co-exists with lateral ankle instability, then a valgus calcaneal osteotomy is recommended.

Tarsal tunnel syndrome

Definition
An entrapment neuropathy of the tibial nerve or its branches as it passes through the tarsal tunnel.

Incidence
An uncommon cause of heel/foot pain.

Causes
- unknown
- trauma
- local swellings within the tarsal canal (varicosities, bony prominences, ganglion cysts, lipomas)
- heel valgus
- systemic disorders, e.g. RA, diabetes.

History
Pain and numbness in heel and sole of foot exacerbated by activity although not always completely settled with rest. Careful past medical history for medical causes of peripheral neuropathy.

Exam
- reduced sensation—distribution of medial and lateral plantar nerves and calcaneal branches
- atrophy of the intrinsic foot muscles may be noted
- foot eversion and dorsiflexion may exacerbate symptoms
- Tinel's sign (radiation of pain and paraesthesia along the course of the nerve) may be induced by percussion over the course of the nerve.

Differential diagnosis
- plantar fasciitis
- calcaneal/talar process fracture
- lumbar radiculopathy
- peripheral neuropathies
- arthritides.

Investigations
- Plain radiographs may show neuroarthropathy (i.e. Charcot disease) in longstanding neuropathies
- Electrophysiology studies—but negative findings do not rule out the diagnosis
- MRI/USS if suspected mass lesion in tarsal tunnel.

Treatment

Conservative

- NSAIDs
- immobilization of ankle
- orthotics to decrease pronation
- low dose neurotropic medications, e.g. amitryptiline.

Surgical

Reserved for those in whom diagnosis is secure and have not responded to conservative management. Decompression (tarsal tunnel release)—incise along course of tibial nerve from proximal to medial malleolus to origin of abductor hallucis. Open flexor retinaculum and fascia of abductor hallucis origin fully. Non-weight bearing 4/52 then mobilize.

Complications: iatrogenic injury to the nerve or posterior tibial artery could have significant deleterious effects on foot function. Failure to adequately release the retinaculum along entire course may lead to treatment failure.

Prognosis: surgical decompression relieves pain in 50–75%. Re-do procedures less successful.

Tibialis posterior tendon dysfunction

Definition
A spectrum of pathology that compromises the function of the tibialis posterior tendon. Inflammation, degeneration and/or rupture of the tendon with associated ligamentous degeneration ultimately lead to secondary changes in foot and ankle shape and functional deficits.

Risk factors
Obesity, hypertension, middle age, female sex, diabetes, collagen disorders, previous ankle fracture, injury or surgery (medial), local steroid injection, seronegative arthritides.

Symptoms and signs
Initially pain ± swelling medially at the ankle and into the foot. Usually no clear history of trauma. As valgus progresses, impingement of the fibula on the calcaneus causes pain laterally.

Look for characteristic medial heel wear of shoes. Observe gait. View from behind to assess valgus deformity of hindfoot and 'too many toes sign' due to forefoot abduction. Also assess medial longitudinal arch and see if all these deformities are flexible or rigid.

Assess strength of heel inversion whilst palpating tendon. Ask patient to perform single leg heel rise—usually impossible in stage 2 or 3 disease.

Staging of disease
- 1: synovitis with intact tendon
- 2: ruptured tendon with flexible deformities
- 3: ruptured tendon with rigid deformities
- 4: valgus angulation of talus in ankle motice.

Differential diagnosis
- Of acquired flat foot: neuropathic (Charcot) foot, degenerative change of ankle, talonavicular or tarsometatarsal joints
- Of medial ankle/foot pain: tarsal tunnel syndrome, Deltoid ligament strain, AVN head of talus or navicular.

Investigations
Plain radiographs abnormal in only 50%. May show uncovering of talar head, abnormal talo-metatarsal angles or arthritic changes at ankle, subtalar and talonavicular joints. MRI can image the tendon directly.

Management

- Conservative—rest, NSAIDs, well-fitted footwear, orthoses (corrective for flexible deformity, accommodative if rigid), cast immobilization (stage 1 disease)
- Surgical options: synovectomy, debridement and repair of the tendon, flexor tendon transfers (e.g. FDL), calcaneal osteotomy, arthrodesis for painful stage 3 or 4 disease.

For further reading see Myerson[1].

Reference

1 Myerson MS. Adult acquired flatfoot deformity. Treatment of dysfunction of the posterior tibial tendon. *J Bone Joint Surg Am* 1996;**78**:780–92.

Bursitis of Achilles tendon insertion

Inflammation of one of the bursae adjacent to the Achilles tendon—the retrocalcaneal bursa, anterior (deep) to the tendon or the subcutaneous bursa, posterior (superficial) to the tendon. Bursitis may co-exist with degeneration of the tendon (tendinosis) or inflammation of the paratenon (peritendonitis).

Incidence Common, especially in physically active individuals.

Causes
- repetitive abrasion by poorly fitting shoes
- high level of athletic activity
- inflammatory disorders, e.g. gout, rheumatoid
- Haglund's deformity: prominent postero-superior calcaneal tuberosity.

History
Chronic posterior heel pain. May be unilateral or bilateral, may have noticed a lump (a 'pump bump'). Ask regarding recent change in activity level or footwear, and for evidence of underlying inflammatory disorder.

Examination
- Local tenderness and warmth superficial or deep to the tendon
- Possible palpable bony mass at the affected site
- Ensure tendon is intact (calf squeeze test).

Differential diagnosis
- Peritendonitis of Achilles tendon
- Achilles tendon rupture
- Achilles tendinosis
- Calcaneal injury/fracture
- Arthritis of ankle joint.

Investigations
- Plain radiographs—?Haglund's deformity
- Blood markers—ESR, CRP—if suspicion of generalized inflammatory disorder
- MRI.

Management—conservative
- NSAIDs
- Rest—may require a period of cast immobilization if severe
- Ice treatment
- Heel rises
- Change of footwear to some with absent or cushioned back
- Graduated stretching techniques for the Achilles/calf muscles
- Steroid injection generally not recommended because of risk of tendon rupture.

Management—surgical
- Removal of Haglund's deformity
- Debridement of Achilles tendon
- Excision of implicated bursa.

Prevention
Well-fitting shoes, careful stretching prior to exercise.

Complications
Chronic pain, rupture of Achilles tendon.

Peritendonitis of the Achilles tendon

Inflammatory change in the paratenon—the soft tissue sheath that surrounds the Achilles tendon. May co-exist with tendinosis (degenerative change of the tendon itself).

Risk factors
Physical exertion in context of poor running technique/footwear, biomechanical abnormalities, e.g. over pronated foot. Increasing age. Inflammatory conditions, e.g. rheumatoid, SLE. Diabetes. Steroids.

Incidence
Reported to be as high as 10% in runners.

History
May be a precipitating change in activity level or training regime. Gradual onset of posterior ankle pain and stiffness particularly when mobilizing. May reduce with exercising or applying heat but recurs. More acute onset suggests a rupture.

Exam
Swelling, thickening and tenderness of the tendon with palpable crepitus. Presence of calf atrophy indicates chronicity. Nodules within the tendon imply an underlying tendinosis.

Differential diagnosis
- Achilles rupture (may be co-existent)
- Bursitis of Achilles tendon insertion
- Achilles tendinosis
- Calcaneal stress fracture
- Bone tumour.

Investigations
- Primarily a clinical diagnosis
- Plain radiographs—may show soft tissue swelling, calcifications, calcaneal avulsion fractures or Haglund's deformity
- USS—useful if rupture suspected. Will show inflammation in paratenon
- MRI—can show any degenerate change in the tendon (tendinosis)
- If other suggestive features, consider investigation for underlying medical condition, e.g diabetes mellitus, rheumatoid.

Treatment—conservative
- Rest, often for several weeks. May require cast immobilization
- NSAIDs
- Physiotherapy to improve strength and flexibility of calf muscles
- Appropriate shoes ± customized orthoses to control the foot position if biomechanics not optimized
- Weight loss if obese
- Corticosteroid injection generally contraindicated.

Treatment—surgical

Release ± excision of paratenon: release is performed on the dorsal, medial and lateral aspects of the tendon. Avoid anterior sheath as may compromise blood supply. Running may begin 6–10 weeks after surgery.

Prognosis

'Excellent' results reported in ~75% with conservative treatment, with mean recovery time 5 weeks. Surgical outcomes variable.

Prevention

Good stretching, footwear and training programme.

Complications

Chronic pain, tendon rupture.

Rupture of Achilles tendon

Complete or partial discontinuity of the Achilles tendon. Commonly 5cm proximal to insertion into the os calcis at the point of the 'vascular watershed' although can happen at any point in its length.

Epidemiology

Peak age 30–50yrs. M:F ~4:1

Risk factors

- Acute physical exertion, often unaccustomed
- Previous rupture
- Underlying tendinosis
- Recent steroid injection around tendon
- Systemic medication—steroids and quinolone antibiotics have been implicated.

History

Sudden sensation of or even audible snap in back of the heel whilst undertaking physical activity. Immmediate severe pain. Patient may believe they have been hit or kicked. Difficulty walking/climbing stairs/standing on tiptoes. Previous rupture or non-specific heel pain (suggestive of underlying tendinosis).

Exam

- Local soft tissue swelling/bruising
- Palpable gap at the site of rupture
- Degree of active plantarflexion does not excluded the diagnosis (intact deep flexor tendons) but power would be subnormal
- Simmond's test: with the patient prone calf muscles are squeezed— induced plantarflexion should be comparable with normal side, reduced if rupture.

Differential diagnosis

- Peritendonitis of Achilles tendon
- Ankle or calcaneal avulsion fracture
- Musculotendinous junction tear
- Gastrocnemius/soleus muscle tear.

Investigations

- Plain radiograph—to exclude fracture
- USS to confirm clinical diagnosis and estimate gap between tendon ends (if <5mm may indicate low re-rupture rate with non-operative treatment[1])
- MRI—for neglected/longstanding cases may provide useful information.

Treatment

Conservative

Regimes vary—below is a guideline

- Initial immobilization in gravity equinus cast for 3–4 weeks
- Progressively decrease amount of plantarflexion over next 3–4 weeks until plantigrade position achieved
- Weight-bearing plantigrade cast for final 3–4 weeks
- Total time in cast 9–12 weeks
- Refer to physiotherapy for progressive mobilization and strengthening
- Heel lift in shoe for 6–8 weeks after casting.

Surgery

- May be performed as an open or percutaneous technique
- End-to-end repair may be augmented with plantaris or peroneal tendons or gastrocnemius fascia (but usually reserved for re-rupture or late-presenting cases)
- Surgery reduces re-rupture rate from 12.6 to 3.5%, but at the cost of a significantly higher number of complications (wound dehiscence, infection, sural nerve damage)[2].

References

1 Kotnis R, David S, Handley R, *et al.* Dynamic ultrasound as a selection tool for reducing Achilles tendon reruptures. *Am J Sports Med* 2006;**34**:1395–400.

2 Khan RJK, Fick D, Keogh A, *et al.* Treatment of acute Achilles tendon ruptures—a meta-analysis of randomized, controlled trials. *J Bone Joint Surg Am* 2005;**87**:2202–10.

Plantar fasciitis

Definition
Degenerative change of the plantar fascia (sole of foot).

Epidemiology
Common in adults, usually in 3rd–5th decades.

Most common cause of heel pain.

Pathogenesis
It develops with repetitive **tensile overload** of the soft tissue attachments to the plantar aspect of the heel.

Pathology
Chronic degeneration at the origin of the plantar fascia. It is a degenerative and not an inflammatory condition. Central part of the deep fascia is attached to the medial plantar tubercle of the os calcis.

Aetiology
Idiopathic, obesity, prolonged standing, trauma, unaccustomed exercise. Possibly—pes planus or pes cavus.

Symptoms
Gradual onset of pain at the origin of the plantar aponeurosis, which is worse in the morning or after rest and increases with weight bearing. A relative heel cord contracture increases the symptoms and pain is more distal than in other causes.

Examination
Assess ankle and foot profile. Establish if the point of maximal tenderness is related to the medial calcaneal tuberosity. Increased with dorsiflexion of toes which tensions the plantar fascia. Tenderness over the medial longitudinal arch may occur.

Differential diagnosis
Heel pain triad—plantar fasciitis, posterior tibial tendon dysfunction and tarsal tunnel syndrome. Other causes of heel pain are calcaneal apophysitis, gout, pseudogout, Paget's disease, inflammatory arthritides or enthesopathies, heel fat pad atrophy and tumours.

Investigations
- Radiology—standing AP and lateral radiographs. 'Saddle sign' is present in 60% of cases of heel pain—radiolucency proximal to plantar calcaneal spur indicating fatigue of the calcaneal tuberosity. Heel spurs are not in the plantar fascia as is commonly thought but are found in the origin of the short flexors. A 45° medial oblique view is useful to diagnose a stress fracture. An axial view: may detect an occult bone tumour
- Bone scan—in planstar fasciitis there is a focal increase in uptake at the origin of the fascia

• Other—chronic cases may require screening to exclude metastatic and inflammatory conditions including HLA B27 if spondyloarthropathy is suspected.

Natural history

Usually a self-limiting condition.

Management

• *Non-operative treatment*: heel cord and plantar fascia stretching— physiotherapy, cast treatment, orthotics (valgus insole), night splints, analgesics and NSAIDs, intralesional steroid, extracorporeal shock wave therapy and oral steroids. A medial arch support that tilts the heel into varus may be helpful in treatment of plantar fasciitis in patients with pes planus. Steroid injection—injection of 0.1–0.2ml of corticosteroid from the medial side of the heel.
• *Operative treatment*: after failure of non-operative treatment (<5%). Most common procedure is a plantar fascia release. Excision of the plantar spur which is located at the origin of the FDB and not that of the plantar fascia is sometimes recommended.

For further reading, see Cullen and Singh[1] and League[2].

References

1 Cullen NP, Singh D. Plantar fasciitis: a review. *Br J Hosp Med* 2006;**67**:72–6.
2 League AC. Current concepts review: plantar fasciitis. *Foot Ankle Int* 2008;**29**:358–66.

Hallux valgus

Definition: Lateral deviation of the great toe at the MTPJ with medial deviation of the 1st metatarsal.

Aetiology

Family history in up to 65% of patients. Metatarsus primus varus (medial deviation of the 1st metatarsal), *acquired* hallux valgus from narrow shoe wear and splayed foot (weak intrinsics with increasing age). Common in patients with hyperlaxity syndrome or acquired laxity due to RA, gout or injury.

Anatomical factors

Distal metatarsal articular angle (DMAA), intermetatarsal angle (IMTA), hallux valgus angle (HVA), congruency of the MTPJ and interphalangeal angle (IPA).

Prevalence: Occurs in up to 30% of individuals. Females affected more than males.

Normal angles

Normal—IMTA <15°, HVA <9°, no incongruency, DMAA <100°.

Classification

- *Mild*—IMTA 15–20°, HVA 9–11°, no incongruency
- *Moderate*—IMTA 20–40°, HVA 11–18°, incongruence
- *Severe*—IMTA >40°, HVA >18°, incongruence.

History

Family history, age of onset, progression, shoe wear, main complaint (pain vs appearance), site of pain, activity level and expectations of surgery. Usually presents with pain over medial aspect of MTPJ. May have discomfort due to impingement of second toe.

Examination

Gait—look for normal push-off. Foot inspection—presence of a large bunion, great toe deformity at MTPJ and IPJ, lesser toe deformities, overriding and under-riding of lesser toes, pronation of the foot, site of pain. Ankle and subtalar movements, plantar callosities, metatarsal–cuneiform movement (if proximal procedures required) MTPJ, evidence of pain on movement. MTPJ (hallux rigidus). Neurovascular assessment.

Differential diagnosis: Gout, fracture malunion, congenital deformity.

Radiology

Weight-bearing AP and lateral views to measure angles. HVA, IMTA, DMAA, MTPJ congruency, evidence of degenerative changes of 1st MTPJ and IPJ, angulation of the 1st metatarsal cuneiform joint, relative lengths of the 1st and 2nd metatarsals. Position of the sesamoids.

Hallux valgus management

Non-operative treatment: always consider first. Wider shoes supplemented with a wide toe-box to prevent rubbing of the bunion, Metatarsal head pads, toe spacers for lesser toes, prescription shoes.

Operative options: surgery aims to establish a congruent 1st MTPJ with sesamoid realignment, correct IMTA and HVA. Resect medial eminence (bunion) and retain the 1st MTPJ motion and foot biomechanics.

Indications: failure of non-operative treatment, progressing deformity and pain, restricted function, cosmesis (controversial).

Groups: (1) congruent MTPJ, (2) incongruent or subluxed MTPJ, (3) hallux valgus with arthritis of MTPJ.

The wide array of surgical procedures indicates that there is disagreement on the best surgical procedure.

Soft tissue and bony procedures

Congruent MTPJ—Chevron and Mitchell's with or without distal soft tissue procedures.

Incongruent joint—treatment depends on the severity.
- Mild—Chevron osteotomy, Mitchell's osteotomy, distal soft tissue procedure
- Moderate—Mitchell's osteotomy, distal soft tissue and proximal osteotomy
- Severe—Scarf osteotomy, 1st MTPJ arthrodesis, proximal osteotomy

Osteotomies

Silver procedure—an exostectomy *with* removal of the painful medial eminence. High chance of recurrence.

Chevron—'V' type osteotomy at level of metatarsal neck with the centre of the metatarsal head used as the apex. The dorsal cut is at 60° to the metatarsal base and should avoid damage to the plantar vascularization. The dorsal cut is 45° to the cortex. Allows displacement to 50% of the width of the metatarsal head. Used to treat mild–moderate hallux valgus. The osteotomy is stable and may correct DMAA. Maximum displacement (30%). AVN occurs in up to 20% of cases.

Mitchell's—for moderate to severe deformity. Osteotomy proximal to metatarsal neck at the metaphyseal–diaphyseal junction with removal of a wedge of bone. Plantar flexes and medially displaces the distal part. The osteotomy may be potentially unstable and may require fixation. Shortens the 1st ray, altering the biomechanics of the foot. May lead to secondary metatarsalgia.

Scarf—consists of a horizontal cut and two transverse cuts allowing for a wide range of angular corrections. The procedure allows for medial and lateral translations, IMTA or DMAA correction, lowering/elevation of the metatarsal head, shortening/elevation of the 1st metatarsal. The procedure is technically difficult and has a learning curve. Internal fixation is required.

Akin's—medial closing wedge osteotomy at the level of the proximal phalanx base. Used to correct hallux interphalangeus. Always performed with a definitive hallux valgus procedure. Requires internal fixation usually with staples.

Basal osteotomy—for moderate to severe deformities. May be combined with other hallux valgus procedures. DMAA must be <20°. There is no shortening of the 1st metatarsal. Less commonly performed compared with other distal osteotomies.

- Opening wedge—when 1st MT shorter than the 2nd
- Crescentic proximal—closing wedge (shortens the metatarsal and is used when the 1st metatarsal is much larger than the 2nd)
- Crescentric shelf—basal osteotomy of choice as it provides good stability and avoids transfer metatarsalgia.

Complications

Recurrence, failure to correct the deformity, hallux varus and transfer metatarsalgia, AVN of metatarsal head. Non-union of the osteotomy.

Adolescents: up to 30% rate of recurrence postcorrection. This may be due to inadequate soft tissue release and failure to correct alignment.

For further reading, see Coughlin[1].

Reference

1 Coughlin MJ. Hallux valgus. *Instr Course Lect* 1997;**46**:357–91.

Hallux rigidus

Definition Degenerative changes at the first MTPJ.

Epidemiology Most common joint affected by OA in the foot. Occurs in 1 in 40 people >50yrs. Twice as common in women. Rare in children.

Adolescent—Localized lesions. Adult—generalized arthrosis.

Cause

Antecedent trauma, Osteochondral defect 1st metatarsal head, congenital elevation of the 1st metatarsal, RA, gout.

History

Insidious onset of pain and stiffness of the great toe increased on walking, running and wearing high-heeled shoes. Burning and paraesthesia. Leading to continuous pain.

Examination

Initial swelling and tender 1st MTPJ. Reduced dorsiflexion. Later, dorso-medial osteophyte (loss of motion, skin irritation), elevated (and long) first metatarsal.

Pseudohallux rigidus—nodular swelling of the proximal FHL limiting hallux dorsiflexion. FHL becomes constricted within its fibro-osseous tunnel; motion is restored on ankle plantarflexion.

Differential diagnosis Gout, RA, pseudohallux rigidus.

Radiology

Joint space narrowing, widening and flattening 1st metatarsal head and base of proximal phalanx, subchondral sclerosis and cysts, formation of dorsal osteophytes at the metatarsal head and proximal phalanx.

Management

Non-operative treatment: aimed at reducing MTPJ movement and relieving dorsal pressure. Metatarsal bar or rocker bottom shoe, NSAIDs, manipulation under anaesthetic (MUA) and intra-articular steroid injection, and cushioned shoe wear.

Operative options: indication is the failure of non-operative treatment.
• *Adolescents:* osteotomy of the base of the proximal phalanx—require preoperative 30° plantarflexion.
• *Adults:*
  • Cheilectomy for treatment of hallux rigidus will relieve only the dorsal impingement (dorsal spur and 1/3 metatarsal head)
  • Arthrodesis—following failed cheilectomy or where advanced degenerative changes are present
  • Arthroplasty—excise base of proximal phalanx
  • Keller's procedure—for the elderly.

For further reading, see Mann[1].

Reference

1 Mann RA. Hallux rigidus. *Instr Course Lect* 1990;**39**:15–21.

Hammer toe deformity

Definition
Abnormal fixed flexion posture of PIPJ of lesser toe with hyperextension of MTPJ and DIPJ. Associated with a contracture of the FDL tendon.

Associated
Long second metatarsal, high heels and narrow shoes. RA, diabetes mellitus, crossover deformity. Iatrogenic—postplantar release.

Epidemiology
Most common is the *2nd metatarsal*. May accompany a hallux valgus.

Differential diagnosis
Interdigital neuroma, claw toe, mallet toe and MTP synovitis.

History
Pain on plantar aspect of the metatarsal head, dorsum of the proximal phalanx and apex of the toe, deformity worse on walking (hammer toes are accentuated on weight bearing when the intrinsics are relaxed).

Examination
Callus formation over dorsum of PIPJ ± volar tip of the toe. Distinguish between a supple and fixed hammer toe (DIPJ remains supple). When there is contracture of the FDL tendon, then plantar flexion of the ankle will straighten the toe with dorsiflexion worsening the deformity. ± Subluxation of the stability of MTPJ hyperextension.

Management
Non-operative treatment: pads over corns and daily stretching of PIPJ. Hammer toe straightening orthotics + taping of toe to prevent further deformity.

Operative treatment: surgery indicated for disabling pain. Flexibility of the deformity determines techniques used, correct hallux valgus first.
- Flexible and mild deformity of PIPJ alone—isolated tenotomy of the FDL tendon, Girdlestone flexor-to-extensor transfer
- Moderate deformity and fixed contracture at PIPJ—arthroplasty, arthrodesis
- Severe deformity—partial proximal phalangectomy (poor cosmesis), MTPJ head arthroplasty (DuVries)
- MTPJ involvement—release EDL tendon, dorsal MTP capsule ± collateral ligaments. For dislocations, MTP resection arthroplasty
- DIPJ with nail deformity—consider amputation distal phalanx.

For further reading, see Coughlin[1].

Reference
1 Coughlin MJ. Lesser toe abnormalities. *Instr Course Lect* 2003;**52**:421–44.

Claw toe deformity

Hyperextension at the MTPJ and flexion at the PIPJ and DIPJ.

Pathogenesis

Imbalance between the extrinsic extensor tendons (which indirectly extend the MTPJ) and the intrinsics (which flex the MTPJ). The deformity results from simultaneous contraction of extensors and flexors and leads to the metatarsal fat pad being pulled distally through its attachment to the proximal phalanx.

Associated

Pes cavus and its neurological associations.

Differential diagnosis

Hammer toes (± MTPJ hyperextension).

Precipitating conditions

Age, RA, diabetes mellitus, post-traumatic compartment syndrome, polio, HSMN, CVA.

History

Pain under metatarsal heads, deformity, callosities, catching of the toes on walking and neurological symptoms.

Examination

- Neurological examination of the upper and lower limbs and look for a cavus foot. Is the deformity correctable? Assess flexibility of toes with ankle in planti–dorsiflexion; if the claw toe deformity disappears with plantiflexion then the deformity is considered flexible. Determine the degree of MTPJ hyperextension and PIPJ flexion. Look for trophic changes of the foot
- Assessment during gait: does the clawing become worse during the stance/swing phase?
- Swing phase weakness: may indicate weak ankle dorsiflexors and overcompensation of toe extensors
- Stance phase weakness: may indicate weak triceps surae and overcompensation of the long toe flexor.

Treatment

Non-operative treatment: corn pads, metatarsal pads and wide toe box in shoe wear.

Operative options: surgical correction depends on the size of the deformity and flexibility of the joints.
- Flexible claw toe implies that there is no contraction of the MTPJ or PIPJ—FDL tenotomy or Girdlestone flexor to extensor tendon transfer with capsulodesis of MTPJ
- Clawed hallux—Robert Jones tendon transfer
- Fixed claw toe

- MTPJ subluxation: MTPJ soft tissue release—extensor tenotomy, release of collateral ligaments ± shortening at the base of the proximal phalanx to aid reduction of MTPJ
- MTPJ dislocation: Stainsby procedure/DuVries metatarsal head arthroplasty with release of EDL, dorsal capsule and MCL
- PIP deformity: PIPJ fusion or resection arthroplasty (removing distal third of the proximal phalanx)
- Arthrodesis MTPJ: for severe or recurrent deformity, or when associated with neurological disturbance of forefoot.

Stainsby procedure: V–Y dorsal incision over MTPJ (single) or web space (multiple). Extensor tenotomy, remove 3/4 proximal phalanx and reduce fat pad under the metatarsal head. Suture distal extensor tendon end to the flexor tendon. Stabilize with a K wire.

For further reading, see Coughlin[1].

Reference

1 Coughlin MJ. Lesser toe abnormalities. *Instr Course Lect* 2003;**52**:421–44.

Lesser toe deformities

Common problems often leading to pain, deformity and problems with footwear. May be an associated hallux valgus which should be corrected first.

Aetiology

Constrictive footwear which restricts the normal movement of the lesser toe joints impeding intrinsic muscle function.

Examination

Is the deformity correctable? Presence of callosities, neurovascular status, subluxation of the MTPJ, presence of hallux valgus or tight FDL?

Deformities

Hammer toe: flexion at the PIPJ ± hyperextension of the MTPJ and DIPJ. Usually acquired. Often flexible early and fixed contracture late. See section on hammer toes (see 📖 p. 363) for treatment.

Mallet toe: flexion contracture of the DIPJ. Patients complain of toe stubbing which may lead to toe-tip pain.

Treatment—*operative options*: flexible FDL tenotomy at DIPJ. Fixed—DIPJ fusion and FDL tenotomy or terminal phalangectomy for severe deformities with abnormalities of the nail.

Claw toe: hyperextension at the MTPJs and flexion at the PIPJ and DIPJ. Usually involves several toes and may be associated with a neurological deformity. Non-operative treatment should be attempted—a deep and wide toe-box shoe, corn padding, and soft metatarsal pads. See section on claw toes (see 📖 p. 364) for operative treatment.

Curly toes: Flexion at both the PIPJ and the distal DIPJ, malrotation of one or more toes. A common disorder in childhood. May be related to contracture of the FDL and FDB tendons.

Treatment—reassurance of parents and initially non-operative. Operative options for pain, progression of deformity and problems with footwear or walking. FDL/FDB tenotomy (age 3–4yrs) or with a severe deformity Girdlestone tendon transfer is preferred.

Overlapping 5th toe: a dorsal adduction deformity of the 5th toe. There may be malrotation with EDL contracture. The deformity is often familial and bilateral. Often asymptomatic but can cause difficulty with footwear, dorsal toe pain, callus or a bunionette.

Treatment—most *treated non-operatively* with strapping. *Operative options* include DuVries correction, Butler's procedure or the Lapidus procedure.

Bunionette deformity: soft corn over the dorsal aspect of the 5th toe.

Classification:

- Enlargement of the MT head
- Lateral bowing of 5th metatarsal
- Wide 4–5th IMTA. A symptomatic plantar callus is secondary to plantar flexion of the fifth MT.

Treatment:

Non-operative initially—wide footwear, metatarsal pads and chiropodist treatment. Soft tissue surgery is unlikely to be successful.

Operative options for type 1: Chevron osteotomy, for type 2–3: midshaft medial displacement oblique osteotomy.

For further reading see Coughlin[1] and Harmondson and Harkless[2].

References

1 Coughlin MJ. Mallet toes, hammer toes, claw toes, and corns. Causes and treatment of lesser-toe deformities. *Postgrad Med* 1984;**75**:191–8.

2 Harmonson JK, Harkless LB. Operative procedures for the correction of hammertoe, claw toe, and mallet toe: a literature review. *Clin Podiatr Med Surg* 1996;**13**:211–20.

Ingrown toenails

Also known as onychocryptosis.

Epidemiology

Common in adolescents and young adults. Usually affects the hallux but other nails may be involved. Bilateral on occasion.

Pathology

Nail plate penetration of the lateral nail fold. A sharp spike of nail presses against the soft tissues and lateral nail fold. Excessive inflammatory response with granulation tissue that grows over the nail.

Aetiology

Tight-fitting shoes, poor foot care, inappropriate nail cutting (longitudinal).

Causes

Pain especially on wearing shoes, bacterial/fungal infection.

Management

Non-operative treatment: regular soaking and foot washing, well-fitting shoes, education on nail cutting (transversely), use of cotton wool pledgets under the nail to encourage outward growing and chiropodist referral.

Operative options: failure of non-operative treatment, recurrent infection, pain. The nail can be removed by avulsion of the whole nail or wedge resection of the involved side of the nail. Complications include recurrence and persistent infection. If simple avulsion fails, ablation of the nail bed should be considered. This can be achieved either chemically or surgically. Chemical ablation can be achieved with phenol. Surgical removal usually involves a Zadek's procedure. Two-stage procedure: in the presence of infection, the 1st stage involves removal of the nail to allow resolution of infection and a 2nd stage Zadek's procedure.

For further reading, see Rounding and Bloomfield[1].

Reference

1 Rounding C, Bloomfield S. Surgical treatments for ingrowing toenails. *Cochrane Database Syst Rev* 2005(**2**):CD001541.

The diabetic foot

Foot disease is common in type 1 and type 2 diabetes. The diabetic foot refers to a spectrum of diseases that include ulcers, bone or joint changes, and infection. The effect of the peripheral neuropathy is to impair protective sensation in the foot, and abnormal pressure may lead to callosities and formation of ulcers[1]. Healing is compromised by arterial and microvascular insufficiency. Infection can develop.

Prevalence 15–20% of patients with diabetes develop foot ulcers.

Assess general health status and establish control of diabetes.

Locally examine
- Shape of foot (bunions/pressure areas)
- Bunions, pressure areas
- Perfusion of the foot
- Sensation
- Movements (pain)
- Ulcers (clean or sloughy, do they probe to bone?)
- Evidence of gangrene.

Regular monitoring and self-management is key to successful management.

Investigation This should include:
- X-ray
- Doppler US
- Ankle–brachial pressure index (ABPI)
- MRI—to establish if there is osteomyelitis, and if so the extent.

Treatment

Non-surgical
- Optimize diabetic control
- Regular inspection and careful chiropody
- Well-fitting footwear with deep, wide toe-box and custom-moulded insole
- Prompt antibiotics for infection
- Total contact casting may be needed.

Surgical
- Debridement and active wound management (microbiology and appropriate antibiotic treatment)
- Local excision of osteomyelitis
- Ray amputation
- Partial foot amputation (Lisfranc or Chopart amputation)
- Below-knee amputation.

All patients with complications as a result of diabetes require multidisciplinary care by GPs, physicians, surgeons, nurse practitioners and community healthcare professionals.

Reference
1 Rathur HM, Boulton AJM. Recent advances in the diagnosis and management of diabetic neuropathy. *J Bone Joint Surg Br* 2005;**87**:1605–10.

Adult trauma

📖 Fractures are illustrated in the Appendices. See 📖 p. 606.

Assessment of the injured patient

Prompt assessment and treatment of trauma patients can save lives. The first 'Golden Hour' is the most important in serious trauma.

The ATLS (Advanced Trauma Life Support) approach is systematic and prioritizes life-threatening injuries. In 1976 an orthopaedic surgeon crashed his light aircraft into a field in Nebraska, USA. His wife died, 3 of his 4 children received critical injuries. So appalled was he at their local treatment he convened multidisciplinary groups to collate management protocols which form the basis for the ATLS manual (published by the American College of Surgeons). All doctors receiving major trauma should receive ATLS training, based around the 'ABCs':

Airway with cervical spine control
- Stabilize neck with a hard collar, sandbags and tape
- Open airway with jaw thrust if patient unconscious. Clear airway with suction or Magill's forceps to remove obstructions
- Maintain with orotracheal or nasotracheal airway if required.
- Give 100% oxygen.

Breathing
Is the patient breathing spontaneously? Look for signs of pneumothorax, open or sucking chest wound, flail chest: treat immediately. Consider also massive haemothorax and ruptured diaphragm. Ventilate if necessary.

Circulation
- Assess, establish IV access, arrange for urethral catheter
- If compromised look for external haemorrhage (apply elevation and pressure), signs of abdominal bleeding, pelvis instability (unstable pelvic injury with decompensated hypovolaemia in the absence of another cause mandates emergent pelvic external fixation)
- Consider also cardiac tamponade if signs of chest injury.

Now go back and reassess ABCs, again treating each significant injury before progressing down the algorithm.

Order *Trauma Series* of radiographs (chest, AP pelvis, cervical spine). Then continue as follows:

Disability
Patient able to talk?

Conscious level—*AVPU*: **A**lert, responding to **V**erbal stimuli, **P**ainful stimuli, **U**nresponsive.

Exposure
Remove all clothing.

Check for hypothermia, give warmed fluids and blankets/Bair hugger©.

Take an *AMPLE* history: **A**llergies, **M**edications, **P**ast medical history, **L**ast meal, **E**vents of injury.

Secondary survey

Head to toe examination with log roll (examine spine, perform rectal examination).

Give tetanus booster/Ig, antibiotics (for open fractures), analgesia as appropriate.

Arrange for definitive treatment of injuries, involving appropriate teams early.

Resuscitation of the injured patient

Principles of haemorrhagic shock resuscitation have been shaped by the wars of the 20th century:

- First World War—W.B. Cannon recommended delayed fluid resuscitation until cause of shock repaired surgically
- Second World War— crystalloids and blood used extensively
- Korean and Vietnam wars—volume resuscitation and early surgery recognized as key to surviving traumatic injuries.

In *hypovolaemic shock* rapid fluid loss results in multiple organ failure due to inadequate circulating volume and tissue perfusion unless recognized and treated early[1]. Volume losses up to 1.5litres may be well compensated in a fit young patient:

	Class I	Class II	Class III	Class IV
Blood loss (ml)	Up to 750	750–1500	1500–2000	>2000
% Volume loss	Up to 15%	15–30%	30–40%	>40%
Pulse	<100	>100	>120	>140
BP (mmHg)	Normal	Normal		
Pulse pressure (mmHg)	Normal or ↑			
Respiratory rate	14–20	20–30	30–40	>35
Urine output (ml/h)	>30	20–30	5–15	Negligible
CNS/mental status	Slightly anxious	Mildly anxious	Anxious, confused	Confused, lethargic
Fluid replacement	Crystalloid	Crystalloid	Crystalloid and blood	Crystalloid and blood

Careful monitoring of urine output and vital signs essential ± CVP catheter.

Dilutional coagulopathy a risk in massive fluid replacement requiring addition of FFP and platelets.

Reference

1 Graham CA, Parke TR. Critical care in the emergency department: shock and circulatory support. *Emerg Med J* 2005;**22**:17–21.

Soft tissue injuries

Closed fracture

Guidelines abound for wound management in open fractures, but less is written about closed soft tissue injuries. Recognition is critical; soft tissue response to blunt injury involves microvascular/inflammatory processes with local tissue hypoxia/acidosis. Incisions through compromised tissue predispose to wound breakdown and deep infection. Splinting, cryotherapy, compression and delayed surgery help limit further soft tissue injury and reduce complications[1]. Tscherne classification (opposite) is useful in assessing closed tibial shaft fractures.

Loss of skin wrinkles and palpable landmarks suggests moderate to severe swelling, loss of or delayed capillary refill indicates severe. Fracture blisters fall into two groups: clear fluid-filled and blood-filled. Both represent dermoepidermal cleavage injury; epidermis not viable in latter. Incision through blood-filled blister at higher risk of wound complication, so best avoided if possible.

Significant crush injury may institute a syndrome of muscle ischaemia, rhabdomyolysis and severe metabolic derangement requiring aggressive fluid rescuscitation ± renal support or dialysis.

Open fracture

Soft tissue assessment by operating surgeon for:
- Neurovascular status ± angiography
- Degree of soft tissue injury: classify according to Gustilo and Anderson[2]. Strictly done after wound excision but can estimate at this stage for planning
- Requirement for plastic surgeon input (IIIB/C injuries),

Photograph and cover wound, give IV antibiotics[3] ± tetanus prophylaxis and take to theatre (emergency) for definitive wound management:
- *Extension* to explore all affected tissue planes
- *Excision* of all contaminated and non-viable tissue
- *Irrigation*
- *Stabilize* fracture (reduces infection rate, improves tissue oxygenation)
- *Dress* to prevent contamination but allow fluid to leak away.

A vacuum dressing may be useful after wound excision, but in IIIB/C injuries definitive plastic surgical coverage within 72h produces lower rates of flap failure and deep infection, shorter time to union and shorter inpatient stay[4].

Tscherne classification of closed fractures and soft tissue injury

- C0: little or no soft tissue injury
- CI: superficial abrasion, mild to moderately severe fracture configuration
- CII: deep, contaminated abrasion with local contusional damage to skin or muscle, moderately severe fracture configuration
- CIII: extensive skin contusion or crushing or muscle destruction, severe fracture.

Compartment syndrome (see 📖 p. 402) can be considered the worst form of closed soft tissue injury.

References

1 Tull F, Borrelli J. Soft-tissue injury associated with closed fractures: evaluation and management. *J Bone Joint Surg Am* 2003;**11**:431–8.
2 Gustilo RB, Anderson JT. Prevention of infection in the treatment of one thousand and twenty-five open fractures of long bones: retrospective and prospective analyses. *J Bone Joint Surg Am* 1976;**58**:453–8.
3 Patzakis MJ, Harvey JP Jr, Ivler D. The role of antibiotics in the management of open fractures. *J Bone Joint Surg Am* 1974;**56**:532–41.
4 Godina M. Early micro-surgical reconstruction of complex trauma of the extremities. *Plast Reconstr Surg* 1986;**78**:285–92.

Burns

Majority thermal, also chemical and electrical. Hand burns common.

Damage depends on temperature and duration of burning; 3 categories:
- Superficial partial thickness (heal 7–14 days)
- Deep partial thickness (heal 14–21 days but scar contracts)
- Full thickness (will not heal unless small and by secondary intention).

Local oedema reaches peak at 24–36h (splint hand to prevent secondary contractures). Burned tissue contracts—may restrict breathing, distal circulation or cause muscle compartment syndrome requiring emergent full-thickness escharotomy.

Management

Initially ATLS (risk of inhalational injury with airway oedema; intubate early).

Burns >20% need fluid replacement; assess % body surface area by:
- Palmar hand surface (including fingers) = 1%
- Rule of Nines—head 9%, upper limbs 9%, anterior lower limb 9%, posterior lower limb 9%, trunk anterior 18%, trunk posterior 18%, genitals 1% (child—head 18%, upper limbs 9%, anterior lower limbs 7%, posterior lower limbs 7%, anterior trunk 18%, posterior trunk 13%).

Then give 4ml/kg Hartmann's solution per % burnt body surface area in first 24h (half given in the first 8h, rest over 16h).

Cling film useful emergency dressing (superficial partial thickness the most painful). Avoid ointments and silver sulfadiazine (makes wound depth assessment difficult due to discoloration).

Re-examine superficial partial thickness burns after 48h as may become deep; otherwise allow to heal. Treat definite full thickness with excision and grafting. Deep partial thickness burns controversial; whether to graft depends on site and extent.

Chemical burns

Acids, alkalis (penetrate deeper), petroleum products. Brush off any dry powder, then copious irrigation with water for minimum 30min.

Electrical burns

Deep tissue damage can occur, with skin appearing normal over deep muscle necrosis. Rhabdomyolysis causes myoglobin release and acute renal failure. As part of ATLS, push IV fluids aiming for large diuresis of 1.5–2ml/kg/h.

Head injury

Severe head injury often accompanies multiple injuries including fractures. Usually secondary to RTA but also falls, assault, occupational and leisure/recreational injury. Should be identified and managed appropriately as part of ATLS (D=disability)[1].

Primary brain injury (haemorrhage, axonal shearing)

Occurs at time of injury.

An orthopaedic surgeon receiving major trauma must prevent and treat secondary brain injury due to:

- Hypoxia
- Hypovolaemia and cerebral hypoperfusion
- Intracranial haematoma causing ↑ICP (CPP = BP–ICP)
- Other causes of ↑ICP: cerebral oedema, hypercapnia
- Epileptic fits (check blood glucose and gases, treat with IV diazepam ± phenytoin)
- Infection (prophylactic antibiotics for open fractures).

Consider cervical spine injury in all cases.

Assess conscious level with Glasgow Coma Scale (Table 9.1).

Identification of skull fracture with plain films important (significantly increases chance of intracranial haematoma) but must not delay CT scan if obvious severe injury[2].

Indications for CT scan, which should proceed only after adequate resuscitation and stabilization (may require intubation and ventilation):

- Skull fracture with GCS <15/15 or any neurological abnormality
- Deteriorating GCS (especially <12)
- Neurological deficit
- Multiple injuries requiring general anaesthetic and orthopaedic surgery
- Continuing symptoms or emerging signs after admission for observation.

Seek advice from neurosurgeon early for severe head injury; may recommend osmotic diuresis with mannitol to decrease ICP and 'buy time' to arrange transfer for definitive management (burr hole or craniotomy) or ICP monitoring.

In children <2yrs old, abuse is a common cause of head injury especially if subdural haematoma or retinal haemorrhage (involve paediatric team immediately).

For severe head injury with likely transfer to ITU/HDU, rigid internal or external fixation of fractures is advised to aid nursing care.

Table 9.1 Glasgow Coma Scale (GCS)

Eye opening	Best motor response	Best verbal response
	6 Obeys commands	
	5 Localizes pain	5 Orientated
4 Spontaneous	4 Withdraws to pain	4 Confused
3 To verbal commands	3 Decorticate (flexes)	3 Inappropriate
2 To pain	2 Decerebrate (extends)	2 Incomprehensible sounds
1 No response	1 No response	1 No response

Minimum score = 3, unconsciousness when no eye response and score <8.

References

1 Wyatt J, Illingworth R, Clancy M, et al. Oxford Handbook of Accident and Emergency Medicine, 2nd edn. Oxford: Oxford University Press, 2003.
2 The Royal College of Surgeons of England. Report of the Working Party on the Management of Patients with Head Injuries. London: The Royal College of Surgeons of England, 1999.

Chest trauma

Thoracic trauma carries an overall mortality of 10%, with chest injuries causing one quarter of all traumatic deaths. Prompt diagnosis and treatment is therefore essential. Can be broadly divided into blunt and penetrating depending on mechanism; however, approaches are similar and begin with ATLS.

Immediately life-threatening injuries should be identified as part of the primary survey: summarized by **ATOM FC**:

- **A** *irway obstruction*—foreign bodies, laryngeal injury, SCJ dislocation. Establishing a patent airway is the first priority
- **T** *ension pneumothorax*—a 'one-way valve' leak allows gas into pleural space which cannot leave
    - **Signs**—respiratory distress, tachypnoea, tachycardia, hypotension, hyper-resonance to percussion, unilateral absence of breath sounds, tracheal deviation *away* from the affected side, neck vein distension
    - **Management**—immediate decompression by insertion of a large bore needle into 2nd intercostal space in the midclavicular line of affected side. Then insert closed chest suction tube
- **O** *pen pneumothorax (sucking chest wound)*—caused by large defects of chest wall. With each breath, air passes through hole rather than into the lung. Ventilation therefore compromised leading to respiratory failure
    - **Management**—cover defect with sterile dressing secured on 3 sides, producing flutter-valve effect. Then insert formal closed chest suction tube on same side remote from wound. Definitive closure may be necessary after adequate resuscitation
- **M** *assive haemothorax*—cause of both respiratory impairment and haemodynamic shock
    - **Signs**—respiratory distress, shock, dullness to percussion, decreased air entry, whiteout seen on CXR
    - **Management**—restore blood volume by rapid crystalloid/ blood infusion through 2 large-bore cannulae. Decompress chest via closed chest suction tube. If 1500ml drained immediately or continued blood loss >200ml/h, thoracotomy indicated
- **F** *lail chest* –when ˅2 ribs broken in ˅2 places causing segment of chest wall to move independently; respiratory compromise exacerbated by pain ± underlying pulmonary contusions. May require intubation and ventilation
- **C** *ardiac tamponade*—bleeding between fibrous pericardium and myocardium, impairing cardiac output
    - **Signs**—may be subtle, include: shock, muffled heart sounds, raised JVP (Beck's triad). Transthoracic echocardiogram may diagnose (but significant false (–)ve rate).
    - **Management**—urgent thoracotomy or needle pericardiocentesis if no thoracic surgeon available.

Secondary survey

- *Simple pneumothorax*—usually requires decompression via a chest drain. **Always** drain a simple pneumothorax in a patient who is to be intubated or transported via air ambulance (may become tension, especially under positive pressure ventilation)
- *Pulmonary contusion*—respiratory failure may develop over time and require ventilatory support
- *Blunt myocardial injury*
  - **Signs**—hypotension, ECG changes (multiple ventricular ectopics, atrial fibrillation, bundle branch block and ST changes). Transthoracic echocardiogram indicated
  - **Management**—monitor for sudden dysrhythmia (risk decreases after first 24h)
- *Traumatic diaphragmatic rupture*—associated with both blunt and penetrating trauma and polytrauma (chest, pelvis, spleen and liver). May present late with respiratory compromise, pleural collection or intestinal obstruction/strangulation. CXR or CT for diagnosis, though sensitivity ~66% with laparoscopy as gold standard. Mandates surgical repair
- *Multiple rib fractures*—may cause significant respiratory compromise due to pain. Appropriate analgesia or intercostal blocks, adequate monitoring mandatory.

Chest drain insertion

- Palpate for 5th intercostal space (~nipple level) just anterior to mid axillary line
- Position patient's arm above head to expose area
- Surgically prepare and drape, infiltrate skin and deep tissues with local anaesthetic. Discard the trocar if the set has one
- Make a 2–3cm transverse incision and use forceps to bluntly dissect over top of the inferior rib
- Clear and pierce pleura, dilate hole with forceps, and finger sweep to clear any adhesions
- Use forceps to guide tube into chest and suture skin either side. Suture drain to skin and reinforce with 'sleek' tape
- Connect tube to the underwater-seal apparatus at ground level, look for fogging of tube and 'swinging' of water in the drain container to confirm expulsion of air from pleural space with respiration
- Obtain a check CXR to identify drain tip.

Abdominal injuries

The primary danger of abdominal injury is life-threatening haemorrhage (ATLS: C = circulation).

History
- Blunt injury—was patient restrained in vehicle, ejected, did an airbag deploy?
- Penetrating injury: time of injury, type of weapon.

Examination
Haemodynamically stable or decompensated?
- Inspection:
  - penetrating injuries, bruises, seatbelt marks, evisceration
  - blood at urethral meatus, scrotal or perineal haematoma to suggest urethral injury
- Palpation:
  - localized or generalized tenderness
  - rectal exam: high riding prostate (urethral injury), sphincter tone (spinal injury), gross blood (viscus perforation).

If patient is haemodynamically unstable with evidence of abdominal injury then proceed to *immediate* laparotomy.

Accurate clinical assessment may be compromised by co-existent alcohol intoxication, brain or spinal cord injury, or injury to adjacent structures such as the ribs or pelvis.

Investigations
- *CXR* for pneumoperitoneum, though unlikely to be visible on supine trauma film
- *FAST scan:* focused assessment with sonography for trauma
  - rapid, non-invasive tool for detecting abdominal free fluid, splenic and liver injuries
  - 86–97% sensitive (significant false (−)ve rate)
  - Poor for bowel, diaphragmatic and pancreatic injuries
- *CT scan*
  - high specificity and sensitivity
  - accurate at detecting free fluid and organ injury to guide decision for laparotomy
  - time consuming and requires transfer to poorly controlled environment so suitable only for haemodynamically **stable** patient
- Diagnostic peritoneal lavage
  - Now very rarely performed in the UK
- Retrograde urethrography
  - Must be performed before urethral catheterization if urethral injury is suspected.

Indications for laparotomy

- Blunt abdominal trauma in a haemodynamically unstable patient
- Hypotension with penetrating abdominal wound
- Bleeding from the stomach, rectum or genitourinary tract from penetrating trauma
- Gunshot wounds traversing the peritoneum
- Evisceration
- Free air, retroperitoneal air or diaphragmatic injury on CT.

Urogenital injuries

Include injuries to bladder, urethra and external genitalia. Usually associated with pelvic fractures and polytrauma; bladder ruptures in 6%, urethral rupture in 2% and combination of both in 0.5% of pelvic fractures[1].

Preliminary assessment

- ATLS protocol on all
- Appropriate analgesia
- Physical examination must precede urethral catheterization and include inspection of external genitalia, perineum and digital rectal examination
- Characterize associated fractures for stability on plain X-rays
- If haemodynamically stable—abdominal/pelvic CT with IV contrast indentifies pelvic (bladder, rectum) and abdominal organ injury (liver, bowel, spleen)

Urethral injuries

Urethra in males is more fixed and prone to injury than in females.

Two levels of injury with different mechanisms:
- Posterior (membranous urethra)—high energy pelvic ring fractures
- Anterior (bulbar and pendulous urethral segments)—straddle injury.

Signs and symptoms of urethral injury

- Blood at the urethral meatus
- Gross haematuria
- Inability to pass urine
- Perineal or scrotal bruising
- 'High riding' prostate
- Inability to pass a urethral catheter.

Management

- Patient should be discouraged from passing urine if rupture of urethra is suspected (may aggravate extravasation of urine)
- Retrograde urethrogram
- One gentle attempt to place a urethral catheter in suspected urethral injuries is acceptable[2]. If any resistance proceed to retrograde urethrography to delineate the urethral injury. If urethral rupture, place a large suprapubic cystostomy tube and plan for later surgical exploration
- If urethra is intact do retrograde cystogram to exclude bladder injury.

Bladder injuries

Mechanisms

- Blunt trauma (75%)
- RTA with pelvic fracture
  - Rapid deceleration injury (e.g. seatbelt injury with full bladder in the absence of pelvic fracture)
- Penetrating trauma
- Gunshot or knife wounds
  - Bony spicule from fractured pelvis.

Types of bladder rupture
- Extraperitoneal rupture—(most common), the peritoneum is intact and urine escapes into the space around the bladder
- Intraperitoneal rupture—the peritoneum over the bladder is breached allowing urine to escape into the peritoneal cavity.

Symptoms and signs
The classic triad of:
- Suprapubic pain and tenderness
- Difficulty or inability in passing urine
- Haematuria.

Investigations
- Retrograde cystography or CT cystography
  - Exclude urethral injury before Foley catheterization
  - Bladder is distended with contrast and cystogram can be obtained
  - A postdrain film is obtained to exclude posterior bladder perforation.

In extraperitoneal perforations, extravasation of contrast is limited to surrounding the bladder. In intraperitoneal perforations, loops of bowel may be outlined by the contrast.

Treatment
- Intraperitoneal—laparotomy and suturing of bladder rupture
- Extraperitoneal
  - If urethral catheter is passed, leave the catheter for 2–3 weeks until the bladder is healed + antibiotics
  - If there are combined bladder and urethral injuries then a suprapubic catheter should be placed (via open approach) along with repair of the bladder.

Injuries to scrotum and testis

Blunt trauma, with crushing of the genitals, may cause damage to scrotum and testis. Scrotal swelling after trauma suggests a ruptured testis or ruptured pampiniform plexus of veins.

Clinical examination shows a haematocele which is non-transilluminant (transilluminant = hydrocele). US examination effective in diagnosing ruptured testis, which requires urgent surgical exploration.

References
1 Cass AS. *Genitourinary Trauma.* Boston: Blackwell Scientific Publications, 1988.
2 McAninch JW. In: Walsh PC, Retik AB, Vaughan ED, *et al.,* eds. *Campbell's Urology,* 8th edn. Saunders: Philadelphia, 2002:3703–14.

Vascular injuries

Extremity vascular injuries may be caused by blunt (RTA, falls from height, crush injury) or penetrating trauma (stab, bullet, blast injuries) or be iatrogenic during emergency or elective surgery.

Common association is with fracture and/or dislocations around knee, elbow, femoral and humeral shafts. These injuries may also be complicated by nerve injury or compartment syndrome.

Arterial injury types range from kinking, spasm or intimal flap to laceration, segmental loss and arteriovenous fistula (if adjacent vein is injured).

Initial management

- Fluid resuscitate and identify associated life-threatening injuries
- Direct pressure (pad and bandage) to external bleeding (avoid direct use of arterial clamps which can damage vessels and nerves). Likewise tourniquets are best avoided as they occlude collateral vessels
- Adequate analgesia
- IV antibiotics if open fracture, tetanus cover as indicated, dress and cover wound
- Bloods to include cross-match, FBC, U&E ± CPK, ABG, coagulation screen, urinalysis (check for myoglobinuria)
- Appropriate radiographic evaluation.

Examination

Reliable signs of vascular injury

- Pain, pallor and paraesthesia
- Cold limb
- Absent or reduced pulse to palpation ± Doppler ultrasonography
- Expanding haematoma, bruit, thrill
- Active bleeding.

Less specific signs of vascular injury

- Proximity of wound to major vessels
- Non-expanding haematoma
- Anatomically related nerve injury
- History of haemorrhage/shock.

ABPI: ratio is obtained by systolic pressure in the ankle (for suspected lower limb vascular injury) divided by systolic pressure in the arm:

- if ABPI is >0.85 to 0.90, close observation
- if ABPI is <0.85, arteriography is indicated.

Ongoing management

Prompt reduction of fracture may restore inflow to the limb.

Once diagnosis of vascular injury is established, involve vascular surgeons early. Where possible, rapid stabilization of associated fracture or joint disruption with external fixation or other device is indicated prior to vessel exploration and reconstruction. Often the location of the vessel injury is obvious, e.g. brachial artery injury over supracondylar fracture, and can be directly explored; in other situations an on-table arteriogram may be indicated.

After any significant period of ischaemia, strongly consider prophylactic fasciotomy(s) following revascularization.

NB: have a high index of suspicion for compartment syndrome (see 📖 p. 402) in crush injuries. In this condition, if you wait for the pulses to disappear irreversible ischaemic damage is likely to have occurred.

Pelvic fractures with haemorrhage are a special situation. If external fixation (to reduce and tamonade the intrapelvic volume) fails to control blood loss then selective embolization with angiography of feeder vessels is indicated.

Knee dislocation

The incidence of popliteal artery injury in knee dislocations is ~20% (common in anterior dislocations)[1]. Tenderness, swelling and ecchymosis in the popliteal fossa indicate prompt exploration and repair (should be done within 6–8h).

Arteriography should be performed in knee dislocations with questionable circulation, even when there are satisfactory distal pulses restored after reduction[2].

References

1 Kennedy JC. Complete dislocation of knee joint. *J Bone Joint Surg Am* 1963;**45**:889.
2 Canale SR, Beaty J, eds. *Campbell's Operative Orthopaedics*, 11th edn. St Louis: Mosby Elsevier, 2007.

cord injuries

Incidence
Highest in young males in their 2nd and 3rd decades.

Types
Incomplete
- Central cord syndrome: most common. Greater loss of upper limb motor function than lower limb motor and sacral function.
- Anterior cord syndrome: loss of motor function and pain and temperature sensation blow injury
- Posterior cord syndrome: very uncommon. Loss of vibration and light touch sensation along with loss of proprioception
- Brown–Sequard syndrome: uncommon injury. Ipsilateral loss of motor function, light touch, proprioception and vibration sense, and contralateral loss of deep pain and temperature sense.

Complete—no cord function below level of the injury.

Aetiology
- Trauma (usually blunt)
- Associated with multiple injuries
- Co-existence of spinal cord injury and traumatic brain injury.

All patients with multiple injuries must be assumed to have an unstable spinal injury. The spine must be protected until formally cleared.

Primary injury is as a result of initial trauma. It involves one or more of the following mechanisms—compression, contusion, distraction, laceration, shear and missile injury.

Secondary injury is as a result of the molecular and cellular events that lead to further tissue trauma. It includes ischaemia, intracellular calcium influx, free radical-associated lipid peroxidation and glutaminergic toxicity. Apoptosis has also been observed. Goal of treatment is aggressive early treatment and prevention of secondary injury mechanisms.

Acute care
Management at scene
- Assess and resuscitate according to ATLS principles
- Assume there is a spinal injury in the case of any serious accident, presence of multiple injuries or in the unconscious patient
- Prevent further injury by protecting the spine
  - Avoid moving unless necessary. If patient head to be moved, keep head in neutral position, immobilize entire spine and 'log roll' if required.
  - Apply hard cervical collar and transfer to spine board (taking care to use log roll technique)
  - Fully immobilize cervical spine with collar, sandbags and straps.
  - If intubation required maintain cervical spine in neutral position by applying gentle in-line traction
  - Transport swiftly to hospital.

Management in hospital

- Assess and resuscitate patient according to ATLS guidelines
- Adequate perfusion and oxygenation crucial for optimal recovery and to prevent secondary injury
- Assess for spinal shock (loss of somatic motor, sensory and sympathetic function and unopposed vagal parasympathetic vasodilation after spinal cord injury leads to relative hypovolaemia and hypotension)
  - Hypotension without tachycardia
  - Skin warmth and hyperaemia
  - Complete anaesthesia and flaccid paralysis below level
  - Absent tendon reflexes
  - Urinary retention
  - Severity and duration correlate with the severity and level of injury
  - Treatment of spinal shock involves use of vasopressor agents (dopamine, dobutamine and noradrenaline)
- Hypotension from spinal shock is much less common than that due to hypovolaemia and is considered only after adequate volume replacement and other sources of ongoing bleeding are excluded
- Early restoration of spinal alignment is important—postural reduction or traction
- The use of methylprednisolone is controversial—consult local spinal cord injury unit for advice, many do not use it at all
- Skin care: turn patient every 2h between supine, right and left lateral positions. Can use Stoke Mandeville bed (turns patient electronically)
- Catheterize to decompress the bladder
- Consider anticoagulation
- Complete secondary survey
- Surgery. Early vs late decompression and stabilization remains controversial but deteriorating neurology associated with persistent spinal cord compression is a widely accepted indication for early surgery.

Prognosis

Ultimate outcome depends on multiple factors, including concomitant musculoskeletal and brain injuries. Degree of residual motor function is important. Recovery of spasticity in an incomplete lesion may be >1yr.

For further reading, see Bracken et al.[1] and Fehlings and Phan[2].

References

1 Bracken MB, Shepard MJ, Holford TR, et al. Administration of methylprednisolone for 24 or 48 h or tirilazad mesylate for 48 h in the treatment of spinal cord injury. Results of the Third National Acute Spinal Cord Injury Randomised Controlled Trial. *JAMA* 1997;**277**:1597–604.
2 Fehlings MG, Phan N. Spinal cord and related injuries. In: Brinker MR, ed. *Review of Orthopaedic Trauma*. Saunders 2001:348–50.

Sprains

A sprain is an injury to the ligaments around a joint. This commonly occurs at the ankle joint.

Some or all of the fibres of the ligament may rupture, producing a varying degree of joint instability. A ligament which appears grossly intact may have been stretched beyond its elastic range causing permanent plastic deformation; it is now functionally incompetent.

History
- Timing and mechanism of injury
- Position of joint during injury, e.g. inversion/eversion of the ankle
- Location of pain
- Ability to weight bear after injury
- Previous functional ability and history of injuries.

Examination
- Examine joint for evidence of swelling, bruising, haemarthrosis, tenderness
- Palpate for bone or soft tissue tenderness; feel for fracture crepitus
- Examine for and document neurovascular status
- Assess range of joint movement and compare with contralateral side
- Assess stability of joint by performing appropriate special tests.

Investigations
X-ray to exclude fracture. US or MRI to exclude rupture.

Management
- RICE: rest, ice, compression bandage, elevation
- Analgesia.

A ligament sprain associated with ongoing, symptomatic functional incompetence may require repair or advancement, e.g. Brostrum lateral ankle ligament advancement.

Dislocations

Defined by joint surfaces which are completely displaced and no longer in contact. Examples:
- High energy injuries, e.g. RTA dashboard impact causing hip dislocation
- Fracture–dislocation, e.g. bimalleolar ankle fracture with talar shift
- Developmental, e.g. hip dislocation in newborn, knee dislocation in Larsen's syndrome
- Neurological, e.g. subluxation (partial dislocation) and dislocation of hip in CP or high level spina bifida
- Prosthetic, e.g. THR dislocation
- Malalignment, e.g. patellar instability.

In cases of traumatic dislocation, ask about:
- Mechanism of injury and speed of impact if RTA
- Previous dislocations; may be recurrent if bone or soft tissue restraints incompetent
- Associated injuries, especially if history of high energy transfer or dislocation consistent with this
- Ligamentous laxity, e.g. Marfan syndrome, Ehlers–Danlos variants if recurrent or low energy mechanism.

Examine for
- Obvious deformity of joint with displaced bony landmarks
- Decreased and painful range of joint movement
- Characteristic limb position, e.g. leg shortened, rotated with hip dislocation
- Other injuries, especially abdominal, chest, spine and head
- Neurovascular injuries, e.g. traumatic knee dislocation.

Investigations
- X-rays: for diagnosis and to look for associated fractures (a trauma series of views may be indicated)
- CT scan to look for bony fragments within joint if associated fracture suspected, e.g. hip dislocation with posterior rim fracture of acetabulum
- MRI to visualize soft tissue structures sometimes required.

Management
- Resuscitation: ATLS protocol for high energy injury
- Prompt joint reduction—this is a true orthopaedic emergency. Have low threshold for X-ray, e.g. to exclude femoral neck fracture prior to pulling a dislocated hip, which may be best done in operating room under image intensifier once patient stabilized. Less critical for, for example, dislocated ankle where restoration of vascularity to foot mandates immediate reduction in the Emergency department
- Stabilize associated fractures
- Soft tissue considerations; primary or delayed closure for open injuries after thorough wound debridement, plastics coverage where necessary.

Complications

- Vascular and neurological injury
- AVN: especially femoral head, scaphoid in transscaphoid perilunate wrist dislocation, talar body AVN in case of talar neck fracture
- Heterotopic ossification, especially with associated head injury; consider prophylaxis with oral indomethacin
- Joint stiffness, contracture or persistent instability
- Secondary OA.

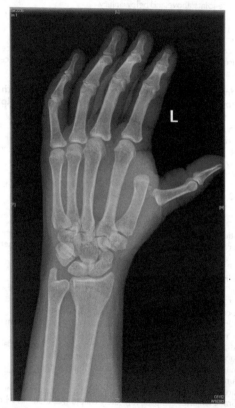

Fig. 9.1 Dislocated thumb metacarpophalangeal joint.

Fractures

General approach to all fractures

- History to include mechanism of injury, areas of pain indicating associated injuries, neurovascular symptoms, joint symptoms above and below suspected fracture. Also ATLS AMPLE history.
- Radiographic evaluation
  - Always 2 good quality orthogonal views
  - Image joints above and below injury
- CT scan useful to delineate fractures poorly seen on plain films, e.g. some foot fractures, tibial plateau and for preoperative planning of hardware placement perpendicular to fracture lines
- MRI scan for soft tissue injuries (or USS, e.g. suspected quadriceps rupture) and in fractures equivocal on plain films, e.g. undisplaced femoral neck fracture.

Open fractures require careful evaluation for which the following classification (Gustilo and Anderson[1]) is helpful

- Grade I: skin opening <1cm, clean, little soft tissue damage
- Grade II: >1cm long, extensive soft tissue damage, minimal to moderate crush
- Grade III: extensive soft tissue damage including skin, muscle and neurovascular structures, severe crushing component includes farmyard injuries.
  - IIIA adequate soft tissue bone coverage, gunshot wounds
  - IIIB periosteal stripping and bone exposure usually with contamination
  - IIIC vascular injury requiring repair and neurological injury.

The critical difference between IIIA and IIIB is that sufficient tissue for closure remains after wound excision (debridement) in the former.

Treatment

- Local irrigation and photograph if necessary
- Cover with poviclone-iodine-soaked sterile dressing and avoid repeated exposure
- Temporary stabilization with traction or splint/plaster of Paris
- IV antibiotics (Gram (+)ve cover with cephalosporin and Gram (−)ve cover with aminoglycoside if contaminated)
- Gross contamination, farmyard injuries and suspected clostridial infections require high dose penicillin in addition
- Tetanus booster if indicated or immunoglobulin for severe contamination
- Prepare for emergency debridement in operating theatre within 6h (Grade I injuries can probably safely wait longer than this with antibiotic cover).

Perioperative fracture considerations

- Thromboprophylaxis—DVTs common in the fracture population; particularly lower limb and pelvis fractures
- Fat embolism syndrome—typically after pelvic or femur fractures with symptom onset at 24–72h. Hypoxia, confusion, petechiae and tachycardia occur. Treatment principally supportive (oxygen); previously common in young males with femoral shaft fracture, less so now with early intramedullary stabilization
- Heterotopic ossification—associated with head injury, acetabular fractures, periarticular elbow surgery. Prophylaxis includes low dose indometacin 25mg daily for 6 weeks. Local radiation postoperatively (800rads) can also be used. Usually develops at 3–6 months
- All surgery with an implant requires prophylactic antibiotic cover; typically broad spectrum with a cephalosporin, but follow local guidelines.

Reference

1 Gustilo RB, Anderson JT. Prevention of infection in the treatment of one thousand and twenty-five open fractures of long bones: retrospective and prospective analyses. *J Bone Joint Surg Am* 1976;**58**:453–8.

Stab wounds

Knife injuries usually, but also glass, screwdrivers, etc. When penetrating object removed the skin contracts so wound appears smaller than original blade. Depth greater than length, difficult to assess externally. Very little force can produce deep injury.

In any laceration, establish

- Site and extent of any associated haemorrhage
- Whether nerve or tendon damage
- Likely depth and path of wound. Probing in Emergency room may give false impression of true depth; have low threshold for formal exploration in operating theatre.

Abdominal and chest wall stabbings require particularly careful assessment. Chest and neck wounds require CXR in search of pneumo/haemopneumothorax. For abdominal stab wounds CT may be required if suspected penetration into peritoneum. Diagnostic peritoneal lavage may be a useful adjunct but is not accurate enough to be used exclusively and is rarely performed in the UK today. Haemodynamic instability with abdominal stab injury mandates emergent laparotomy.

Stab wounds of the chest without evidence of intrathoracic injury can be appropriately managed with limited observation and follow-up inspiratory and expiratory radiographs after 6h[1].

Emergent management

- Cardiopulmonary resuscitation according to ATLS
- Continuous pressure to control bleeding (not tourniquet)
- Temporarily cover sucking chest wound with 3-sided flap dressing
- Tetanus booster or immunoglobulin ± antibiotic cover
- Antibiotic prophylaxis if closed suction chest tube insertion indicated[2].

Definitive management depends on location and extent of wound. Abdominal and chest injuries should be explored if indicated with general and cardiothoracic teams, respectively. For limb injuries, exploration indicated if significant contamination or evidence of tendon, nerve or vessel injury. The assistance of a plastic or vascular surgeon may be advisable.

References

1 Brown PF 3rd, Larsen CP, Symbas PN. Management of the asymptomatic patient with a stab wound to the chest. *Southern Med J* 1991;**84**:591–3.
2 Cant PJ, Smyth S, Smart DO. Antibiotic prophylaxis is indicated for chest stab wounds requiring closed tube thoracostomy. *Br J Surg* 1993;**80**:464–6.

Gunshot wounds

Widespread availability of civilian firearms and a constant level of global conflict require a clear understanding of these injuries[1].

Wounding potential depends on the amount of kinetic energy the projectile can impart to its target, which is dependent on:

- *Velocity* primarily: E (kinetic energy) = $1/2mv^2$ so increased velocity has more dramatic effect on energy than changes in mass
- *Terminal ballistics*—the behaviour of the projectile in its biological target.

The traditional distinction of firearms into high and low velocity is somewhat arbitrary; nonetheless high velocity bullet wounds (all military rifles) are four times as lethal as low velocity (most handguns).

Mechanisms of injury

- Primary missile injury; permanent and temporary cavitation
- Shockwaves causing rupture of hollow gas-filled organs, e.g. bowel, bladder
- Secondary projectiles from fragmentation of bone as well as bullet
- Discharge gasses exiting the barrel pass into wound track if close range
- Contamination from clothing or other material drawn into wound.

Management

Modern strategy continues to evolve; in First World War 90% of gunshot wounds became infected with streptococci, a major cause of death. Antibiotics and rapid evacuation from the battlefield challenge the traditional military practice of extensive and aggressive debridement of all tissue in the zone of injury; modern high energy weapons leave large exit wounds which provide decompression[2]. Adequate wound drainage must be achieved, but the following are reasonable recommendations:

- Resuscitation according to ATLS protocol
- Tetanus prophylaxis and appropriate IV antibiotics
- Debridement of all grossly necrotic tissue, bony fragments and foreign material
- Pulsed lavage may be useful for wound cleansing
- All lead shot (shotgun wounds) does not need removal.

Wound may be primarily closed if it is <6h old, appropriate antibiotics have been given and there is no gross contamination. Otherwise leave open with a view to delayed primary closure if appropriate.

References

1 Bulstrode C, Buckwater J, Carr A, et al., eds. *Oxford Textbook of Orthopaedics and Trauma.* Oxford: Oxford University Press, 2002.

2 Fackler M, Breteau JP, Courbil LJ, et al. Open wound drainage versus wound excision in treating the modern assault rifle wound. *Surgery* 1989;**105**:576–84.

Polytrauma

Look for common patterns in the multiply injured patient with significant energy transfer:

- Falls from height—calcaneal, other limb and spinal fractures
- Head injury and associated C-spine/thoracic spine fractures
- Lap belts and thoraco/lumbar spine fracture and abdominal visceral injuries
- Pelvic fracture and urological, gynaecological, colorectal and spinal injury
- Ejection from vehicle following RTA signifies high risk of multiple and severe injuries.

Such patients require the immediate attention of a dedicated trauma team—including anaesthetist, orthopaedic and general surgeons, emergency department doctors and specialist nursing staff. Triage is necessary first if multiple polytrauma patients. Decision making in the 'Golden Hour' is critical, with resuscitation starting immediately and sequentially according to the ATLS ABC protocol in the 'Platinum 10 minutes'.

Monitored patient resuscitation and stabilization is the key to initial management and may include early surgical intervention for haemorrhage if not responding to resuscitation. Do not focus on a mangled extremity before ABC management (life before limb). The extent of polytrauma may not become apparent until secondary survey which may be delayed by life-saving interventions. Beware later of distracting injuries and missing smaller fractures. Also beware compartment syndrome and other missed but serious injuries in the unconscious patient.

Imaging in polytrauma

- X-ray evaluation of spine is necessary in unconscious patient. Lateral C-spine film is initial but not definitive series (AP and peg views)
- USS—consider in resuscitation room to assess for free fluid in the abdomen
- CT—used for head, spine, chest, abdomen and pelvic evaluation.
- MRI if spinal cord injury

NB: the role of CT/MRI must be carefully evaluated in polytrauma patients, as clinical deterioration is not uncommon in the scanner where monitoring and ongoing resuscitation are difficult. Once there, try to image all relevant areas, e.g. CT head; include spine views.

Definitive management

Life-threatening injuries are initially treated by neurosurgical, cardio-thoracic, general surgical/vascular and (pelvic) orthopaedic teams as appropriate. This may involve urgent transfer. Subsequent priorities then include orthopaedic (including spine), maxillofacial, ophthalmic and non-haemorrhagic visceral injuries requiring surgery. Sometimes differing injuries of equal importance may be dealt with by parallel surgical teams at the same time, e.g. maxillofacial and lower limb orthopaedic injuries.

Multiple fracture management

Assuming ATLS protocol and resuscitation performed initially, then trauma and orthopaedic priorities include:

- Unstable pelvic fractures with associated haemorrhage
- Fractures with vascular injury compromising limb viability
- Compartment syndrome
- Open fractures
- Debridement of devitalized or severely contaminated tissue
- Long bone fractures (lower limb stabilized before upper limb)
- Unstable spinal fractures with or without neurological deficit
- Dislocated joints and intra-articular fractures.

NB: pelvic fractures are associated with life-threatening haemorrhage, but always consider other bleeding sources and whether the fracture pattern is unstable before proceeding to external fixation. Nonetheless given the correct indications, this is potentially a life-saving manoeuvre.

Damage control orthopaedics

Early stabilization of long bone fractures (typically femoral shaft) is generally a good thing but caution is required in the polytraumatized patient. Analogous is a bath of finite capacity into which is poured perhaps a certain level of preinjury morbidity followed by any number of chest, abdominal, head and long bone injuries. Add in systemic hypoperfusion from haemorrhage and there is not much room left for definitive treatment without the bath overflowing; embolization of marrow products during intramedullary nailing, for example, is a potent factor in the development of adult respiratory distress syndrome (ARDS), systemic inflammatory response syndrome (SIRS) and later end-organ failure. This is the concept behind so-called damage control orthopaedics, doing the minimum (which may involve temporary external fixation) to stabilize fractured long bones until adequate resuscitation (measured by end-points such as BP, urinary output, heart rate, base deficit and serum lactate levels) has been achieved.

Compartment syndrome

Increased pressure in a closed fascial space causing muscle ischaemia[1]

The insult occurs at the capillary bed level, where increased pressure in the muscle compartment causes venous collapse, increased capillary pressure and extravasation of fluid. As pressure rises the muscle becomes ischaemic, but large arterial vessels passing through the compartment remain patent due to their high intraluminal pressures and thick walls. If you wait for the '5 Ps' (pulselessness especially) you will miss the boat. The cardinal clinical sign is pain on passive stretching of an involved muscle.

Muscle ischaemia progresses rapidly to necrosis with subsequent fibrosis and disabling contractures. Long-term changes become inevitable 4–6h into an evolved compartment syndrome, becoming irreversible after 12h. Thus decompression is required as an emergency.

Presentation

Lower leg and forearm flexor compartments are the most common sites by far, but the syndrome can occur anywhere that muscles are bound in fascial envelopes. Usually seen with fracture, e.g. tibial shaft, supracondylar elbow, but may be minimal trauma without fracture. Also seen after reperfusion in crush injuries when pressure released and inflow restored. A tight circumferential cast or dressing may precipitate or exacerbate the condition.

Patient complains of pain unresponsive to strong analgesia and resists movement, in particular passive muscle stretching (finger or toe extension). The involved compartment is tightly swollen. Paraesthesia may also be a feature.

Management

The diagnosis is a clinical one unless the patient is obtunded, otherwise unconscious or has an anaesthetic limb block, in which case measurement of compartment pressures is indicated. Guidelines suggest pressures within 30mmHg of diastolic or 30–40mmHg absolute are indicative for fasciotomy[2] (normal resting muscle pressure 0–12mmHg).

Split dressings and casts to skin and review. Maintain a low threshold for decompressive fasciotomy(ies) and a high index of suspicion.

The patient is taken to theatre as an emergency. Fasciotomy incisons must be full length since the skin is itself a constricting layer. The fascial envelopes of all involved muscle compartments must be released and the fracture, if present, stabilized. Skin wounds are left open for delayed closure or later grafting.

When treatment is delayed due to transfer, crush injury or failed revascularization then fasciotomy may introduce infection (to necrotic tissue) or precipitate release of myoglobin into the circulation, causing renal compromise. Fasciotomy under these circumstances carries little chance of muscle recovery; it should be done acutely or probably not at all.

References

1 Bulstrode C. Compartment syndrome. In: Bulstrode C, Buckwater J, Carr A, *et al.*, eds. *Oxford Textbook of Orthopaedics and Trauma*. Oxford: Oxford University Press, 2002:2412–7.
2 McQueen MM, Court-Brown CM. Compartment monitoring in tibial fractures: The pressure threshold for decompression. *J Bone Joint Surg Br* 1996;**78**:99–104.

Fractures in the elderly

Fractures occur in the elderly because of skeletal fragility; peak bone mass is achieved at the end of skeletal maturation and consolidation in early adulthood, after which there is a steady deterioration in bone density which is more marked in women. Since peak bone mass can no longer be influenced in the elderly, efforts to reduce fracture risk must centre on falls prevention strategies and optimization of bone mass by dietary and pharmacological manipulation of bone turnover.

Around 310 000 fractures occur each year in elderly people in the UK. The cost of providing social care and support for these patients is estimated at £1.7billion[1]. Most common are fractures of the hip, vertebrae and distal radius[2].

Many elderly fracture patients have complex medical problems. For those requiring operative fracture fixation or prolonged immobilization a thorough medical ± anaesthetic assessment with prompt treatment is mandatory. Postoperative care should include identification of risk factors for and secondary prevention of further fractures.

Common causes of falls in the elderly
- Mechanical
- Medication
- Arrhythmias
- CVA
- Metabolic
- Syncope.

Secondary prevention[3]
- Falls assessment
- Bone densitometry (DEXA scanning)
- Medication review
- Patient awareness
- Calcium and vitamin D supplements ± bisphosphonates according to DEXA scan result and local protocol
- Home assessment.

When and which other specialties should be involved
- Physiotherapy
  - Liaise closely throughout; 'motion is the lotion' particularly in this group. Postoperative instructions as to what can and cannot be done must be crystal clear; this is the responsibility of the operating surgeon
- Occupational therapy
  - Inform early during admission if discharge home likely to be problematic due to reduced mobility and function postoperatively
- Acute medical team
  - If patient becomes acutely medically unwell during admission
  - For medical stabilization and optimization prior to surgery
  - Patient with complex medical co-morbidity likely to be affected by operation

- Anaesthetist
  - Once decision has been made to manage fracture surgically
  - If patient has previous adverse reaction to anaesthetic
  - If patient felt to be an anaesthetic risk
- Ortho-geriatrician
  - Should see all elderly patients admitted to the orthopaedic ward
  - Manage day to day medical conditions and make recommendations for further investigations and management
- GP
  - Should be informed of all admissions
  - On discharge all patients with suspected osteoporotic fractures should be referred to their GP for assessment ± treatment (secondary prevention) unless a pathway for this exists within the admitting hospital.

References

1 Woolf A, Akesson K. Preventing fractures in elderly people. *BMJ* 2003;**327**:89–95.
2 The British Orthopaedic Association. *The Care of Patients with Fragility Fracture.* London: BOA, 2007.
3 Lord S, Sherrington C, Menz HB. *Falls in Older People: Risk Factors and Strategies for Prevention.* Cambridge: Cambridge University Press, 2001.

Adult hand injuries

- The hand is central to normal function and cosmetically is second only in importance to the face
- Post-traumatic stiffness which elsewhere might result in minimal loss of function can be devastating in the hand, so a core principle in managing injuries is to maintain motion
- The PIPJs are the functional pivots of the hand; stiffness here is particularly poorly tolerated
- Angular deformity generally better tolerated than rotational
- Key factors in assessment are hand dominance, occupation, age, co-morbidities; all affect treatment options
- Examine for neurovascular injury, rotational and angular deformity and range of movement.

Soft tissue injuries to digits

- In absence of neurovascular injury a clean wound may be sutured primarily
- If nerve injury detected refer for consideration of acute repair
- Nail bed injuries are important and often neglected (common paediatric injury; finger caught in drawer or car door)
  - Failure to treat results in deformed nail growth
  - If terminal phalanx fracture, this is an open injury
  - Treatment is accurate repair of nail bed and reinsertion of nail plate as temporary spacer to prevent adhesions.

Injuries to distal phalanx

- A tuft injury results from a crush force to the distal phalanx
  - Treatment is management of the soft tissue injury
- Mallet finger results from forcible flexion of an extended finger
  - Following injury the patient is unable to extend finger fully
  - The deformity is caused by bony or tendinous rupture of the extensor tendon insertion
- Both injuries managed in a hyperextension splint (mallet splint)
- Rugger jersey finger is an avulsion fracture of the FDP
  - Most common in the ring finger, but much rarer than mallet finger
  - Treatment is surgical repair.

Other phalangeal and metacarpal injuries

- In absence of rotational deformity most closed phalangeal shaft fractures treated with buddy strapping and early mobilization
- If fracture is intra-articular (± dislocation) consider ORIF if significant displacement (>1mm).
  - If <1mm and joint is stable, treat non-operatively
  - Volar fracture dislocations more unstable than dorsal
  - DIPJ more tolerant of stiffness than PIPJ or MCPJ
- MCPJ dislocations usually easily reduced and stable following reduction

- Metacarpal neck fractures commonly a punching injury
  - Fracture of 5th metacarpal is the 'boxer's fracture'
  - Angulation of up to 50° well tolerated (treat with buddy strap ± volar slab or metacarpal brace), but check rotation
  - Reduce and fix if rotated or multiple metacarpals fractured
  - Less angulation is acceptable in 2nd and 3rd metacarpals.

Injuries to the thumb

- Bennett's is a fracture dislocation of the base of the 1st metacarpal
  - May result from punching with thumb inside the palm of hand
  - X-rays show small medial fragment (with attached ligaments) and a subluxed CMCJ
  - Fracture is easily reduced, but difficult to maintain reduction
  - Treatment is by closed reduction and pinning (or ORIF if unable to maintain reduction in plaster
- Rolando is an intra-articular fracture of 1st MCPJ with at least three fragments (T or Y shape)
  - Treated with ORIF if displaced and not too fragmented
- Thumb dislocation
  - Treat as for MCPJ dislocation
- Skier's thumb an acute injury to the ulna collateral ligament (UCL)
  - Results from forced abduction to thumb base
  - UCL resists laterally directed forces; injury results in weak pinch grip
  - Diagnosed by stress testing ± local anaesthetic
  - If grossly unstable suspect complete rupture of the UCL ± interposition of adductor aponeurosis (Stener lesion) which prevents healing; needs operative repair.
  - If only mild instability treat as sprain in thumb cast.

Compartment syndrome

- May present after any injury to the hand
- Symptoms are increasing pain and reduced movement
- Hand typically held with metacarpal extended and IPJ flexed
- Treatment is decompression of the 10 compartments through a midline volar and 2 dorsal incisions.

Traumatic amputation

- Always consider re-implantation for thumb as reconstruction results inferior. Also any digital amputation in child and when multiple digits lost
- Warm ischaemia time for distal amputations (no muscle) <12h
- Warm ischaemia for more proximal amputations is <8h
- Polytrauma, severe crush, atherosclerosis and mental instability are contraindications for re-implantation.

Adult wrist injuries

Scaphoid fractures

- In adults the scaphoid is the most commonly fractured carpal bone
- Mechanism of injury is violent hyperextension of the wrist
- Scaphoid most commonly fractures through its waist
- Blood supply arises from the distal pole through an end artery; therefore, waist fractures associated with subsequent AVN
- Symptoms/signs include pain maximal in the anatomical snuff box (bounded by EPL, APL and EPB), weakness of pinch grip and pain on axial compression of the thumb
- X-rays should include AP, lateral and 2 oblique views ('scaphoid series')
- These fractures are notoriously missed at presentation, which is critical as union rates fall off rapidly if not immobilized at this stage. Common strategy is to cast if clinical signs in absence of radiographic confirmation and repeat views at 2 weeks. If no fracture seen then and signs resolved mobilize
- Much interest in more sophisticated imaging (CT, MRI, bone scan) for earlier, more accurate diagnosis of minimally displaced scaphoid fracture and for ongoing signs in absence of fracture on plain film
- Can treat minimally displaced fracture in a scaphoid cast (includes thumb, though no definite benefit over one which does not) until clinical and radiographic union (6–8 weeks, though may be considerably longer). For displacement >1mm or perhaps patient choice, consider operative fixation, either percutaneously or after open or arthroscopically assisted reduction
- Complications are AVN, delayed or non-union with secondary wrist instability and/or OA
- Fractures of the other carpal bones are uncommon, usually managed in cast.

Carpal dislocations

- Carpal dislocations represent significant soft tissue injuries to the wrist, yet they can be missed as a 'sprain' with disastrous results to the patient
- The scaphoid bridges the proximal and distal carpal rows and so dislocation of either row results in rotation or fracture of the scaphoid
- Lunate and perilunate dislocations result from forced dorsiflexion of the wrist. The lunate remains attached to the radius and the rest of the carpus dislocates (perilunate dislocation). If the carpus spontaneously reduces it may lever the lunate out anteriorly (can cause median nerve compression)
- The forces directed through the scaphoid can result in a fracture through the waist (trans-scaphoid perilunate dislocation)
- Mayfield et al.[1] described the different zones of disruption (bone and soft tissue) as the injury force passes around the lunate
- Gilula's arcs are helpful (if disrupted) to diagnosis; on an AP wrist radiograph, the proximal and distal carpal row joint spaces should decribe separately distinct, parallel arcs

- Other radiographic signs are diminished height of the carpus and a lunate which appears triangular ('sector shaped') instead of quadrilateral on the AP view
- Treatment is urgent reduction which may be achieved closed (traction to the wrist in extension, followed by palmar flexion with simultaneous pressure over the displaced bone(s)) or open. Fix/repair bone/soft tissue disruption as required to restore stability to wrist
- Complications include AVN of the lunate (Kienbock's disease), median nerve injury and wrist stiffness or ongoing instability.

Herbert screw

The Herbert screw is the original and best known of the variable pitch devices ideal for achieving compression across a fracture involving a small, difficult to access bone. Timothy James Herbert from Sydney, Australia was originally a UK surgeon (trained under Alan Apley) but left these shores in the 1970s when NHS jobs were scarce and hard to come by in Orthopaedics. The first batch of the screws which made his name was fashioned on a lathe from regular Steinmann pins in the garage of an engineering student at the University of New South Wales.

Reference

1 Mayfield JK, Johnson RP, Kilcoyne RK. Carpal dislocations: pathomechanics and progressive perilunar instability. *J Hand Surg Am* 1980;**5**:226–41.

Adult forearm injuries

The forearm is made up of the radius and ulna bound together by the interosseous membrane. Primary function is pronation and supination which requires radius to rotate over the ulna; injury to either can block rotation.

Isolated injury to either bone is uncommon as the two form a closed chain; if only one is fractured look critically at the joints either ends for signs of disruption. Eponyms abound.

Closed management of shaft fractures is difficult and requires adherence to all the tenets of Charnley's text, now sadly out of print, on the subject: generation of hydrostatic pressure in soft tissues to maintain reduction achieved by 3-point moulding of a well-fitting cylindrical cast. Often disruption and interposition of soft tissues and the tendency of the forearm to swell mandate open reduction and internal fixation.

Damage to the median nerve (especially the anterior interosseus branch), ulnar and radial nerves is common; the sensory and motor function of each must be carefully tested and documented prior to any intervention. Compartment syndrome is also relatively common in the forearm, especially with a 2-level fracture, e.g. elbow and forearm.

Combined fractures of radius and ulna shafts

- Fractures usually occur at about the same level in each bone
- Injury usually clinically and radiologically obvious
- Treatment is operative, for anything other than minimal displacement, to achieve anatomical reduction. Plate fixation in adults.

Galeazzi fracture–dislocation

- Radius fracture in association with dislocation of the DRUJ; injury forces pass out through bone and soft tissue in the closed chain
- Always examine wrist and elbow with any forearm injury and order true AP and lateral wrist radiographs if isolated radius fracture. DRUJ injury is otherwise easily missed
- Operative treatment to restore length and rotation to the radius; if this is achieved the radioulnar dislocation should spontaneously reduce but may require temporary pinning to restore stability.

Monteggia fracture–dislocation

- Displaced ulna fracture in association with radial head dislocation
- Examine for tenderness over the radial head. On any elbow radiograph a line up the long axis of the radial neck should pass through the centre of the capitellum. If it runs eccentrically there is subluxation; if it misses there is dislocation
- Treatment is operative for anatomical reduction of the ulna which should achieve closed reduction of the radial head, unless the soft tissues (capsule and annular ligament) are disrupted and interposed
- If radial head dislocation is missed, subsequent reduction is much harder and may be impossible mandating excision of the radial head.

Isolated ulna fracture (night stick fracture)

- A direct blow to the arm raised in self-defence (hence the name)
- Can usually manage non-operatively in cast, though non-union is not uncommon and can steer towards plate fixation if significant displacement

Distal radial fractures

- Extremely common, especially as insufficiency fracture
- Incidence increases with age and correlates with OP
- Distal radial fractures may be extra-articular (Colles' or Smith's) or intra-articular (Barton's)
- There is currently enthusiasm for operative management of these fractures with specialized locking plates applied via a volar approach. Usage runs far ahead of proper evidence of benefit over classical treatment methods of closed reduction and casting ± supplementary K wire fixation, external fixation and low profile dorsal plates.

Colles' fracture

Abraham Colles, an Irish Professor of anatomy and surgery, in 1814 described the clinical deformity of an extra-articular fracture of the distal radius with dorsal displacement of the distal fragment, as a low energy injury in the elderly. He trained under Sir Astley Cooper in London, walking >8 days from medical school in Edinburgh for the privilege.

Smith's fracture ('reverse Colles')

Robert Smith, another Irish Professor of surgery, described a flexion compression injury of the distal radius with volar displacement of the distal fragment in 1847. This occurs in a younger age group and is intrinsically less stable.

Barton's fracture dislocation

John Barton (you've guessed it, Irish surgeon) in 1835 described an intra-articular fracture of the distal radius in which the dorsal or volar rim of the radius is displaced with the carpus.

- Volar tilt of the distal fragment is much more common than dorsal tilt
- Displaced intra-articular fractures require anatomical reduction to prevent the development of early arthritis. Usually done with a volar plate in buttress mode.

Adult elbow injuries

Most result from a fall onto an outstretched hand.

A positive fat pad sign on a lateral X-ray indicates the presence of a lipo-haemarthrosis and a likely undisplaced fracture which may otherwise be occult, particularly if the posterior fat pad is visible.

Elbow injuries are associated with marked stiffness, so avoid prolonged immobilization.

Elbow dislocation
- 90% posterior or posterolateral
- Examination reveals disruption of the equilateral triangle formed by the olecranon and the epicondyles (this positional relationship is preserved in supracondylar fractures)
- Treatment is closed reduction—traction on slightly flexed arm with thumbs behind the olecranon pushing it forward
- Test stability postreduction
- ORIF required if the elbow is unstable with associated epicondylar fracture or an incarcerated fragment prevents closed relocation
- Complications include neurovascular injury, compartment syndrome, chronic instability and myositis ossificans
- The combination of elbow dislocation with coronoid fracture, radial head fracture and medial/lateral epicondyle injury is the 'terrible triad'; indicates severe injury with almost inevitable instability.

Olecranon fracture
- Two types are common
  - Multifragmentary fracture from a fall onto the elbow
  - Oblique traction injury resulting from a fall onto the hand
- Treatment
  - Undisplaced fractures are treated in cast for 2 weeks followed by gentle mobilization
  - Displaced fractures require an ORIF (tension band wire biomechanically very sound)
  - Highly comminuted fractures with an intact triceps mechanism are treated non-operatively with early mobilization
- Complications include ulnar nerve injury, stiffness and non-union, and the development of secondary OA.

Radial head fractures
- Often associated with ligamentous injury to the elbow
- Examine the forearm for tenderness, which may indicate concomitant rupture of the interosseous membrane (Essex–Lopresti injury)
  - Signifies risk of DRUJ disruption with progressive proximal migration of the radius
  - An indication for radial head replacement (as a temporary spacer) if the fracture is not reconstructable

- Aspiration of elbow haemarthrosis and injection of local anaesthetic will relieve pain and facilitate assessment of motion and stability
- Treatment for small fracture fragments with no block to elbow rotation is collar and cuff with early mobilization
- Larger, displaced fragments may require ORIF with mini screw/plate fixation; severe fragmentation mandates radial head excision ± radial head replacement
- Complications include stiffness, chronic wrist pain and secondary elbow OA.

Tension band principle

To convert a longitudinal tensile force (in this case, concentric triceps contraction) into an eccentric compressive force across the reduced fracture.

Adult humerus injuries

Proximal humeral fractures

- Common fractures associated with OP
- Result from a fall onto an outstretched arm
- Fracture lines occur through the greater and lesser tuberosities, the humeral shaft and the humeral head
- Fracture described by number of displaced fracture parts[1]
- Most treated non-operatively in elderly; fixation into osteoporotic bone often unrewarding (though locking plate technology may widen indications for fixation in future)
- In younger patients consider reattachment of a displaced greater tuberosity (essentially a rotator cuff injury)
- Four-part fractures have significant chance of developing AVN (~30%) which is main determinant of outcome; may require shoulder arthroplasty in elderly
- Complications include neurovascular injury (brachial artery, axillary nerve and brachial plexus), shoulder stiffness, non-union, secondary arthritis and AVN.

Humeral shaft fractures

- Fracture may be transverse, spiral or comminuted
- Treatment is usually in a hanging cast then functional brace as moderate degrees of malalignment or shortening (up to 3cm) are functionally well tolerated
- Fixation (see opposite for indications) generally best with plate; humeral nails have high complication rate
- Complications
  - Nerve injury, particularly radial nerve in the spiral groove and to a lesser extent in distal third (Holstein–Lewis fracture)
  - Non-union, may require fixation ± bone grafting.

Distal humeral fractures

- May be unicondylar, bicondylar, supracondylar or intercondylar
- Supracondylar fractures rare in adults; unstable injuries which generally require fixation
- Intercondylar fractures the most common:
  - A fall drives coronoid into trochlea splitting the two condyles apart
  - Intra-articular fracture (requires anatomical reduction). Principle to reconstruct articular surface (lag condylar fragments back together with screws) and reattach both to diaphysis (with one or sometimes two plates). An extensive procedure, may need osteotomy of ulna to access the fragments and elbow joint
  - If highly comminuted and/or poor bone quality then treatment ranges from early mobilization (bag of bones philosophy) to primary total elbow replacement
  - Complications are neurovascular injury, stiffness and secondary OA
- Unicondylar fractures usually require ORIF with 2 cancellous lag screws.

Indications for open reduction and internal fixation of humeral shaft fractures

- Open injury
- Polytrauma
- Floating elbow (associated both bone forearm fracture)
- Floating shoulder (rare)
- Associated elbow or shoulder dislocation, to facilitate early mobilization
- Lower limb injury mandating use of crutches
- Radial nerve palsy occurring after manipulation of fracture
- Pathological fracture (usually metastases)
- Segmental fracture (a relative indication for nailing if middle third)
- Delayed or non-union.

Reference

1 Neer C. Displaced proximal humeral fractures: part I. Classification and evaluation. 1970. *Clin Orthop Relat Res* 2006;**442**:77–82.

Adult shoulder injuries

Clavicle fractures
- Result from direct blow to clavicle, common cyclist injury
- Most common site of fracture is junction of middle and outer 1/3
- Proximal fragment elevated by pull of sternomastoid
- Examine to exclude neurovascular injury, pneumothorax or ipsilateral limb or rib injury
- Treatment classically non-operative with broad arm sling, early motion and assumed low rate of non-union
- Recent randomized controlled trial (RCT[1]) supported plate fixation of displaced midshaft fractures in active adult patients (better function and lower rate of non-union)
- Non-union is a rare complication, most common in outer 1/3 fractures.

Sternoclavicular dislocation
- Uncommon injury
- Anterior more common than posterior
- Diagnosis clinical as injury is difficult to detect on X-ray (CT better)
- Anterior dislocation usually managed non-operatively
- Posterior dislocation requires reduction ± fixation
- Complications include injury to the great vessels and pneumothorax.

Acromioclavicular dislocation (see also 📖 p. 290)
- Usually results from fall onto the shoulder
- Injury types listed opposite
- Treat types I–III non-operatively; if residual functional weakness then CC ligament may be surgically reconstructed (variety of options). More severe types require reduction and fixation/reconstruction
- Complications include long-term weakness or discomfort and secondary OA.

Shoulder dislocation
- See section on shoulder instability and dislocation (see 📖 p. 280)
- In young adults the anterior glenoid rim and glenohumeral ligaments are disrupted (Bankart lesion); in older adults the rotator cuff usually ruptures

Scapula fractures
- Result from high energy trauma, so look for other injuries
- Scapula blade injuries heal well with a sling and analgesia
- Scapula neck fractures generally managed the same unless concomitant fracture of clavicle resulting in a floating shoulder (mandates fixation).

Classification of ACJ injuries

- Type I—sprain of acromioclavicular ligament only. ACJ intact
- Type II—ACJ ligaments and joint capsule disrupted but coracoclavicular ligaments intact. ACJ subluxed
- Type III—ACJ dislocation with clavicle displaced superiorly and coracoclavicular ligaments ruptured
- Type IV—clavicle displaced posteriorly into or through trapezius muscle (posterior displacement confirmed on axillary radiograph)
- Type V—ACJ dislocation with extreme superior elevation of clavicle and complete detachment of deltoid and trapezius from distal clavicle
- Type VI—ACJ dislocation with clavicle displaced inferior to acromion and coracoid process.

Reference

1 Canadian Orthopaedic Trauma Society. Nonoperative treatment compared with plate fixation of displaced midshaft clavicular fractures. A multicenter, randomized clinical trial. *J Bone Joint Surg Am* 2007;**89**:1–10.

Soft tissue disorders of the neck

Soft tissue disorders that result in neck and shoulder girdle symptoms include dermoid cysts, lipomas, lymph nodes, thyroid lesions, thryoglossal cysts, brachial cysts, pharyngeal pouch anomalies, carotid artery aneurysms and soft tissue tumours. The most common soft tissue disorder of the neck in adults is an injury to soft tissues following trauma.

Whiplash

The term 'whiplash' refers to any injury of the cervical spine other than an unequivocal fracture. It is also known as cervical sprain.

Epidemiology

People who sustain this type of injury often seek compensation—350 000 people submit claims for a whiplash injury each year.

Mechanism

The problem usually arises with a rear end collision where there is rapid extension and flexion of the neck.

Clinical

Neck pain, interscapular and lower back pain are common presenting symptoms. Limb paraesthesia or weakness may occur. Symptoms usually develop within 48h of the injury. Psychological symptoms (depression, anxiety) are commonly associated with the physical injury.

Clinical signs are often absent. Spinal tenderness, muscle spasm, reduced range of movements and neurological findings are found occasionally.

Investigations

Usually none required. Lateral and anteroposterior X-rays of the cervical spine at the time of the injury may be requested if clinically indicated. An MRI scan is useful if with persistent neurological symptoms or signs.

Prognosis

Approximately 85% of patients have full resolution of symptoms within 3 months of the injury and of those who have symptoms beyond this period, 86% will still be symptomatic at 2yrs. 70% reach steady state by 1yr and 97% by 2yrs[1,2].

Management

Early physiotherapy is important. Analgesia, NSAIDs and muscle relaxants can be used.

Medico-legal reporting

The expert's primary duty is to the court. Most cases are settled out of court, but there are a few where arbitration in the High Court is required. The expert writing the report will be called to give evidence in such a case. The final prognosis is determined 2yrs after the causative event.

References

1 Watkinson A, Gargan MF, Bannister GC. Prognostic factors in soft tissue injuries of the cervical spine. *Injury* 1991;**22**:307–9.

2 Squires B, Gargan MF, Bannister GC. The fluctuation in recovery following whiplash injury: 7.5-year prospective review. *Injury* 2005;**36**:758–61.

Adult spine injuries—cervical spine

General principles

History: mechanism of injury is important.

Examination: spinal tenderness, thorough neurological examination especially perianal sensation and rectal tone. The use of the Canadian C-Spine rules or the NEXUS low risk criteria[1] can help decide whether imaging is required.

X-rays: AP and lateral, peg view for C-spine series, CT scan good for bony detail, MRI scan for soft tissue detail.

Cervical injuries: 50% occur due to RTAs, usually in young males, and often alcohol is involved.

Upper cervical spine

Occipital condyle fractures

Rare, secondary to axial loading. Three subtypes:
- 1 and 2 are stable and treatment requires a hard collar for 6–8 weeks
- 3 is unstable and requires a halo jacket for 8–12 weeks or ORIF.

C1 (Jefferson's) fracture

Secondary to axial loading

Treatment depends on displacement 12–16 weeks in a halo jacket or fusion if unstable (>6.9mm combined overhang of lateral masses on open mouth view).

C1/C2 rotary subluxation (torticollis)

Aetiology—upper respiratory tract infection, trauma or inflammatory arthritis

Treatment depends on cause: if traumatic, traction and a halo jacket for 8–12 weeks, if atraumatic then physiotherapy and NSAIDs.

C2 odontoid fractures

10% of all cervical spine fractures, High incidence in the elderly. Three subtypes:
- 1: fracture of tip of dens—hard collar for 6 weeks
- 2: base of dens—controversial, high rate of non-union. If displacement <5mm then halo jacket for 12–16 weeks; if >5mm then surgical treatment (atlanto-axial arthrodesis or direct anterior screw fixation)
- 3: into body of C2—halo jacket for 12–16 weeks.

Traumatic spondylolisthesis of the axis (hangman's fractures)

Classically distraction and extension, now most often due to direct trauma to the face and head in RTAs and falls, mostly an injury of discs and ligamentous structures. Treatment depends on type; 95% unite by non-operative treatment. Three subtypes.
- 1: undisplaced—hard collar for 8–12 weeks
- 2: translated/angulated—halo jacket for 12–16 weeks
- 3: with dislocated C2/3 facet joint—ORIF.

Complications: often a missed injury.

Lower cervical spine

Mechanism of injury
- Vertical compression leads to burst fractures

- Extension injury
- Flexion injury leads to:
  - unilateral facet dislocation
  - bilateral facet dislocation (1% risk of ruptured disk requires an MRI prior to reduction)
  - tear drop fracture
- 1/3rd missed at presentation.

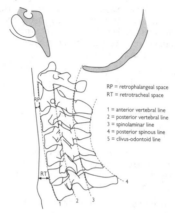

RP = retrophalangeal space
RT = retrotracheal space

1 = anterior vertebral line
2 = posterior vertebral line
3 = spinolaminar line
4 = posterior spinous line
5 = clivus-odontoid line

Fig. 9.2 Anatomy of the cervical spine.

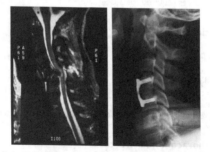

Fig. 9.3 (a) Sagittal MRI shows a C4–5 dislocation with cord impingement caused by the displacement of the spinal column and a retropulsed C4–5 disc. (b) Treatment consisted of emergency anterior C4–5 discectomy with interbody fusion and plate fixation.

Reproduced from Hakim, Clunie, Haq, *Oxford Textbook of Rheumatology*, with permission from Oxford University Press.

Reference

1 Stiell IG, Clement CM, McKnight RD, *et al.* The Canadian C-Spine rule versus the NEXUS low risk criteria in patients with trauma. *N Engl J Med* 2003;**349**:2510–8.

Adult spine injuries—thoracolumbar spine

RTAs are the most common cause of thoracolumbar fractures in developed countries, whereas in developing countries the most common cause is falls. OP is a major risk factor for thoracolumbar fractures.

The spectrum of injuries is related to the type and severity of the forces and the direction in which they are applied to the spine. Distraction, flexion, extension, rotation, shear forces or a combination of these forces can be applied. If sufficient force is applied, bone and/or ligaments or joints fail and fractures and dislocations occur.

These injuries are frequently overlooked because of patient intoxication, multiple injuries and head injuries.

Clinical

Patients with thoracolumbar fractures present with pain, deformity and neurological deficits (sensory changes, weakness, abnormal reflexes, bladder and bowel dysfunction).

Look for bruises, abrasions, swellings, local tenderness, deformity and neurological deficits. These fractures are associated with other fractures and visceral injuries (10–15% of patients with spinal injuries); these injuries must be excluded by doing a systematic examination.

Thoracic injuries have a high risk of cord injury due to:
- Poor blood supply
- Narrow canal
- Very high forces required to cause fracture
- Associated chest injuries.

Investigations

Radiology
- X-rays: initial investigation should include AP and lateral views of spine
- CT scan: to exclude or define bony injuries. In assessing stability, it may be helpful to consider the Denis classification based on a three column theory of the spine (Fig. 9.4). Stability only occurs if at least two of the three columns are intact
- MRI scan: useful in documenting soft tissue, spinal cord or nerve root injuries and distinguishing old and new fractures (insuffiency fractures).

Types of thoracolumbar fractures

1. Compressive flexion (wedge fracture)
Description: anterior column fails in compression and if force great enough posterior column and middle column may also fail.

Management: bed rest and thoracolumbar orthosis as these fractures are normally stable.

2. Distractive flexion (seatbelt or Chance fracture)
Description: all 3 columns may fail as a result of flexion about an axis at or anterior to the anterior longitudinal ligament. Stability depends on

magnitude of forces and structures involved, osseous, ligamentous or both. Neurological injury occurs occasionally.

Management: posterior instrumented fusion.

3. Lateral flexion
Description: unilateral failure of 2 or 3 columns under compressive load. There may be contralateral facet fracture or dislocation.

Management: with minimal collapse of vertebral body, the injury can be treated in a thoracolumbar orthosis. For any significant change in vertebral alignment, a correction and instrumented fusion is indicated.

4. Translational (shear fracture)
Description: these injuries result from shear forces, in either the sagittal or coronal plane. Displacement can be anterior, posterior or lateral. Neurological injuries are common.

Management: most, certainly any fracture with >25% translation, require reduction and instrumented fusion.

5. Torsional flexion (slice fracture)
Description: the forces in these fractures cause anterior and middle column compression and rotation, and posterior element failure due to torsion and rotation. Vertebral body fractures, and there may be a facet fracture—dislocation. Neurological injury common.

Management: reduction and instrumented fusion.

6. Vertical compression (burst fracture)
Description: there is a loss of vertebral body height due to failure of the anterior and middle columns with compression. Posterior elements may also fail. Neurological injury is uncommon.

Management: reduction (ligamentotaxis) and posterior instrumented fusion. In highly unstable fractures anterior stabilization may be necessary.

7. Distractive extension
Description: these fractures occur as a result of failure of the anterior column under tension and posterior column under compression. Rare injuries. Seldom associated with neurological injury.

Management: rest and thoracolumbar orthosis.

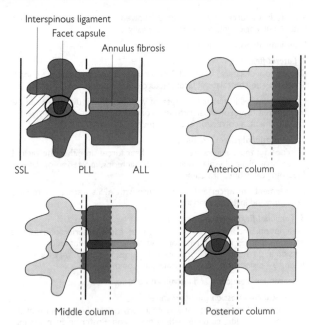

Fig. 9.4 The three anatomic columns: SSL = suprasinus ligament; PLL = posterior longitudinal ligament; ALL = anterior longitudinal ligament.

Reproduced from Bulstrode et al., *Oxford Textbook of Orthopaedics and Trauma*, with permission from Oxford University Press.

Fractures of the pelvic ring in adults

Infrequent, ~3–4% of all fractures. Commonly high energy trauma—RTAs and falls from significant height in young, and low energy falls from standing height in elderly. Anticipate other injuries with high energy transfer; up to 40% have retroperitoneal or intra-abdominal source of blood loss.

Classification

Multiple different systems exist. Simplest and most useful is the Tile classification:

- Type A—pelvic ring stable
- Type B—rotationally unstable ring disruption
- Type C—vertically unstable ring disruption.

Type A injuries include iliac wing fractures, pubic rami fractures, avulsion injuries around the periphery of the pelvis.

Type B injuries include the anterior–posterior compression or 'open-book' and the lateral compression type fractures, in which the posterior part of the ring is usually at least partially stable in the vertical plane.

Type C injuries include the vertical shear or 'Malgaigne' fractures, with fractures of the pubic rami and sacrum or SIJ, and superior displacement of the hemipelvis. Typically associated with massive bleeding.

Management

- Primary evaluation should be that of C in the ATLS protocol.
- Resuscitation may require massive transfusion so coagulopathy and need for FFP should be anticipated.
- AP pelvic radiograph as part of primary survey
- Call for senior input early.

Presence of an unstable pelvic ring injury with haemodynamic compromise requires careful search for another source of bleeding from associated injury. If none is found with an unstable pelvic fracture pattern and compromised circulation immediate external fixation is indicated to restore alignment and reduce intrapelvic volume. Ongoing haemodynamic compromise should prompt consideration of emergent surgical exploration and packing or angiographic embolization.

Temporizing measures if external fixation not immediately available include reducing pelvic volume by using a pelvic binder and skeletal traction for vertically unstable injuries.

Once stabilized, definitive work-up includes pelvic inlet and outlet views ± CT scan to plan operative fixation according to fracture type.

Most type A fractures can be managed non-operatively.

Associated pelvic injuries

- Urethral injury occurs in up to 15% of males, classically with type C and some type B injuries. Signs can include blood at the urethral meatus, a high riding prostate on rectal exam and 'straddle' type injuries. Any suspicion mandates retrograde urethrography prior to catheterization, which could cause contamination of the pelvic fracture
- Bladder rupture in up to 15% of major fractures
- Vaginal laceration
- Rectal injury (rare: ~1%).

Complications

- Mortality 3–20% dependent on associated injuries and blood loss.
- Neurological deficit: up to 33%, predominantly with major posterior injuries, usually lumbosacral plexus (L5, S1) or femoral nerve
- DVT 30–50%
- PE 5–7%
- Infection
- DIC
- ARDS/fat embolus
- Chronic pain
- Gait abnormality
- Sexual dysfunction.

For further reading, see Burgess et al.[1] and Gruen et al.[2].

References

1 Burgess AR, Eastridge BJ, Young JW, et al. Pelvic ring disruptions: effective classification system and treatment protocols. *J Trauma* 1990;**30**:848–56.
2 Gruen GS, Leit ME, Gruen RJ, et al. The acute management of hemodynamically unstable multiple trauma patients with pelvic ring fractures. *J Trauma* 1994;**36**:706–11.

Adult acetabular fractures

The acetabulum (derived from Latin for 'vinegar cup') is best considered to sit as an inverted 'Y' between anterior and posterior columns[1]. Violation of these requires big energy transfer (or very osteopenic bone); significant association with other lower limb fractures, pelvic and visceral injury. Exclude open injury which may communicate with bowel and require temporary defunctioning stoma. Pelvic vascular and sciatic nerve injury also possibe.

Classification

Based on anatomical configuration; involvement of the superior pelvic columns and acetabular walls[1]. Some types disrupt integrity of the pelvic ring.

Elemental (or simple) fracture types: ~20%

- Posterior wall
- Anterior wall
- Posterior column—involvement of strut running from posterior superior iliac spine (PSIS) to ischium
- Anterior column—involvement of strut running from ASIS to pubis
- Transverse—fracture line traverses the acetabulum creating a ring disruption with superior and inferior fragments.

Combination (or associated) fracture types: ~80%

- Posterior column and wall
- Posterior wall and transverse
- T shaped—combination of transverse and a vertical fracture through inferior fragment
- Two column—disruption of both pelvic struts
- Anterior column and posterior hemitransverse.

Investigations

- AP pelvis radiograph
- Judet views (45° oblique iliac and obturator views)
  - Rotate patient, not X-ray beam
  - Iliac view shows posterior column and anterior wall
  - Obturator view shows anterior column and posterior wall
- CT ± 3-D reconstruction useful better to define fracture patterns and intra-articular fragments
- Pelvic angiography may be necessary in an unstable patient.

Management

Resuscitation and detailed secondary survey are mandatory prior to definitive management of the acetabular injury.

Principles of management to restore congruency between the femoral head and acetabulum with a stable reduction of the fracture[2]. For marginal wall fractures without intra-articular fragments, simple closed reduction may suffice. Often there has been fracture–dislocation at the hip joint; reduction of the femoral head is an emergency to restore vascularity. When the column(s) are significantly disrupted operative reduction and stabilization is indicated, except perhaps in the elderly where prolonged skeletal traction may be considered.

Surgical exposure is via an ilioinguinal, iliofemoral or Kocher–Langenbeck posterolateral approach. Direct open reduction and internal fixation is required for stable and concentric reconstruction.

Complications
- Infection 3–4%
- DVT (30%) and PE
- Sciatic nerve injury 2–3%
- Femoral head AVN 3–9%
- Heterotopic ossification
- Secondary OA.

References
1 Letournel E, Judet R. *Fractures of the Acetabulum*, 2nd edn. Berlin: Springer Verlag, 1993.
2 Matta JM. Fractures of the acetabulum: accuracy in reduction and clinical results in patients managed operative within 3 weeks after the injury. *J Bone Joint Surg Am* 1996;**78**:1632–45.

Adult femoral injuries: shaft, subtrochanteric and supracondylar fractures

Shaft fracture

Common injury frequently associated with major trauma. Management revolutionized by antegrade locked, reamed intramedullary nail fixation (with an anatomically contoured implant inserted 'closed' via the piriformis fossa). Advantages of early mobilization (cf. prolonged traction) reducing risk of embolic phenomena and other associated morbidity, 95–99% union rate for closed fracture with low rates of infection or malunion. Open injuries uncommon and serious.

Definition

>5cm below lesser trochanter and >8cm above knee joint.

Assessment

ATLS protocol. 1–3 units blood may be lost even with closed femoral fracture.

Radiographs should include whole femur for ipsilateral neck fracture (2–5%) or supraconylar fractures. Arteriogram if ABPI <0.9 (neurovascular injury uncommon).

Treatment

Thomas splint in A&E for comfort and to reduce blood loss; now a temporizing device only. Convert to skeletal traction 10–15lb if theatre not available within 24. Intramedullary (IM) nailing within this window optimal to reduce incidence of fat embolism syndrome—multisystem disorder, especially dysfunction of pulmonary system and CNS (previously commonly seen in young adult femur shaft fractures treated definitively by traction).

External fixation less well tolerated around the femur. Indicated possibly in severe open fracture (though primary wound excision and nailing with early definitive cover is safe for shaft fracture) and polytrauma to temporize if patient requires further rescuscitation, sometimes after other long bone nailing.

Thigh compartment syndrome is uncommon. If ipsilateral tibial shaft fracture ('floating knee') fix femur first (to allow patient to sit up if becomes too unwell to tolerate second nailing).

Indications for retrograde nailing[1]

- Distal extra-articular fracture
- Ipsilateral femoral neck and shaft fracture; allows separate implant for optimal neck fixation, though reconstruction nail often preferred now (has a large diameter proximal entry hole for a screw to go across the neck fracture)
- Obesity where access to piriformis fossa (entry point for antegrade nail) difficult
- Pregnancy, to reduce radiation exposure to fetus

- Associated acetabular or pelvic fracture requiring different proximal incision
- Associated open knee injury
- Shaft fracture above knee replacement or below a hip replacement.

Subtrochanteric fracture

One located between the lesser trochanter and 5cm down shaft.

Bimodal incidence; typically young adult high energy trauma (initial management as for shaft fracture to resuscitate) or older pathological fracture (metastatic disease, osteopenia). Psoas and abductors tend to pull proximal fragment strongly into flexion and abduction which is difficult to correct; hence traction classically '90–90', i.e. hip and knee flexed 90° but high rate of malunion if used as definitive treatment.

Treatment

Intramedullary nail effective and has some mechanical advantage over a plate/screw device; precluded if fracture extends into entry point in piriformis fossa. Fixed angle device (blade plate, dynamic condylar screw or a specifically contoured proximal femoral locking plate) then preferred. Consider primary bone grafting if medial wall fragmented. All methods have ~10% failure rate, usually poor reduction ± loss of medial buttress.

Supracondylar (distal femoral) fracture

Common in the elderly, requires evaluation of co-morbidity to establish whether surgical treatment safe; majority managed this way. Relatively high rate of associated vascular injury mandating frequent and careful checks; absent pulses despite adequate reduction and splintage an indication for exploration (those that return if initially absent warrant an arteriogram in search of an intimal tear).

Half are intra-articular fractures of which majority intercondylar; aim to restore articular congruity and two-column condylar stability. Prolonged immobilization worsens inevitable knee stiffness.

Non-operative treatment

Long leg cast or skeletal traction—reserve for elderly immobile patient.

Operative treatment

- Plate and screws: blade plate (technically diffcult), dynamic condylar screw, contoured distal femoral locking plate (which has particular advantages in porotic bone to reduce risk of sequential screw pull-out)
- Retrograde intramedullary nail. Entry point via knee joint through roof of intercondylar notch
- External fixation. For severe/open injuries.

Reference

1 Wolinsky P, Tejjmani N, Richmond JH, et al. Controversies in intramedullary nailing of femoral shaft fractures. J Bone Joint Surg Am 2001;**9**:1404–14.

Adult femoral injuries: periprosthetic fractures

Femur
The femur is most common site for periprosthetic fractures around a total hip (1% rate after primary, 4% after revision) or knee replacement.

Hip
For hip fracture, classification of Masri et al.[1] guides treatment:

A Trochanteric fracture—non-operative if undisplaced

B Around stem
- B1: prosthesis well fixed—extramedullary fixation, i.e. plate with screws ± cables
- B2: prosthesis loose, good bone stock—revise to a long-stemmed prosthesis which bypasses and fixes fracture
- B3: prosthesis loose, poor bone stock—long stem revision; either uncemented or cemented into impacted bone graft and passing at least 2 canal widths distal to fracture. Consider extramedullary strut grafting to supplement construct.

C Fracture so distal to stem that implant can be ignored

Knee
A similar classification by Rorabeck and Taylor[2] guides treatment for fracture around a knee implant:

Undisplaced fracture, stable prosthesis: non-operative

Displaced fracture, prosthesis stable
- Plate and screws as for supracondylar
- Fracture ± grafting
- Retrograde femoral nailing an option if prosthesis slot will allow nail entry.

Loose prosthesis
- 1 stage: long-stemmed revision, allograft–implant
- Composite or tumour prosthesis
- 2 stage: fix fracture then revise implant.

References
1 Masri B, Meek R, Duncan C. Periprosthetic fractures evaluation and treatment. *Clin Orthop Rel Res* 2004;**420**:80–95.
2 Rorabeck C, Taylor J. Periprosthetic fractures of the femur complicating total knee arthroplasty. *Orthop Clin North Am* 1999;**30**:265–77.

Adult hip injuries

Hip dislocation

Associated with high velocity RTA (dashboard injury) and fall from height.

Fractures of femoral head, neck and acetabulum are associated.

Soft tissue injuries (degloving, open wounds) and co-existent abdominal, chest, head and neck injuries are common; manage initially as per ATLS guidelines.

Definitive management

- Emergent reduction after resuscitation, but beware displacing a missed femoral neck fracture
- A gentle attempt at reduction in the Emergency room under sedation and image intensification may be justified, but better done in the operating room under general anaesthetic
- If it is possible to obtain a preoperative CT scan without significant delay or compromise to patient safety, this is of great value for:
  - Locating acetabular rim fractures (± intra-articular fragments requiring removal) which may require fixation for capsular reattachment and stability
  - Delineating associated femoral head or neck fractures.

Thus, if closed reduction is unsuccessful, the preoperative CT scan will inform planning of the appropriate approach to deal with these associated injuries.

Complications

- AVN of femoral head
- Thromboembolism
- Sciatic nerve injury
- Retained bone fragments in joint
- Heterotopic ossification; consider prophylaxis
- Joint incongruence ± instability
- Secondary OA.

For further reading, see Bulstrode et al.[1].

Reference

1 Bulstrode C, Buckwater J, Carr A, et al., eds. Oxford Textbook of Orthopaedics and Trauma. Oxford: Oxford University Press, 2002.

Adult knee injuries

Knee dislocations

Rare but severe and potentially limb-threatening injury; usually high energy (RTA).

35% anterior (displacement of tibia relative to femur) hyperextension injury; 25% posterior (dashboard injury); 20% lateral, medial or rotatory and 20% occult, i.e. relocate spontaneously at time of injury. 30% will be open. 40% associated popliteal vessel injury; intact pulses do not exclude so measure ABPI. 25% rate of neurological damage; the bundle is relatively tethered behind the proximal tibia.

Manage by emergent reduction; interposed soft or associated fracture may mandate open procedure. Any vascular injury the priority after rapid skeletal stabilization with (joint-spanning) external fixator. Adequate pro-phylactic fasciotomies mandated for secondary re-perfusion injury.

Injury implies rupture of all ligamentous structures; should be repaired/ reconstructed early unless low demand or significant co-morbidity.

Proximal tibio-fibular joint dislocation

Classically a parachute injury with axial force applied to knee flexed to 80°. Closed reduction usually successful. Neuropraxia of common pero-neal nerve usually transient.

Acute patellar dislocation

Valgus load to flexed, axially loaded knee causes lateral patellar disloca-tion (similar to mechanism for ACL injury).

Ruptures the medial patellofemoral ligament, but vogue for acute repair/recon-struction discouraged by recent RCT evidence of no benefit. After reduction and plain films consider MRI if any suspicion of associated osteochondral fracture; fix early as cartilage swelling complicates delayed reattachment. Otherwise long leg cast or hinged brace.

Traumatic ligamentous injuries

Medial collateral injuries

Usually direct blow with valgus stress; any rotational force will probably injure cruciates too. Vast majority heal with non-operative brace manage-ment; exception where repair indicated is with associated PCL injury.

Lateral collateral injuries

May involve other lateral stabilizers that make up the 'posterolateral corner'; isolated injuries again treated non-operatively.

Cruciate ligaments

Anterior injury common, posterior much less so but perhaps under-diagnosed. See section on ligamentous knee injuries in non-traumatic conditions (see p. 328).

Extensor mechanism injuries

Quadriceps tendon rupture is common in elderly, often through degenerate tendon. Follows direct blow or forced contraction with foot planted. Tendon avulses from superior pole of patella causing palpable gap, though may be partial rupture; USS then useful.

Manage with operative repair if unable to SLR, drill holes through patella with heavy non-absorbable sutures. Late presentations require more complex reconstruction.

Patellar tendon avulsion: usually from inferior pole of patella in younger age group; skeletally immature may pull off an osteochondral sleeve which contains chondral surface of the patella. Midsubstance ruptures rare. See Knee injuries in children (see 📖 p. 580).

Patellar fractures: typically male aged 20–50 following direct blow or axial load to flexed knee.

Patterns: transverse (50–80%), stellate (30%), longitudinal (12%) marginal (pole), or osteochondral. Significant displacement is an articular step of 2mm or separation >3mm.

Treatment depends on extensor mechanism; if intact (able to SLR supine or actively to extend lying on side) then non-operative with cylinder cast or brace for 4–6 weeks. Otherwise operative; variety of techniques but longitudinal K wires with 'cerclage' figure of 8 acts as a tension band (converts eccentric tensile force with quads contraction into compression).

Haemarthrosis

Primary (spontaneous) in absence of trauma. Consider bleeding disorders, warfarin, vascular tumours/malformations, e.g. PVNS. Recurrent haemarthroses cause secondary OA.

Treat by correcting underlying clotting abnormality ± acute aspiration, also chemical or mechanical synovectomy.

Secondary to trauma. 80% ACL injury, 10% patellar dislocation, remainder include peripheral meniscal tears, capsule tears, osteochondral/osteophyte fractures.

Aspirate for pain relief and to examine; inspect for fat globules indicating fracture. Arthroscopy indicated if locked knee which may indicate osteochondral fracture or incarcerated meniscus.

Adult leg injuries

Tibial plateau fractures

Common fracture (1% of all; 8% in elderly), intra-articular by definition, high rate of associated injuries:
- Meniscal tears (in up to 50%)
- Collateral or cruciate ligament rupture (especially younger patients)
- Neurovascular injury and compartment syndrome with higher energy injuries (popliteal trifurcation tethered behind, and peroneal nerve laterally).

Schatzker classification useful; descriptive and higher grade corresponds to severity. Types I–III lower energy, IV–VI high energy severe injuries:
- Type I: lateral split (in young bone which resists compression. Often lateral meniscal tear that slips into displaced fracture)
- Type II: lateral split-depression
- Type III: pure lateral depression (older age group)
- Type IV: medial split or split-depression; medial tibial plateau bigger and stronger so more force transferred to fracture. Associated also with avulsed intercondylar eminence and ACL rupture; associated soft tissue injury often the issue with this type which may indicate the knee has dislocated and spontaneously reduced
- Type V: bicondylar, i.e. both plateaus involved (usually significant axial load)
- Type VI: tibial condylar fragments separated from shaft by metaphyseal fracture ± fragmentation.

Management
Order CT in addition to plain films to characterize fracture, establish extent of displacement and for operative planning where indicated.

Non-operative if undisplaced or low demand/significant co-morbidity: early mobilization in cast brace.

Operative guidelines (vary):
- >4mm depression of articular surface
- Significant varus/valgus instability
- Options include: percutaneous fixation ± arthroscopy to clear incarcerated meniscus and confirm reduction, open reduction with elevation of depressed fragment(s) via split or creation of a metaphyseal window (recent trial indicates synthetic bone graft better results than autogenous iliac crest), external fixation.

A recent RCT[1] showed benefits of circular frame management over open reduction and plate fixation for bicondylar fractures (V, VI).

Tibial shaft fractures

The most common long bone fracture of which up to a quarter will be open—described in graphic detail by legendary Parisian barber–surgeon Ambroise Paré (1510–1590) who sustained such an injury when kicked by his own steed and remarked upon 'pain that it is not possible for a man to endure greater without death'.

Tibial fracture is the most common cause for **compartment syndrome**.

Closed injuries with minimal displacement can be managed in a moulded above-knee cast with early conversion to a functional patella tendon-bearing

(Sarmiento[2]) cast; beware those with an intact fibula which tend to angulate into varus. Reamed intramedullary nailing facilitates early mobilization but carries operative risks.

Open fractures require emergent debridement (see Fractures 📖 p. 396) followed by stabilization. Much is written about these injuries; safe to fix after adequate wound excision with IM nail[3] (reamed or unreamed) or plate with early definitive soft tissue cover as required. This is the so-called 'fix and flap' method; requires early liaison with a plastic surgeon.

Absolute indications for surgery: open fracture, vascular injury, compartment syndrome, polytrauma. **IM nailing** suitable for most diaphyseal fractures with rotation and length controlled by locking bolts. **Plating** has a role in periarticular fractures; new specifically contoured locking plates popular. **External fixation** is safe for open fractures; higher rates of malunion and re-fracture if used for definitive management.

Complications

- Delayed or non-union (high energy injury, displacement, fragmentation, infection)
- Malunion
- Compartment syndrome (3–20%)
- Infection (<2% after IM nail, increases in open injury with severity)

Tibial pilon (plafond) fractures

Involve weight-bearing articular surface of distal tibia. Paucity of local soft tissue cover with precarious microcirculation so swelling can be massive, minimal ligamentotaxis effect, with traction and vascularity a serious issue. Mechanism of injury generally low energy rotational force or high energy axial compression (driving talus into tibial plafond). The classification of Ruedi and Allgower is useful:

- I   Undisplaced articular fracture
- II Significant articular displacement but fragmentation minimal
- III Significant fragmentation of articular surface and metaphyseal disruption with impaction.

but was based mainly on relatively low energy fractures in skiers. More severe injuries later recognized as behaving badly after early open reduction and plating. Recommended to span ankle joint with external frame ± fibula plating to maintain length while allowing soft tissues to recover over prolonged period. Then well-planned anatomical reconstruction of articular surface and stable fixation to shaft.

Complications

- Wound breakdown and infection
- Mal/non-union, pain, stiffness, instability
- Secondary OA.

References

1 Canadian Orthopaedic Trauma Society. Open reduction and internal fixation compared with circular fixator application for bicondylar tibial plateau fractures. Results of a multicenter, prospective, randomized clinical trial. *J Bone Joint Surg Am* 2006;**88**:2613–23.

2 Sarmiento A. A functional below-the-knee cast for tibial fractures. *J Bone Joint Surg Am* 1967;**49**:855–75.

3 Gopal, S. Majumder A, Batchelor GB, *et al.* Fix and flap: the radical orthopaedic and plastic treatment of severe open fractures of the tibia. *J Bone Joint Surg Br* 2000;**82**:959–66.

Adult ankle injuries

The ankle joint comprises articulations, with associated ligaments (see Fig. 9.5), between distal tibia and fibula (interosseus syndesmosis), talus and tibia (medial and lateral ligament complexes), os calcis/talus and fibula (calcaneofibular and anterior talofibular ligaments).

Relatively small disruptions of the articular contours and soft tissue restraints can adversely affect transmission of load; increased joint contact stresses (same load over a reduced area of contact) lead inevitably to OA.

Injuries divided into those that directly disrupt load-bearing surface of distal tibia (**pilon fractures**—discussed in Adult leg injuries, see 🕮 p. 436) and those that compromise stability and alignment of the ankle (medial, lateral and posterior malleolar fractures and ligament ruptures).

Ankle fractures

The most common are lower limb fractures, especially seen in young male sportsmen and middle-aged overweight females.

The simplest descriptions comprise the number of malleoli fractured (medial, lateral and posterior), extent of displacement and whether the joint is congruent, subluxed or frankly dislocated.

The Lauge–Hansen classification is complex and relates position of foot at time of injury (first word) and direction of deforming force (second word) to the actual fracture pattern.

Simpler and more widely used in practice is the Weber system. The higher the fibula fracture, the greater the energy transfer and soft tissue disruption with a greater propensity for instability:

Level of fibula fracture relative to tibiofibular syndesmosis
- A Below
- B At the level of
- C Above (less stable, may require temporary fixation).

Examination: should focus on distinguishing bone and soft tissue tenderness. Check for proximal fibular tenderness indicative of a Maisonneuve fracture (probably extensive disruption of the tibio-fibular interosseous membrane).

X-rays: AP mortise (15° internal rotation) and lateral views. Look critically for fracture lines and presence of talar shift.

Management
Initial:
- Protect soft tissue envelope—a clinically dislocated or grossly deformed ankle mandates immediate reduction prior to radiographs
- Plaster backslab in optimally reduced position for comfort and elevate.

Definitive
Goal is to achieve a congruent, stable joint; bone union; viable and intact soft tissue envelope; motion for cartilage nutrition and early return to function.

Non-operative treatment in cast or suitable brace for stable injury patterns—operative for the rest. Consider first the soft tissues upon which vascularity and therefore healing depend.

After 24h from time of injury swelling may mandate a prolonged period of rest and elevation before safe surgery. Severe, highly unstable injuries require temporary external fixation to hold reduction while allowing soft tissues to settle.

Guidelines for suitable operative management according to Weber type

Lateral malleolus fixation
- Type A: 1/3 tubular plate, tension band wire or locking plate for very low fracture
- Type B: lag screws plus neutralization plate, posterior antiglide plate
- Type C: lag screws plus neutralization plate, bridging plate if multifragmentary to maintain length and correct rotation.

Medial malleolus: usually 2 partially threaded screws or screw and wire

Posterior malleolus: if fragment >25% joint surface, fix with (cannulated) lag screw(s).

Syndesmosis: if disruption (diastasis) suspected, stress the inferior tibiofibular joint under anaesthetic ('hook' test) and fix with temporary screw as indicated.

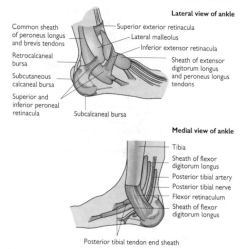

Lateral view of ankle

Common sheath of peroneus longus and brevis tendons
Retrocalcaneal bursa
Subcutaneous calcaneal bursa
Superior and inferior peroneal retinacula
Subcalcaneal bursa
Superior exterior retinacula
Lateral malleolus
Inferior extensor retinacula
Sheath of extensor digitorum longus and peroneus longus tendons

Medial view of ankle

Tibia
Sheath of flexor digitorum longus
Posterior tibial artery
Posterior tibial nerve
Flexor retinaculum
Sheath of flexor digitorum longus
Posterior tibial tendon end sheath

Fig. 9.5 Ankle anatomy.
Reproduced from Hakim, Clunie, and Haq, *Oxford Handbook of Rheumatology*, with permission from Oxford University Press.

Lauge–Hansen classification

Supination–adduction	1. Transverse fibular fracture or tear of lateral ligaments
	2. Vertical medial malleolus fracture
Supination–external rotation (of talus in mortise)	1. Disruption of anterior tibiofibular ligament ± avulsion of anterolateral tibia (Tillaux fragment)
	2. Spiral/oblique fracture of distal fibula at syndesmosis
	3. Disruption of posterior tibiofibular ligament or fracture of posterior malleolus
	4. Fracture of medial malleolus or deltoid ligament rupture
Pronation–abduction	1. Transverse fracture of medial malleolus or deltoid ligament disruption
	2. Rupture of syndesmotic ligaments or avulsion fracture
	3. Short horizontal/oblique fibular fracture above syndesmosis
Pronation–external rotation	1. Transverse fracture of medial malleolus or deltoid ligament disruption
	2. Disruption of anterior tibiofibular ligament ± avulsion fracture
	3. Short oblique fracture of fibula above syndesmosis (if proximal = *Maisonneuve* fracture)
	4. Rupture of posterior tibiofibular ligament or avulsion of posterolateral tibia
Pronation–axial compression (pilon)	1. Fracture of medial malleolus
	2. Fracture anterior margin of tibia
	3. Supramalleolar fibula fracture
	4. Transverse fracture of posterior tibial surface

Paediatrics

Paediatrics

Paediatric orthopaedics

Cerebral palsy: introduction

Heterogeneous group of non-hereditary, UMN impairment syndromes caused by chronic brain abnormalities affecting mainly movement and posture. Although the cerebral lesion is non-progressive, musculoskeletal deformities and impairment are progressive in the growing child.

Incidence

- The most common cause of physical disability in children
- 1–3 per 1000 live births
- In children weighing <1500g at birth the rate is 70 times higher than those >2500g.

Aetiology

- Prenatal (30%)—maternal infection (toxoplasmosis, rubella, cytomegalovirus, herpes, syphilis); maternal exposure to alcohol/drugs; congenital brain malformations
- Perinatal—birth weight <2500g with prematurity (25–40%); anoxia (10–20%)
- Postnatal (10%)—meningitis, head injury, immersion, intracerebral haemorrhage.

Pathophysiology

- Weakness is caused by UMN lesion that also results in loss of voluntary movement and early onset of fatigue
- Spasticity is a feature of all lesions of the pyramidal system. Spasticity in a muscle is mediated via a stretch reflex that is hyperactive. Tendon reflexes are brisk, and clonus may appear
- Contracture. As muscles do not follow the growing pace of bone (i.e. they are not stretched for more sarcomeres to form), the muscle–tendon unit is shortened, leading to contractures
- Deformity probably follows muscle imbalance, though it also occurs in hypotonic neuromuscular disorders.
- Reduced weight bearing or wheelchair dependence lead to OP which is increasingly a problem into adulthood. Similarly contracted joints with secondary deformity develop OA in later life.

Classification

- Spastic (most common, 60%). Increased muscle tone, hyperreflexia, slow and restricted movement. Contractures typical.
- Dystonic (20%). Basal ganglia involvement. Slow, writhing involuntary movements. Choreiform athetosis. Movements increase with emotional tension and disappear in sleep.
- Ataxic (10%). Involvement of cerebellum. Weakness, coordination difficulties, tremor, difficulty in fine or rapid movements
- Hypotonic
- Combined (spasticity occurs in 30% of CP types other than spastic).

Cerebral palsy: general management and GMFCS

Definition

A non-progressive lesion of the immature brain (static encephalopathy) causes a disorder of movement and posture which is permanent but not unchanging. Progressive musculoskeletal pathology results in the vast majority[1].

Common patterns of involvement are hemiplegia (unilateral arm and leg), diplegia (predominantly both legs) and total body involvement—formerly known as quadriplegia but revised to emphasize loss of truncal muscle balance and systemic problems such as gastro-oesophageal reflux, poor vision, hearing, seizures, etc. All children with hemiplegia will walk as will most (±assistive device) with diplegia; those with total body involvement rarely do so except 'therapeutically' in a walker frame.

Management

Therapy in the first decade of life focuses on function; appearance increasingly important in the second, and management of pain (from secondary OA) in the third[1].

Spastic CP is amenable to orthopaedic intervention (dystonic and other forms much less predictably so). Follow a stepwise approach reflecting that children are born without but develop skeletal abnormality. Multidisciplinary assessment and management: physiotherapy, orthotics, carers and occupational therapy (especially for the upper limb) plus orthopaedics (paediatric and spinal), general surgery and urology:

Spasticity management. Botulinum toxin muscle injections, systemic or intrathecal baclofen, selective dorsal rhizotomy. Young children have a wide 'dynamic range' (as described by Tardieu); when involved muscle is stretched rapidly there is an early catch beyond which further stretch (dynamic range) is possible with sustained tension. This responds well to botulinum toxin therapy.

Orthotic prescription, e.g. to support weak muscle (drop foot AFO), to correct foot deformity or preposition for stance (solid AFO), to correct abnormally directed forces on skeleton (ground reaction AFO).

Soft tissue rebalancing. The notion of a weak agonist muscle and overactive antagonist is too simplistic; there is generalized weakness in CP, and overall muscle strength must be preserved. Apparently overactive ankle plantar flexors must be balanced not against the weaker dorsiflexors but against ground reaction forces; failure to appreciate this may lead to a 'crouch gait' due to excessive surgical weakening of antigravity muscles. Muscle rebalancing should be achieved by intramuscular tendon lengthening whenever possible.

Indicated in older children with less dynamic range and more fixed shortening of the muscle–tendon unit. Muscle transfers should be of split tendons to avoid overcorrection.

Correction of fixed bone deformity. Best deferred until child older (~8yrs) but sometimes proximal femoral ± pelvic surgery will be required in children as young as 3 or 4yrs with total body involvement CP and a subluxed hip(s).

Salvage procedures. Arthrodesis, excision arthroplasty, hip replacement.

Gross Motor Function Classification System (GMFCS)

A validated and reliable 5-level functional grading system based on ability to sit and walk. Better describes and predicts motor function than topographical categorization (hemi-, di-plegia etc.):

- Level I: nearly normal level of gross motor function
- Level II: ability to walk independently but limitations in activities such as running or jumping
- Level III: require assistive devices to walk and use a wheelchair for longer distances
- Level IV: can stand for transfers, have minimal walking ability, depend mainly on wheelchair for mobility
- Level V: lack head control; cannot sit independently, stand or walk; are dependent for all aspects of care.

See also p. 445 for further general comments.

Anti-spasticity agents

- Botulinum toxin A (Botox®). Polypeptide chain that irreversibly binds to the cholinergic terminals at neuromuscular junction and effectively inhibits release of acetylcholine from synaptic vesicles. Injected locally to muscles can cause a rapid onset of weakness lasting 3–6 months
- Baclofen. γ-Aminobutyric acid agonist acting peripherally and centrally to spinal cord level to impede the release of excitatory neurotransmitters that cause spasticity. Can be administered orally (large doses needed and sedation is a side effect), intrathecally as a single injection or with a continuous infusion pump.

Reference

1 Graham HK, Selber P. Musculoskeletal aspects of cerebral palsy. *J Bone Joint Surg Br* 2003;**85**:157–66.

Cerebral palsy—hemiplegia

Involvement

Predominantly unilateral upper and lower limb.

Usually normal intelligence and high levels of function.

Problems

Upper limb: elbow flexion, forearm pronation ('folded wing' posture seen especially as child walks), wrist flexion/ulnar deviation, thumb in palm.

Lower limb: distal involvement (common) with drop foot ± equinus ankle, more proximal involvement with hamstring ± psoas overactivity causing 'jump knee'.

Hip subluxation rare but does occur.

Orthotics

Drop foot AFO, ground reaction AFO for more proximal involvement, neoprene or dynamic lycra/neoprene 'second skin' splints for upper limb.

Surgical options

Spasticity management (botulinum toxin) of overactive muscle groups effective in younger child and may delay, and decrease magnitude of, later surgery.

For fixed ankle equinus, gastrosoleus release usually suffices, rarely necessary to release posterior ankle or subtalar joints. Silverskiold's test confirms that both muscle groups tight. Equinovarus foot deformity common; best managed prior to development of fixed bone deformity with suitable soft tissue release and split tendon transfer, usually tibialis anterior, posterior or combination thereof.

Upper limb surgery less commonly indicated on functional grounds as uninvolved side usually dominant, but may be required for cosmesis and modest functional gains. Options include tendon release(s), transfer and wrist arthrodesis.

Lower limb examination in cerebral palsy

Measure and record

Supine:

- Hip flexion range and fixed flexion deformity (**Thomas's test** or prone Staheli method)
- Hip abduction in hip flexion and normal supine extension
- Hip adduction in same positions
- Hip rotation (internal and external) in same positions.

Popliteal angle; flex hip and knee to 90°, then extend knee. 0° corresponds to a fully extended knee.

(Any) Fixed knee flexion with hip extended.

Ankle dorsiflexion knee flexed (so *gastrocnemius* is de-tensioned—*Silver-skiold's test*; this muscle, unlike *soleus* which is under test, crosses the knee joint).

Ankle dorsiflexion knee extended (if dorsiflexion reduces, there is fixed shortening specifically in *gastrocnemius*—a common finding in CP diplegia).

Prone:

- Extend hips from flexion (with legs over end of examining table) until the pelvis lifts up (**Staheli method** for measuring fixed hip flexion)
- Retest hip rotation with knee flexed 90°
- Assess femoral neck version by feeling for greater trochanter with hip in varying positions of (usually internal) rotation. When it is most obvious, the angle made by the leg from the vertical (knee flexed 90°) is a reasonable approximation of femoral neck anteversion
- Rapidly flex knee up to 90° from extension and watch whether and when the buttocks rise, indicating *quadriceps* spasticity (**Duncan–Ely test**)
- Assess angle the foot makes relative to the thigh (thigh–foot axis with knee flexed 90°) as measure of tibial torsion and forefoot alignment
- Also assess hindfoot position (varus/valgus) and correctability viewed from above.

Cerebral palsy—diplegia

Involvement

Predominantly both lower limbs

The majority function at GMFCS levels I, II, III.

Problems

Overactivity in muscles spanning 2 joints causes sagittal plane imbalance, e.g. *rectus femoris*, hamstrings, *gastrocnemii*.

Resulting gait patterns characterized into 4 types by Rodda and Graham: true and apparent equinus, jump knee and crouch.

Torsional bony deformity causes 'lever arm disease'; loss of mechanical advantage, particularly for hip abductors and ankle plantar flexors.

Hip displacement (lateral migration >30% associated with high risk of subluxation/dislocation) is strongly related to GMFCS level (see Table 10.1).

Orthotics

- Hinged or solid AFO
- Ground reaction AFO indicated for crouch gait pattern of hip, knee and ankle flexion. Works to decelerate the leg during stance, moving the ground reaction force forwards passively to extend the knee.

Surgical options

Over-riding principle is to address muscle imbalance and bone deformity at every level (foot/ankle, knee and hip, the spine) simultaneously. This avoids the 'birthday syndrome' where isolated distal correction unmasks more proximal involvement requiring another operation the next year. Worse still, overcorrection at the ankle is a real risk if more proximal contributions not understood and addressed.

3-D instrumented gait analysis (see opposite) very useful before major surgical intervention in unpicking primary from secondary abnormalities. Planned simultaneous multilevel surgery, which may be staged into bony and soft tissue procedures followed by intensive physiotherapy rehabilitation, is best performed by expert teams with a paediatric anaesthetist and intensive care facilities available.

Common *soft tissue* procedures include: psoas (intramuscular) tendon lengthening at pelvic brim, fractional hamstring lengthening, rectus femoris release or transfer (if gait analysis indicates reduced knee flexion in swing phase with this muscle firing out of phase on EMG), gastrocnemius aponeurosis recession (leaving soleus intact).

For *bone*: varus derotation proximal femoral osteotomies for femoral anteversion and hip migration, pelvic osteotomies to improve acetabular coverage, distal femoral extension osteotomies for fixed knee flexion, supramalleolar tibial derotation osteotomies, lateral column lengthening of foot (through os calcis) for PPV with midfoot break.

Table 10.1 Correlation between GMFCS and hip displacement

GMFCS level	Incidence of hip displacement
I	0%
II	15%
III	41%
IV	69%
V	90%

From Soo et al.[1].

Gait analysis

A team, which includes the orthopaedic surgeon and physiotherapist, evaluates the following data:
• Physical examination findings
• 2-D video recording of gait (can be paused, played back and slowed down)
• 3-D kinematics (graphical mapping of limb movements in coronal, sagittal and axial—for rotation—planes)
• 3-D kinetics examining the moments acting across lower limb joints
• Dynamic EMG from superficial or needle electrodes to establish which/whether muscles firing inappropriately out of phase
• Energy cost of walking, using calorimetry or oxygen consumption.

Reference

1 Soo B, Howard JJ, Boyn RN, et al. Hip displacement in cerebral palsy. *J Bone Joint Surg Am* 2006;**88**:121–9.

Cerebral palsy—total body involvement

Involvement

All four limbs and spine.

Some function at GMFCS level III, but majority at IV and V.

Problems

Hip displacement and scoliosis are common and often rapidly progressive (Fig. 10.1). Early hip subluxation may be clinically 'silent', but established dislocation is a potent cause of pain, pelvic obliquity and difficulty with perineal care (limited hip abduction) and transfers. Hence screening with regular pelvic radiographs indicated. Spinal curves are typically long, C-shaped pattern.

Orthotics

More limited role than for ambulant CP children. Standing frames very useful to counteract hip and knee flexion contractures from prolonged sitting, also for emotional well-being and respiratory function.

Bracing is ineffective for spinal deformity, but customized moulded (wheel) chair that supports the trunk optimizes functional use of upper limbs.

Surgical options

Aggressive soft tissue release (hip adductors ± hamstrings, psoas) for early detected hip displacement. For established subluxation reconstruction is with varus derotation femoral osteotomies (bilateral) ± pelvic osteotomy for acetabular dysplasia. The deficiency is usually posterior. Longstanding dislocation with painful femoral head ulceration is difficult to salvage, hence importance of hip surveillance.

For severe spinal curves (>40–50°) a long instrumented posterior fusion (down to the pelvis) may be indicated ± anterior release to obtain correction.

These are major procedures requiring careful preoperative assessment and optimization of respiratory, gastro-oesophageal and other co-morbidities (seizures, poor nutrition, anaemia, etc.).

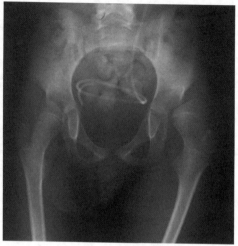

Fig. 10.1 Migrating CP hip.

Skeletal dysplasias

A diverse group of mainly inherited developmental disorders of bone, cartilage and fibrous tissue.

Dysplasia means 'abnormal growth or development'. Disturbed growth occurs as a result of genetic errors of structure or metabolism of certain proteins which lead to altered mechanical properties of developing bones and subsequent deformity.

Rubin's anatomical classification based on bone formation and modelling is simple to recall:

	Overgrowth	Undergrowth
Epiphyseal	Trevor's disease	SED, MED
Physeal	Multiple enchondromatosis	Achondroplasia
Metaphyseal	Hereditary multiple exostoses	Osteopetrosis
Diaphyseal	Diaphyseal dysplasia	Osteogenesis imperfecta

MED = multiple epiphyseal dysplasia; SED = spondyloepiphyseal dysplasia.

Also disorders of:
• **Chromosomes**: Turner's, Down syndrome, Edward's trisomy
• **Lysosomal storage**: Hunter's, Hurler's, Morquio's
• **Connective tissues**: Ehlers–Danlos, Marfan syndromes.

Increasingly molecular biologists are defining the genetic aetiology of these disorders necessitating new categorization based on function of the causative gene, e.g. structural, tumour and cell regulatory, developmental, protein processing[1].

Management

In general terms, parents require education (including dysplasia societies), reassurance and genetic counselling for future offspring. Treatment is multidisciplinary; operative management depends on the specific condition but may include:
• Correction of limb angular deformity ± lengthening
• Decompression of spinal stenosis, e.g. achondroplasia
• Scoliosis correction and fusion, e.g. Marfan syndrome
• Cervical fusion for instability, e.g. Down syndrome
• Telescopic rodding for progressive long bone deformity

Key is to recognize when a syndromal child is deviating from 'normal' for that condition[2]. For example, an achondroplastic child would be expected to have an exaggerated lumbar lordosis, but symptoms of dural compression mandate urgent intervention.

Dwarfism

Said to be **proportionate** if the limbs and trunk are equally affected (e.g. mucopolysaccharidoses). **Disproportionate** dwarfism can be of the short trunk, e.g. spondyloepiphyseal dysplasia, or short limb, e.g. achondroplasia variety. Shortening in the limbs can be more pronounced in different regions (**rhizomelic**–proximal, **mesomelic**–middle segment, **acromelic**–distal).

Below are examples with underlying genetic defect and features:

	Defect/ inheritance	Features
Achondroplasia	FGFR3/AD	Frontal bossing, button nose, trident hands, lumbar stenosis and lordosis
Pseudoachondroplasia	COMP/AD	Normal facies, cervical instability
Spondyloepiphyseal dysplasia	Type II collagen/ AD/XLR	Epiphyseal fragmentation, platyspondyly, odontoid hypoplasia
Kneist's syndrome	Collagen II/AD	Short trunk, scoliosis, dumbbell femur, retinal detachment
Metaphyseal chondrodysplasias		
Jansen's	PTHrP/AD	Hypercalcaemia, metaphyseal expansion
Schmid's	Collagen X/AD	Coxa vara, genu varum
McKusick's	Unknown/AR	Odontoid hypoplasia, ankle deformity
Multiple epiphyseal dysplasia	Collagen II/AD	Short limbed dwarfism, irregular proximal femora (cf. Perthe's), valgus knees
Diastrophic dysplasia	STP/AR	Kyphoscoliosis, ear deformities
Cleidocranial dysplasia	CBFA1/AD	Clavicle aplasia, coxa vara
Mucopolysaccharidoses		Proportionate dwarfism
Hurler's	DS HS/AR	MR, cloudy cornea, poor prognosis
Hunter's	DS HS/XLR	MR, clear corneas
Sanfilippo's	HS/AR	MR, cloudy corneas
Morquio's (most common)	KS/AR	Normal intelligence, skull thickening, wide ribs, beaked vertebrae, flat pelvis, coxa vara, bullet metacarpals

FGFR3 = fibroblast growth factor receptor 3; COMP = cartilage oligomeric matrix protein; PTHrP = parathyroid hormone-related peptide; AD = autosomal dominant; AR = autosomal recessive; XLR = X-linked recessive; CBFA1 = core binding factor alpha 1; DS = dermatan sulphate; HS = heparan sulphate; KS = keratin sulphate; MR = mental retardation.

References

1 Alman BA. A classification for genetic disorders of interest to orthopaedists. *Clin Orthop Rel Res* 2002;**401**:17–26.
2 Cole WG. Bone, cartilage and fibrous tissue disorders. In: Benson MKD, Fixsen JA, Macnicol MF, et al., eds. *Children's Orthopaedics and Fractures*, 2nd edn. Churchill Livingstone, 2002:67–92.

Vascular syndromes

Arteriovenous malformations that are associated with recognizable patterns of deformity. Some of those with orthopaedic relevance are set out below.

Klippel–Trenaunay syndrome

Uncommon disorder, exact prevalence unknown. Defined by presence of:
- Cutaneous capillary malformations of an extremity (port wine stain)
- Congenital venous varicosities
- Skeletal or soft tissue hypertrophy.

Lesions are usually present at birth and increase in size over the first years of life. Usually only one limb is affected (cf. hemihypertrophy). Leg length discrepancy may be present because of the associated hypertrophy of the limb. When associated with an arteriovenous fistula (high-flow lesion) it is known as **Parkes–Weber** syndrome.

Complications
- Lymphoedema
- Ulceration/infection
- Thrombophlebitis
- Kasabach–Merritt syndrome (consumptive thrombocytopenia).

Treatment
- Conservative (compression stockings, pneumatic pumps, anticoagulants, sclerotherapy)
- Epiphysiodesis for limb length discrepancy, soft tissue debulking
- Amputation for severe deformity.

Proteus syndrome

A sporadically occurring hamartomatous disorder with manifold mesodermal malformations. There are characteristic overgrowths (partial or regional gigantism) and subcutaneous lesions that lead to thickening of the soles of the feet. It is exceedingly rare, disfigurement is usually severe.

Maffucci syndrome

A rare genetic disorder, characterized by multiple enchondromas, bone deformities, and dark, irregularly shaped haemangiomas. Treatment is symptomatic.

Clinical findings
- Short stature, arm or leg length inequality
- Haemangiomas
- Enchondromas (usually in the hands) can lead to pathological fractures and deformity
- Malignant transformation (chondrosarcoma) may occur in ~30% of patients.

Metabolic and endocrine abnormalities of the immature skeleton

Rickets

- Syndrome of lack of available extracellular Ca^{2+}, PO_4^- or both, that interferes with physeal growth and mineralization of the skeleton. Literal meaning is 'twisted' bones
- *Causes* include dietary deficiency ± inadequate sunlight exposure, GI disorders, vitamin D-resistant rickets. X-linked hypophosphataemia is most common cause in the developed world with inappropriate phosphate loss in proximal renal tubule
- *Clinical features*: weakness, lethargy, irritability, delay in developmental landmarks, short stature, frontal bossing, long thoracic kyphosis, ligamentous laxity, long bone deformity, e.g. genu varum, repeated fractures
- *Tests*: serum Ca^{2+}, PO_4^-, ALP and PTH levels. Serum vitamin D, urine Ca^{2+} and PO_4^- levels. Genetic testing for X-linked disease
- *X-rays*: osteopenia, 'fuzzy' cortices, irregular widening or cupping of growth plates, Looser's lines (linear radiolucencies extending transversely from one cortex across to the medullary canal), bowing of femur or tibia
- *Treatment*: phosphate and vitamin D.

Renal osteodystrophy

- Bone disease secondary to renal failure
- Glomerular damage leads to phosphate retention and tubular injury causing decreased production of 1,25-dihydroxyvitamin D
- *Clinical* (may have all the features of rickets): bone fragility, calcification of conjunctivae and skin, periarticular calcification and ossification, ligamentous laxity, muscle weakness, slipped capital femoral epiphysis, genu valgum
- *X-rays*: 'salt and pepper' skull (tiny punched out lesions), brown tumours (secondary hyperparathyroidism)
- *Treatment*: endocrinology consultation, fracture treatment with cast or fixation, surgical correction of deformity.

Osteogenesis imperfecta

- Genetic disorder of type I collagen formation causing bone fragility (frequent fractures) and associated hearing, ocular and dental abnormalities
- Sillence[1] classification commonly used (see Table 10.2)
- Treatment for type I is early mobilization after fracture splintage or fixation, delayed union unlikely
- For more severe types III ± IV, bisphosphonate therapy may reduce bone pain and fracture rate
- IM nailing of long weight-bearing bones with telescopic rods after age 2yrs can be effective but is not without complications. Indications are recurrent fractures causing progressive deformity and secondary disuse osteopenia which predispose to ongoing re-fracture. Newer generation Fassier–Duval rods are easier to implant.

Table 10.2 Sillence[1] classification of osteogenesis imperfecta (OI)

OI type	Clinical features	Inheritance
	Normal stature, little or no deformity, blue sclerae, hearing loss in 50% of families. Tendency to fracture reduces markedly at skeletal maturity	
I	Dentinogenesis imperfecta is rare	AD
		AD (new mutations)
		Parental mosaicism
II	Severe form that is lethal in the perinatal period	
		AD
	Progressively deforming form, usually with moderate deformity at birth. Scleral colour varies, often lightening with age. Dentinogenesis imperfect and hearing loss common. Stature very short	AR (rare)
III		Parental mosaicism
	Mild to moderate bone deformity and variable short stature; dentinogenesis imperfecta is common, hearing loss occurs in some families. White or blue sclerae	AD
IV		Parental mosaicism

Idiopathic juvenile osteoporosis

- Rare, self-limited disorder of unknown aetiology characterized by profound reduction in bone mass
- Onset usually 8–14yrs, most resolve within 2–4yrs
- Clinical: back pain, leg pain, marked metaphyseal osteopenia, kyphosis, metaphyseal fractures
- Differential diagnosis: osteogenesis imperfecta, hematological malignancies, thyroid disorders, Cushing's disease, steroid-induced osteopenia.

Osteopetrosis ('marble bone disease')

- Rare metabolic bone disease characterized by diffuse increase in bone density and obliteration of marrow spaces. Osteoclast failure to resorb bone (secondary to carbonic anhydrase deficiency). Bones dense but brittle.
- Treatment: bone marrow transplantation at young age for severe form, high dose vitamin D, γ-interferon. Beware delayed union after fracture and anticipate extreme difficulty drilling/osteotomizing bone.

Reference

1 Sillence DO, Senn A, Danks DM. Genetic heterogeneity in osteogenesis imperfecta. *J Med Genet* 1979;**16**:101–16.

Diseases related to the haemopoietic system 1

von Willebrand's disease (vWD)
Deficiency or abnormality of vWF causes reduced platelet adherence to damaged endothelium. Inherited either AD or AR; affects males and females equally.

Haemophilias
Common forms
Type A
Congenital bleeding disorder affecting 1 in 10 000 males. Deficiency of factor VIII; X-linked recessive inheritance in ~2/3, remainder new mutations. Males affected, female carriers (rarely symptomatic). Severity depends on factor VIII level; 50% of known haemophiliacs are moderate or severe.

Type B (Christmas disease)
Deficiency of factor IX. Less common. Also X-linked recessive inheritance. Similar spectrum of severity to type A.

Clinical findings in general
Usually males with (+)ve family history. Recurrent haemarthroses are painful, cause restricted motion, synovitis and accrue chondral damage. Target joints in order of predilection are knee > shoulder > elbow > ankle > hip > wrist. Increased intraoperative bleeding with routine procedures if not anticipated and corrected.

Investigation
Platelet count, bleeding time, APTT and PT, factor VIII and IX assays are measured; abnormalities vary according to type of deficiency and should be discussed with haematologist.

Prophylaxis
Regular infusions of exogenous clotting factor concentrates and activity modification to prevent joint bleeding.

Treatment
Immobilization for acute haemarthrosis ± washout of joint. Consider also surgical (arthroscopic) or radionuclide synovectomy (radioactive ablation of hypertrophic synovium).

Sickle cell disease (SCD)

Sickle-shaped red blood cells obstruct capillaries leading to ischaemia and acute episodes (*crises*) of bone pain.

Incidence

Trait is common in western Africa. 10% of African-American population carries the HbS gene and 1 in 600 has full homozygous SCD.

Orthopaedic manifestations

Common orthopaedic manifestations are bone pain and/or osteomyelitis, commonly *Salmonella* sp. (cf. *S. aureus* in general population). AVN (femoral or humeral head). Pathological fractures. Septic arthritis. Pneumococcal septicaemia and meningitis. Dactylitis (seen early in life). Growth retardation and skeletal immaturity. Avoid tourniquet for homozygous disease.

Treatment (of crises)

Opioid analgesia. Rehydration. Broad-spectrum antibiotics. Consider transfusion.

Thalassaemias

Definition

Heterogenous group of inherited haemolytic anaemias resulting from mutations affecting globulin synthesis. Patients are usually of Mediterranean descent.

Orthopaedic manifestations

Bone pain and fragility, growth retardation, slipped capital femoral epiphysis (SCFE).

Radiographic findings

OP, widened marrow spaces, thinned cortices, 'hair-on-end' appearance of the skull.

Systemic findings

Tissue fibrosis (due to increased body iron loads), cardiomyopathy, diabetes mellitus, and hypoparathyroidism and hypothyroidism.

Treatment

Early transfusion therapy maintaining haemoglobin >9g/dl, iron chelation, bone marrow transplantation, splenectomy and supportive medical management.

Diseases related to the haemopoietic system 2

Gaucher's disease

AR deficiency of lysosomal enzyme glucocerebrosidase leading to accumulation of its fatty substrate **glucocerebroside** (in bone and elsewhere). Common in Ashkenazi Jews.

Recurrent bone crises (episodes of pain and swelling) without initial radiographic changes. Pain not well controlled despite opiates. Expansion of metaphyses—'Erlenmeyer flask' appearance—at distal femur. Erosion of bone cortices gives 'moth-eaten' appearance. AVN of femoral or humeral head. Bone crises similar to SCD. Pathological fractures.

Niemann–Pick disease

Accumulation of sphingomyelin in reticuloendothelial cells, seen commonly in eastern European Jews. Radiographs: marrow expansion, cortical thinning, coxa valga. Niemann–Pick disease is similar to Gaucher's except it is associated with severe mental retardation.

Eosinophilic granuloma

A uni- or multifocal proliferation of **Langerhans** histiocytes that commonly affects the skeletal system. Multiple form is **Langerhans cell histiocytosis** (formerly known as **histiocytosis** X). Letterer–Siwe disease and Hand–Schüller–Christian disease are different manifestations of the same disease process. The latter classically presents with triad of a skull lesion, exophthalmos and diabetes insipidus; the former is severe and usually fatal.

Incidence

1–5% benign bone tumours. 80% of patients are >10yrs old.

Orthopaedic manifestations

Skull, femur and spine affected most commonly. A cause of vertebra plana (Fig. 10.2). A 'great mimic' (of infection and other tumours).

Differential diagnosis

Ewing's sarcoma, osteomyelitis, lymphoma, leukaemia. Biopsy to confirm; skeletal survey to identify most accessible lesion.

Treatment

Bone lesions benign and usually heal spontaneously. Occasionally steroids or radiotherapy for more severe systemic disease.

Leukaemia

Most common malignancy in childhood. Uncommon presentation to orthopaedic services, but 30% acute lymphoblastic leukaemia presents with bone pain so need to consider as differential diagnosis and look critically at haematological indices. Can also present with osteomyelitis or septic arthritis.

Radiographs may show any of: osteopenia, metaphyseal bands, periosteal new bone formation, geographic lytic lesions, mixed sclerosis and lysis.

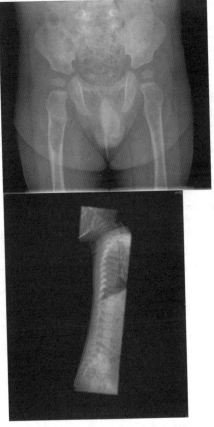

Fig. 10.2 Multifocal eosinophilic granuloma with vertebra plana.

Juvenile idiopathic arthritis

Definition

Arthritis that persists >6 weeks in child/adolescent under age 16yrs. Arthritis of a known cause must be excluded.

~1:1000 children will develop swelling of one or more joints and 50% of these will progress to juvenile idiopathic arthritis (JIA).

Classification

- Systemic (Still's disease): rash, daily high fever, inflamed joints, anaemia, high WCC, hepatosplenomegaly, lymphadenopathy. Highest likelihood of systemic complications and internal organ involvement
- Polyarticular—involvement of ˇ5 joints (both large and small) in the first 6 months of the disease. May be RhF positive
- Oligoarticular—most common type affecting ~50% of JIA patients. Peak incidence between 2nd and 3rd year of life, female predominance. Usually involves a few large joints, commonly knee; single hip joint rarely involved in isolation however.

Clinical findings

Early morning symptoms including stiffness (worse in cold), limp and restricted joint motion with synovitis. In monoarticular disease inflammatory markers may not be raised (if acutely so reconsider infection).

Beware anterior uveitis—inflammation of iris and ciliary body, 80% of that seen in children is associated with JIA. Seen especially with (+)ve ANA disease; need slit lamp eye examination to exclude.

Prognosis—treatment

- Refer to paediatric rheumatology
- Onset <1yr, RhF (+)ve, eye and hip involvement are poor prognostic factors
- Orthopaedic involvement along a spectrum from simple diagnosis and referral to occasional joint washout for severe synovitis, correction of secondary joint or growth deformity, joint replacement for end-stage burnt-out disease. Latter often requires custom small implants in gracile bones
- Physiotherapists and occupational therapists help significantly.

Seronegative spondyloarthropathies

A group of four conditions: ankylosing spondylitis, psoriatic arthritis, reactive arthritis, arthritis associated with inflammatory bowel disease.

Ankylosing spondylitis

Chronic inflammatory disease of axial skeleton. Cardinal symptoms: insidious onset, back pain especially at night with prolonged morning stiffness and progressive loss of spine motion. Exercise may help in pain relief. X-rays demonstrate sacroiliitis with spinal syndesmoses and ankyloses. Presents in young adults 15–25yrs old. Frequent peripheral joint inflammation, acute anterior uveitis, cardiac and pulmonary disease. HLA B27 antigen present in 5–8% of the general population, but in 95% of white and 50% of black patients. Not diagnostic but useful in children and young women with normal X-rays and atypical presentation.

Psoriatic arthritis

Five subtypes: oligoarticular asymmetric (most common), polyarticular symmetric (similar to RA), axial (similar to AS), DIPJ involvement, arthritis mutilans with telescoping digits. All subtypes are usually preceded by cutaneous psoriasis, but in 20% of patients arthritis precedes the psoriasis. Nail pitting and dactylitis are usually present.

Reactive arthritis

Previously called Reiter's syndrome. Triggered by a sexually transmitted infection (*Chlamydia*) or bowel infection (*Yersinia*, *Salmonella*, *Campylobacter*, *Shigella*). Cardinal findings are lower limb oligoarthritis, conjunctivitis and dysuria.

Arthritis associated with inflammatory bowel disease

20% of patients with IBD will develop inflammatory arthritis. Usually peripheral joint inflammation presents with bowel disease activity, while axial joint inflammation flares up irrespective of bowel disease.

All types have overlapping symptoms of axial inflammation, sacroiliitis and enthesitis.

Treatment

- Posture and range of motion exercises
- NSAIDs
- Methotrexate and sulfasalazine help in reducing joint erosions and damage in chronic peripheral joint involvement
- Intra-articular steroids may be helpful. Systemic steroids not usually used
- In psoriatic arthritis and resistant AS, anti-TNF-α agents have yielded promising results
- Antibiotics for reactive arthritis.

Osteomyelitis in children

In children, bone pain + fever = osteomyelitis until proven otherwise.

Acute haematogenous osteomyelitis (usually metaphyseal) responds to appropriate IV antibiotics.
- Empirical antibiotic treatment is reasonable if clinical presentation and imaging consistent with infection, but have low threshold for biopsy (sending samples for culture and histology) before commencing
- Coverage for Gram negatives may be less critical with *Haemophilus* vaccination
- Duration of IV therapy controversial; tailor this and step-down to orals according to culture results and clinical response
- Consider also atypical organisms, e.g. *Kingella kingae* (request appropriate culture media) if indolent presentation and *Mycobacterium tuberculosis*.

Manage operatively if USS or MRI demonstrates a significant abscess/subperiosteal collection or if child fails to respond to non-operative treatment.
- Even with established, chronic osteomyelitis children have excellent healing and remodelling capacity once infection adequately treated, and can resorb extensive sequestra. Preserve periosteum where possible to facilitate this
- Infection near and across a physis carries risk of subsequent growth arrest; warn parents and follow child for longitudinal or angular growth arrest.

Always consider that 30% of **acute leukaemia** presents with bone pain secondary to osseous infiltration. May have elevated CRP and fever, and radiological features mimic those of infection. Request blood film ± haematology review for bone marrow aspirate if FBC shows anaemia or neutropenia.

Consider also **bone tumours** which mimic radiological appearance of osteomyelitis, e.g. eosinophilic granuloma (benign) or Ewing's (malignant); hence the importance of biopsy especially in chronic cases with established bone changes. Send samples for microbiology and histopathology. If indolent presentation consider mycobacterium tuberculosis and request CXR and Heaf or Mantoux skin test.

CRMO

Chronic recurrent multifocal osteomyelitis is an uncommon chronic form of bone disease with a radiological appearance consistent with chronic osteomyelitis. Foci may be epiphyseal and multifocal with sequentially relapsing symptoms. Biopsy cultures are negative and disease may represent an inflammatory process rather than a truly infective one ('RA of bone'). This is, however, a diagnosis of exclusion, requiring negative microbiological cultures (and failure to respond to best-guess antibiotic therapy) and biopsy histology consistent with chronic non-granulomatous infection (presence of plasma cells favours CRMO rather than a neoplastic process). Treat with simple analgesics; consider also steroids, bisphosphonates (in liaison with paediatric rheumatologist).

Septic arthritis in children

Common in children (especially <2yrs); in neonate increased risk of multi-focal infection and whole bone involvement from metaphyseal focus. Can be especially devastating in the hip.

Causes

Primary seeding of synovial membrane (haematogenous or direct puncture) or secondary to adjacent metaphyseal osteomyelitis which ruptures into the joint capsule—shoulder, hip, elbow and ankle joint capsules all overlap the metaphysis and in neonate hip vessels cross the physis (up to 18 months of age) facilitating direct spread. The metaphysis is a common site for infection in children (end arterial loops collect haematogenous bacteria).

In neonates *Staphylococci* and *Streptococci* predominate (*H. influenzae* largely eradicated in developed countries with vaccination). Beware recent emergence of PVL *S. aureus* which elaborates a (Panton–Valentine) leukocidin toxin associated with severe and widespread disease. Consider also *Escherichia coli* and *Pseudomonas* spp. (drug abusers) in older age groups and *Neisseria gonorrhoea* in sexually active adolescents.

Clinical features
- Fever
- Local swelling, erythema, temperature
- Inability to weight bear
- Joint motion severely restricted
- Elevated WCC, CRP, ESR
- 'Pseudoparalysis' in neonate.

Differential diagnosis

Mainly transient synovitis in childhood; see Kocher criteria (see 📖 p. 469) to differentiate for hip.

Long list includes inflammatory arthropathy (JIA), malignancy (including leukaemia), bleeding disorder, PVNS, acute rheumatic fever, Lyme disease, Henoch–Schonlein purpura.

Management
- USS to confirm (purulent) effusion
- Joint aspiration for diagnosis: Gram stain positive in 30–50% only (so negative aspirate microscopy does not exclude), culture in 50–80%. Also WCC $>5\times10^9$/l in aspirate, protein levels less than serum
- Emergent surgical drainage and irrigation of the joint
- Broad-spectrum antibiotics after aspiration, rationalized by culture results.

Complications

- Physeal destruction or bar formation (secondary limb length discrepancy or angular deformity)
- Osteonecrosis
- Joint instability (**always** immobilize hip in spica after washout to prevent secondary dislocation)
- Stiffness or ankylosis secondary to chondrolysis

Kocher criteria for assessment of painful hip in children[1]

- ESR >40mm/h
- Fever
- WCC >12×10^9/litre
- Non-weight bearing.

All 4 criteria = 99% chance septic arthritis; 3 = 93%; 2 = 40%; 1 = 3%.

For further reading see McCarthy et al.[2]

References

1 Kocher MS, Zurakowski D, Kasser JR. Differentiating between septic arthritis and transient synovitis of the hip in children: an evidence-based clinical prediction algorithm. *J Bone Joint Surg Am* 1999;**81**:1662–70.
2 McCarthy JJ, Dormans JP, Kozin SH, et al. Musculoskeletal infections in children. *J Bone Joint Surg Am* 2004;**86**:850–63.

Myopathies

Degenerative skeletal muscle diseases not caused by nerve dysfunction or abnormality of the neuromuscular junction.

Cause progressive weakness and muscle wasting in early childhood. Typically present as 'floppy baby' that goes on to delayed achievement of motor milestones. Aetiology may be hereditary, inflammatory or the result of an endocrine disorder. Cure or effective treatments are generally elusive; tend to be chronic, slowly progressive diseases.

Diagnosis often requires EMG and muscle biopsy in additional to physical signs and blood investigations. Generally function will improve with age though respiratory muscle weakness may cause failure and death.

Examples

Core central myopathy

Muscle biopsy for definitive diagnosis. Congenital hip dislocation occurs, also patella subluxation and scoliosis. It is associated with malignant hyperpyrexia.

Nemaline myopathy

Muscle biopsy; microscopy shows rods at the level of the z lines, type 1 fibres predominate. Associated with slender but strong muscles, facial weakness and nasal speech.

Muscular dystrophy

Definition

A subgroup from myopathies of inherited, non-inflammatory, progressive muscle disorders without a central or peripheral nerve abnormality. All types have progressive muscle weakness, generally in a proximal to distal direction.

Classification

Sex-linked:
- Duchenne's. Defect occurs in the protein dystrophin (cytoskeleton cell membrane component) on short arm of X chromosome (Xp21 region)
- Becker's (same defect)
- Emery–Dreifuss. Defect on long arm of X chromosome (q28 locus).

Autosomal dominant:
- Fascioscapulohumeral (FSHD)
- Oculopharyngeal.

Autosomal recessive:
- Limb-girdle.

Duchenne's muscular dystrophy

Pathophysiology

Low dystrophin leads to sarcolemma membrane instability and leakage of intracellular components. Results in high blood CPK.

Clinical

For Duchenne's affected males are normal at birth and generally walk by ~18 months but all manifest features by age 5yrs. IQ reduced (average 85) compared with normal population (100). Classic gait is waddling (due to gluteus weakness), wide-based with hyperlordosis and toe walking. Tendency to falls without tripping or stumbling.

Test for *Gower's sign* in any male toe-walker under 5yrs; weakness in proximal hip muscles uncovered when child stands up from seated position by 'walking' hands up thighs.

Iliopsoas/tendo-achilles contractures develop. Scoliosis very common and progresses to compromise respiratory reserve. Lose walking ability by 7–13yrs when contractures and scoliosis usually rapidly progressive.

Other findings: absent deep tendon reflexes (<30%), calf pseudohypertrophy resembling 'inverted champagne bottle' (60%) and macroglossia (30%). Cardiopulmonary involvement makes Duchenne's a terminal disease, with death typically by the third decade.

Investigations

- CPK level 50–300 times normal but falls with decrease in muscle mass overtime. Elevation less striking in Becker's. Lactate dehydrogenase and aldolase also raised
- Genetic testing
- Ultrasonography: increased echogenicity in the affected muscles (and corresponding reduction from bone)
- EMG: short-duration, polyphasic action potentials with decreased amplitudes
- Muscle biopsy: variations in fibre size with focal areas of degeneration and elevated CPK.

Orthopaedic management

- Aim is to keep child ambulatory for as long as possible
- Physiotherapy for gait training and transfer techniques, orthotics, serial casting of ankle equinus contracture once established
- A wheelchair is needed in the later stages of the disease
- Steroid therapy used to stabilize muscle strength and preserve pulmonary function, but more recently demonstrated to slow progression of scoliosis. Gene therapy to increase dystrophin may be beneficial in future.

Surgical options

- *Foot deformities*: tendo-achilles lengthening for ankle equinus, tibialis posterior transfer (through interosseus membrane) for equinovarus deformity.
- *Scoliosis*: instrumented fusion while respiratory capacity permits. Cardiorespiratory complications rise dramatically once FVC (forced vital capacity) falls below 30%.

Other dystrophies

Becker's

Similar to Duchenne's but symptoms start later (age 10 or even adulthood) and are less severe.

Emery–Dreifuss

Symptoms in late childhood, again mostly boys. Also involves upper limb muscles.

Fascioscapulohumeral muscular dystrophy

Affects both sexes during teens or early adulthood. Classical 'flat' facies due to facial muscle weakness with inability to whistle or blow cheeks out. Also winging of scapulae causing poor control of shoulder motion which may be improved by surgical fusion of scapula to thoracic wall.

Spinal muscular atrophies

Description
Group of disorders characterized by idiopathic degeneration of anterior horn motor neurons in the spinal cord, medulla and midbrain. Denervation of muscle fibres leads to progressive muscle weakness and wasting, fasciculation and paralysis.

Incidence and inheritance
Relatively rare—1 in 6000 newborns affected and 1 in 40 of population are genetic carriers. AR inheritance. Approximately 95% associated with deletion in the survival motor neuron (SMN) gene on chromosome 5.

Classification
Four types based on age at onset and motor milestones achieved. Diagnosis of types I–III usually made before 3yrs. Type IV is adult onset and much less common.
- Type I: Werdnig–Hoffmann disease (most severe form) presents in first 6 months
- Type II: intermediate and presents after 6 months
- Type III: Kugelberg–Welander disease presents after the age of 2yrs
- Type IV: late onset.

Diagnosis
- DNA testing for absent or mutated SMN gene
- Muscle biopsy—valuable mainly where DNA test is negative
- EMG—to distinguish from other motor neuron diseases.

Clinical
- Predominantly proximal muscle weakness in lower limbs
- Also dysphagia and respiratory compromise, scoliosis, hip dysplasia
- Progessive loss of function; may be rapid around time of accelerated growth spurt or intercurrent illness.

Management
- Genetic counselling
- Physiotherapy and occupational therapy
- Orthotics
- Prompt treatment of respiratory complications
- Surgical treatment of scoliosis or hip subluxation.

Hereditary motor and sensory neuropathies

Charcot–Marie–Tooth disease

Approximately 1:2500 people are affected, men more than women but the latter usually more severely affected. The age of onset varies, depending on inheritance, but usually within first two decades.

Many forms, I–III the main ones with orthopaedic manifestations:
- Type I (hypertrophic demyelinating neuropathy): AD. Slowed nerve conduction and absent deep tendon reflexes
- Type II (axonal neuropathy): variable inheritance. Normal nerve conduction and reflexes
- Type III (Dejerine–Sottas disease): loss of deep tendon reflexes.

Diagnosis
- Clinical features (cavovarus foot and small muscle wasting in hands classical) and family history
- DNA testing—duplication of part of chromosome 17
- NCS.

Clinical features
- Motor deficits more prominent than sensory
- Cavovarus foot, hip dysplasia, peroneal weakness, intrinsic hand muscle wasting, scoliosis.

Treatment
- Physiotherapy helps prevent contracture and stiffness. Orthotics—corrective and accommodative
- Procedures for foot reflect that it is a rigid, progressive deformity; surgical management should address both bone deformity (with osteotomy) and soft tissue imbalance (with release ± muscle transfer) whilst leaving options open for the future. Triple arthrodesis the final solution
- Also intrinsic procedures for hand deformity.

Friedreich's ataxia

- AR inheritance. Frataxin gene implicated
- Onset between 7 and 15 yrs.

Clinical features
Spinocerebellar degeneration occurs with ataxia, wide-based gait and nystagmus. Cardiomyopathy, pes cavus and scoliosis may develop. Motor and sensory defects occur. Often wheelchair bound by 30yrs and death occurs between 40 and 50yrs.

Diagnosis

EMG shows increase in polyphasic potentials.

Orthopaedic manifestations

Pes cavus and scoliosis.

Dejerine–Sottas disease

- AR
- Infantile onset.

Also referred to as type III Charcot–Marie–Tooth disease (see above).

Delayed ambulation, pes cavus, foot drop, glove and stocking pattern of sensory change and spinal deformity are features of this disorder.

For further reading, see Milbrandt and Sucato[1].

Reference

1 Milbrandt TA, Sucato DJ. Pediatric orthopaedics. In: Miller MD, ed. *Review of Orthopaedics*, 4th edn. London: Saunders, 2004:171–2.

Spina bifida

Definition

Congenital neural tube defect in which there is incomplete closure of the neural tube resulting in prolapse of the dural sac containing spinal cord and nerve roots.

- The term spina bifida includes any congenital defect involving insufficient closure of the spine
- **Myelomeningocele** accounts for ~75% of all cases of spina bifida
- Remainder are **spina bifida occulta** (incomplete closure of neural tube but spinal cord and meninges remain in place and skin usually covers the defect) and **meningocele** (meninges protrude through vertebral defect but the spinal cord remains in place).

Incidence and aetiology

Incidence of myelomeningocele ~1:800 infants. Spina bifida occulta occurs in 2–3% of the general population. Risk to subsequent sibling is 1 in 25.

Folic acid supplementation (400mcg daily) to women of child-bearing age (to cover conception to 4 months) and triple test screening in first trimester have decreased incidence.

Also associated with chromosomal abnormality (e.g. trisomy 13), maternal diabetes, intrauterine drug exposure (e.g. carbamazepine), poor perinatal nutrition, folic acid deficiency.

Clinical manifestations

At birth midline defect in posterior elements of vertebrae noted with protrusion of meninges and neural elements into dural sac. Spina bifida occulta may be indicated by a tuft of hair overlying or dimpling of the sacrum; USS useful for confirmation.

Neurological deficit

- Variable motor (including paraplegia) ± sensory deficit. Functional motor level may not exactly correspond to anatomical level of defect
- Neurogenic bladder or bowel causing urinary incontinence and recurrent UTIs. This can develop later in life
- Associated **hydrocephalus** is common—tethering of cord distally can cause cerebellar herniation through foramen magnum (Chiari malformation) resulting in CSF block
- Seizures and meningitis.

Musculoskeletal problems

Deformities related to functional level of lesion, include
- Hip subluxation/dislocation
- Scoliosis
  - Congenital—associated with underlying vertebral anomaly
  - Acquired—related to muscle imbalance (40–60% of those with myelomeningocoele)
- Severe kyphosis (gibbus)
- Contractures: hip abduction and external rotation, fixed knee flexion, ankle equinus and fixed PPV.

Management

Initially neurosurgical repair of defect as indicated and release or correction of associated cord anomalies and hydrocephalus. Survival rates have dramatically improved with introduction of antibiotics and development of neurosurgical techniques.

Subsequent multidisciplinary care includes orthopaedic input with recent shift towards functional rather than radiological/anatomical goals.

Orthopaedic management

- Scoliosis instrumentation for severe curves, preserving lumbosacral level in ambulant children to permit pelvic motion
- Historically aggressive approach to hip relocation replaced by functional one; generally reduce only those ambulators with unilateral migration and low (sacral) level lesion. Muscle transfers no longer performed, contracture release alone indicated for unbalanced pelvis
- Correction of knee deformity, typically valgus with femoral and tibial malrotation, in sacral level ambulators. Correction of deformity restores lever arms for muscle function
- Foot deformities associated with sensory deficit so avoid arthrodeses for risk of pressure ulceration. A supple, deformed but braceable foot is always preferable; choose tendon releases (rather than transfers) and extra-articular bony procedures where indicated. Ponseti method for correction of neonatal congenital talipes equinovarus (CTEV) recently reported good results in this group of children.

For further reading, see Broughton[1].

Reference

1 Broughton NS The orthopaedic management of myelomeningocoele. In: Bulstrode C, Buckwater J, Carr A, et al., eds. *Oxford Textbook of Orthopaedics and Trauma*. Oxford: Oxford University Press, 2002:2479–85.

Poliomyelitis

Definition
A neuromuscular disorder of anterior horn cells, now rarely encountered in the UK and USA (due to vaccination) but still endemic in parts of sub-Saharan Africa and the Indian subcontinent.

Aetiology
Caused by high infectivity enterovirus. 3 serotypes P1, P2 and P3. Type P1 accounted for 85% of paralytic disease prior to the introduction of vaccine. Main route of infection is via GI tract (faeco-oral) in humans.

Clinical
Vast majority (95%) of infections asymptomatic (in immunocompetent host) or result in minor flu-like illness. Fewer than 1% of infections result in flaccid paralysis.

The paralytic stage begins with myalgia and muscle spasms followed by asymmetric, predominantly lower limb, flaccid weakness. Muscle weakness in the presence of normal sensation is characteristic.

Vaccination
Parenteral trivalent inactivated vaccine (Salk vaccine) introduced in 1956 for routine immunization, reduced incidence of poliomyelitis by 90% in USA.

Oral live attenuated vaccine (Sabin vaccine) replaced Salk in 1962. Advantages are that it is cheap, taken orally and excreted in faeces, leading to herd immunity. However, with excretion of live virus there is a small incidence of vaccine-induced paralytic poliomyelitis in non-immunized direct contacts.

In the UK, children currently receive parenteral vaccination as part of the national immunization programme.

Diagnosis
- Serological
- CSF—usually have an increase in WCC and mildly elevated protein
- PCR is technique of choice for identifying serotype and differentiating between wild-type and vaccine-induced poliomyelitis.

Differential diagnosis
Includes: infection by other enteroviruses or flavivirus, tickborne encephalitis, Guillain–Barre syndrome, acute intermittent porphyria, HIV neuropathy, diphtheria, Lyme disease, disorders of neuromuscular junction.

Management

- Acute attack: strict bed rest and analgesia. Physiotherapy to prevent contracture. Ventilatory support as required
- Later: mainstay of treatment is physiotherapy including stretching, muscle retraining and splintage of limbs to prevent deformity. Orthoses may be used to compensate for loss of function and improve mobility. Surgery may be needed to release contractures, stabilize joints or correct deformities (scoliosis).

Postpolio syndrome

Between 25 and 40% with residual disabilities develop new impairments following a period of stability (30–40yrs). This is thought to result from the increased demands placed on the musculoskeletal system in order to compensate for muscular weakness (rather than virus reactivation). They present with new muscle pain and exacerbation of existing weakness or even paralysis.

Connective tissue disorders

Marfan syndrome
- AD disorder
- Disorder of fibrillin.

Clinical features
- Arachnodactyly (spider like fingers—long and slender)
- High arched palate
- Arm span greater than height
- Pectus (chest wall) deformities
- Scoliosis (50%) and spondylolisthesis
- PPV
- Herniae
- Cardiac valve abnormalities—aortic incompetence
- Ocular—superior lens dislocation in 60% of patients
- Dural ectasia and meningocele can occur
- Striking joint laxity.

Orthopaedic management
- Generally non-operative, high recurrence rate after soft tissue correction and significant anaesthetic risks
- Scoliosis and kyphosis may require anterior discectomy with posterior fusion and instrumentation.

Ehlers–Danlos syndrome
- AD disorder
- 11 types (types 2 and 3 most common and least disabling).

Clinical features
- Hyperextensibility of skin with easy bruising
- Joint hypermobility
- Soft tissue calcification.

Treatment
- Physiotherapy
- Orthotics
- Arthrodesis (if indicated; as for Marfan, soft tissue procedures generally fail).

Homocystinuria
- AR disorder
- Inborn error of methionine metabolism resulting in accumulation of intermediate metabolite homocysteine in production of cysteine.

Clinical features

Marfanoid-like habitus but with:

- Stiff joints
- OP
- Inferior lens dislocation
- Mental retardation common
- Heart rarely affected
- Recurrent thromboses.

Diagnosis

Important to differentiate from Marfan as treatable (vitamin B6 and decreased dietary methionine). There is increased urinary methionine (cyanide-nitroprusside test).

Limb length discrepancy: assessment

Discrepancies in limb length are common; up to 1.5cm is usually asymptomatic with no long-term problems. 2–5cm causes an increased tendency to limp, pelvic tilt, low back ache, secondary scoliosis and accelerated degenerative changes in opposite hip (uncovered femoral head). Large discrepancies in upper limbs compensated by positioning, seldom symptomatic.

Aetiology
- Congenital
  - Undergrowth—skeletal dysplasias, PFFD, hypoplasia, e.g. fibular hemimelia
  - Overgrowth—hemihypertrophy
- Acquired
  - Undergrowth—trauma, physeal injury, infection, paralysis
  - Overgrowth—postinfection, congenital NF, vascular malformations, trauma, e.g. after childhood femoral shaft fracture.

History and examination
- Height and weight (plot on chart with percentiles)
- Signs of puberty, e.g. axillary hair, growth spurt, menarche
- Parents' heights (estimate of individual's final height)
- Pelvic tilt; quantify difference in heights of ASIS
- Scoliosis flexible (secondary to pelvic tilt from discrepancy) or fixed
- Blocks under short leg to quantify overall functional discrepancy
- Flex knees and hips to 90° and assess whether difference is in upper or lower leg segment, or both
- Limb alignment; normal, varus or valgus
- Joint ranges of motion, e.g. equinus ankle on short side
- Joint stability, e.g. ACL deficiency common in PFFD, equinovalgus ankle (ball and socket) in fibular hemimelia.

Investigations
X-rays
- Standing long leg film for alignment and length—digital films as accurate as CT scanogram with reduced radiation dose
- Left wrist/hand film to compare bone age with chronological age (Greulich and Pyle atlas analysis).
- Lateral elbow film (Sau-vegrain method) during pubertal growth spurt.

Growth remaining charts, e.g. Anderson data, Eastwood and Cole chart: most congenital and many acquired discrepancies show proportional growth so final difference at maturity predictable from serial measurements 6–12 months apart. Alternatively, use the simpler Paley multiplier method[1]; best is to use a number of methods to reduce risk of error.

Reference
1 Paley D, Bhave A, Herzenberg JE, *et al.* Multiplier method for predicting limb-length discrepancy. *J Bone Joint Surg Am* 2000;**82**:1432–6.

Limb length discrepancy: treatment

Non-operative options:

- *Up to 1.5cm* observe, shoe raise or insert if symptomatic
- *Over 2cm* consider surgery. Up to 5cm can be managed with shoe raise but cumbersome and may predispose to ankle injury.

Surgical options:

- *Shorten or limit growth of long leg*—segmental excision, e.g. closed femoral shortening or timed epiphysiodesis
- *Lengthen short leg*—corticotomy and distraction with monolateral or ring fixator (Ilizarov method)
- *Prosthetic*—amputate foot of short leg and manage discrepancy with prosthesis, e.g. severe fibula hemimelia with ≤3 rays in foot, unstable ankle and large predicted discrepancy (>20–30% of affected limb segment), severe trauma with mangled extremity.

Epiphysiodesis

Surgical physeal ablation. Attractive and fairly reliable option if adequate predicted adult height and sufficient growth remaining. Can use Menelaus method; estimate physes of distal femur and proximal tibia to contribute 9 and 6mm/yr, respectively, assume long bone growth in males stops at 16yrs and females at 14yrs.

Pitfalls: overcorrection, especially if bone age significantly behind chronological; undercorrection after accelerated phase of pubertal growth spurt when long bone further growth is minimal.

Acute shortening

Acute shortening of longer leg quicker, safer and more reliable than lengthening short side: can shorten 4–5cm in femur or 3–4cm in tibia before soft tissue compression and muscle defunctioning prohibitive. Options are open excision of bone or closed technique with intramedullary saw, splitting device and nail stabilization.

Distraction lengthening[1]

Pioneered by G. Ilizarov in Siberia in the 1950s: a low energy cortical fracture (corticotomy) is made with an osteotome; resultant fracture allowed a short (latent) period of consolidation before being stretched (callostasis) in an external frame applied prior to corticotomy. Bone forms by primary intramembranous ossification, can gain up to 20% additional length before complications limit further gains. Can usually lengthen 1mm/day divided into 4 increments, then double lengthening period to calculate additional time in frame for consolidation. Can also correct angular deformity. Minor obstacles, e.g. pin-site infection common; joint contracture, delayed union, neural dysfunction less frequent but more serious.

Tips for limb lengthening in children

- Wait until the discrepancy is 4–5cm before the (first) procedure; this is generally an amount that can be comfortably achieved and beyond this the child will have significant difficulties with ambulation
- Ensure the joints above and below are stable (otherwise bridge with fixator or add a procedure to stabilize) and monitor for subluxation during lengthening. Losses of joint motion or contracture are warning signs.

Reference

1 Aronson J. Limb-lengthening, skeletal reconstruction, and bone transport with the Ilizarov method. *J Bone Joint Surg Am* 1997;**79**:1243–58.

Brachial plexus injuries

The brachial plexus is derived from the anterior rami of the roots of C5, 6, 7, 8, T1 (Fig. 10.3). Injuries to the brachial plexus are an uncommon but often life-changing injury with significant long-term sequelae.

Aetiology and anatomy

Injuries may be open or closed. Closed injuries are most commonly traction injuries, e.g. RTAs in a motorcyclist, or obstetric traction injuries due to shoulder dystocia in the second stage of labour. Other causes include lacerations, gunshot injuries and irradiation.

Pathology

* Neurapraxia—good prognosis, complete recovery should occur
* Rupture—postganglionic, may recover if continuity is restored
* Lesion in continuity—stretching of large segment, no rupture, but peri- and intraneural fibrosis leads to a poor prognosis
* Avulsion—preganglionic root avulsion, poor prognosis.

Classification

Upper trunk, lower trunk, complete, mixed.

Assessment

* Usually a history of high energy injury to upper limb, or of polytrauma
* Complains of painful (deafferentation), weak or insensate upper limb
* Look for position of arm, bruising or swelling (particularly in the supraclavicular fossa), muscle wasting if chronic. Horner's syndrome (ptosis, miosis, anhydrosis) associated with lower root avulsions
* Feel for brachial/radial pulse, Tinel's sign in supraclavicular fossa, sensation and motor power, muscle function and sensory loss (Table 10.3).

Investigations

* CXR—1st rib injury, raised hemidiaphragm (C3, 4, 5 injury)
* MRI—of plexus and cervical spine (?spinal cord injury) may be useful
* Neurophysiology—little value in acute injury, denervation changes after 2–3 weeks. Sensory action potentials preserved in preganglionic avulsions, absent in postganglionic ruptures.

Treatment

* Resuscitation according to ATLS guidelines
* Discuss early with specialist centre
* Treat associated musculoskeletal and vascular injuries
* Early treatment may involve nerve repair, grafting or nerve transfer
* Late treatment: functional splinting, tendon transfers.

Prognosis

Poor prognosis in pan-plexus lesions, those with severe pain, supraclavicular sensory loss, Horner's.

Obstetric brachial plexus palsy

* Traction injury, usually from shoulder dystocia
* 3 main types—upper trunk (Erb's palsy—waiter's tip position), lower trunk (Klumpke's) or whole plexus

- Many show spontaneous recovery, exploration considered if no biceps function at 3 months
- Careful observation of shoulder needed as may show subluxation or dislocation which can develop even after neurological recovery.

For further reading, see Romm and Chu[1].

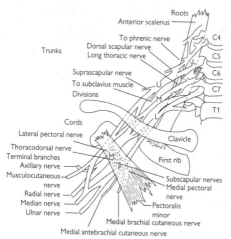

Fig. 10.3 The brachial plexus.
Reproduced from Bulstrode et al., *Oxford Textbook of Orthopaedics and Trauma*, with permission from Oxford University Press.

Table 10.3 Muscle function and sensory loss

Root injured	Functional loss	Sensory loss
C5/C6	Shoulder external rotation, flexion and abduction, elbow flexion, possibly wrist extension	Thumb and index finger
C5/C6/C7	Additionally elbow, wrist, finger and thumb extension	Additionally the middle finger
C8/T1	Finger and thumb flexion, median and ulnar intrinsics	Ring and little fingers
C5/T1	All arm function	All arm sensation

Reproduced from Bulstrode et al., *Oxford Textbook of Orthopaedics and Trauma*, with permission from Oxford University Press.

Reference

1 Romm DS, Chu DA. Learn the Brachial Plexus in Five Minutes or Less, www.ama-assn.org/ama1/pub/upload/mm/15/brachial_plex_how_to.pdf (accessed 18 February 2008).

Upper limb malformations

The upper limb develops during intrauterine weeks 4–8. Heart, eyes, CNS and auditory systems develop at this time so congenital limb malformation mandates paediatrician review for associated anomalies, e.g. VACTERL and TAR syndromes (see opposite) and genetic counselling (many anomalies hereditary so subsequent children may be affected).

Management involves reassurance (condition is not the parents' fault) and consideration of child's future growth and development when timing intervention.

Swanson's classification[1] is a helpful way to think about the range of malformations:

Failure of formation
- Transverse absence
  - Congenital amputations
- Longitudinal absence
  - Radial ray absent/dysplastic
  - Ulnar ray
  - Central ray (cleft hand).

Failure of differentiation (separation of parts)
- Radioulnar synostosis
- Symphalangism, syndactyly
- Camptodactyly (flexion contracture of digit)
- Clinodactyly (valgus deformity of digit).

Duplication
- Whole limb
- Humerus
- Radius
- Ulna
- Digit (polydactyly).

Overgrowth
- Whole/partial limb
- Macrodactyly.

Undergrowth
- Brachymetacarpia
- Brachysyndactyly (with absent pectoral muscle = Poland syndrome)
- Brachydactyly.

Constriction ring syndrome
Generalized skeletal abnormalities
Assessment must include hand or occupational therapy for function. Consider also cosmetic as well as functional importance of the hand. If intervention is planned, do so early for cerebral imprinting.

VACTERL anomalies as follows:

- Vertebral
- Anorectal
- Cardiac
- Tracheo-oesophageal
- Renal
- Limb

TAR—thrombocytopenia with absent radius.

Reference

1 Swanson AB, Swanson GD, Tada, K. A classification for congenital limb malformation. *J Hand Surg* 1983;**8**:693–702.

Torticollis 1

Description
Torticollis (from the Latin *torti* (twisted) and *collis* (neck)) refers to presentation of the neck in a twisted or bent position. It arises as a result of involuntary contractions of the neck muscles, leading to abnormal postures and movements of the head. It is a combined deformity of head tilt and rotation of the cervical spine.

Epidemiology
Torticollis commonly occurs in the 15–30yr age group but may present soon after birth (transient postural torticollis) or during infancy.

Congenital muscular torticollis (CMT) is the most common form of torticollis. It occurs as a consequence of damage to the sternocleidomastoid muscle and is often seen in the first 2 months after birth. There is increased incidence in breech and forceps deliveries and in 1st born. The child presents with head tilted towards the affected side and rotation of the chin to the contralateral side. There are often associated problems such as facial asymmetry, retarded facial growth on the affected side, plagiocephaly and congenital foot and hip problems.

Spasmodic torticollis is a type of dystonia affecting the muscles of the neck leading to involuntary muscle contraction. It often involves the trapezius and sternocleidomastoid muscles which results in abnormal head posture.

Aetiology
Congenital Occipitovertebral anomalies, neck skin webbing.

Acquired Idiopathic, neurogenic (spinal cord and posterior fossa tumours, syringomyelia, bulbar palsies, tumours, ocular problems), inflammatory (pyogenic, rheumatoid, tuberculous) or traumatic (atlantoaxial rotatory subluxation).

CMT is the most common form of the deformity.

Congenital muscular torticollis
Clinical
The child presents with deformity and may have neck pain and an inability to move the head. The head is rotated, pulled to one side, facing upwards or downwards. Passive and active neck movements are restricted. The head is typically held in a position flexed away from the pain. Movements may be intermittent or abnormal posture. The head and neck may be fixed by continuous muscle spasm. A small knot may be palpable in the involved sternocleidomastoid on the involved side—a sternocleidomastoid tumour. A sternomastoid tumour is not a true malignancy but a fibrous mass in one of the sternocleidomastoid muscles, and represents reaction to intrauterine or birth trauma.

Natural history
In most, torticollis resolves in several days to a few weeks. A few will develop neck problems lasting months to years. Persistent neck muscle spasms may require referral to a neurologist or surgeon.

Investigations

- Radiology—plain cervical X-rays are indicated to ensure the deformity is purely due to muscular problem and not a structural problem of the base of skull or cervical spine
- CT scan—used to establish if there is fixed rotation and define bony elements of the skull and cervical spine
- MRI scans—used to detect brain, spinal cord, nerve root and intervertebral disc abnormalities. They are also useful when an inflammatory process, infection or neoplasm is suspected.

Management

Non-operative treatment—gentle, daily manipulation of the neck with stretching exercises. Invasive, but non-operative, options aim to relax the contracted neck muscles and focus on preventing involuntary muscle contraction. These options include local injection of botulinum toxin to paralyse affected muscles or destruction of the nerve supply to affected muscles (selective denervation).

Operative options—surgery is reserved only for a few selective cases. A sternocleidomastoid release is indicated for failure of non-operative treatment. It should be performed after 2yrs of age. It involves division of the lower ends of the two heads of the sternocleidomastoid and over-lying tight fascia. The incision is just superior to the clavicle. Structures at risk are the carotid vessels and jugular vein. Division of the proximal part of the sternocleidomastoid muscle is more difficult and places the spinal accessory nerve at risk. Complications include persistent pain, scar tissue formation, recurrence (usually from inadequate release) and neurovascular injury.

Torticollis 2

Atlantoaxial rotatory subluxation (AARS)

Description: AARS is the most common acquired form of childhood torticollis.

Aetiology: trauma, upper respiratory tract infection (Grisel's syndrome) or following head or neck surgery.

Clinical: child presents with typical 'cock robin' appearance. The head is tilted and rotated. Pain is a feature of this form of torticollis. The deformity may be mobile or fixed. If untreated, head and facial asymmetry may develop.

Investigations

- Radiology—plain radiographs should include AP, lateral and open mouth views
- CT scan—a dynamic CT scan with the head rotated maximally to each side should be done to establish if there is indeed AARS and if there is deformity.

Management

Non-operative—may resolve spontaneously, but if it does not it should be treated with a soft collar and physiotherapy. If it does not reduce with rotation, halter traction is needed, followed by serial monitoring.

Operative options—surgery indicated for failed reduction, persistent deformity or neurological deficits. The subluxation should be corrected and the vertebrae fused to prevent recurrent subluxation.

Further reading

1 Tachdjian MO. Diagnosis and treatment of congenital deformities of the musculoskeletal system in the newborn and infant. *Pediatr Clin North Am* 1967;**14**:307–58.

2 Epps HR, Salter RB. Orthopaedic conditions of the cervical spine and shoulder. *Pediatr Clin North Am* 1996;**43**:919–31.

Scoliosis in children 1

Definition
Deformity of the spine in the coronal plane >10°.

Classification
Two main groups are:
- Postural scoliosis
- Structural scoliosis.

The latter is classified as congenital, idiopathic, neuromuscular and a miscellaneous group.

Congenital scoliosis
Classification
Failure of formation
- Complete hemivertebra: fully segmented
- Semi-segmented or non-segmented: incarcerated or non-incarcerated
- Incomplete or partial vertebra: wedge or butterfly vertebra.

Failure of segmentation
- Unilateral bar or bilateral bar (block vertebra)
- Mixed variety.

Description
Lateral curvature of the spine secondary to developmental vertebral anomalies producing imbalance of longitudinal growth. The hallmark is vertebral anomaly. There is a very high incidence of intraspinal anomalies.

Investigation
MRI is essential. Intraspinal lesions found include diastematomyelia, tethered spinal cord, syringomyelia and low conus. Skin abnormalities (hairy patch, dimple in the midline) may herald a congenital vertebral anomaly. Neurological assessment is essential.

Management
Bracing is not usually successful. Surgical treatment is indicated if non-operative treatment measures fail. Operative options include: posterior *in situ* fusion, a combined posterior hemiarthrodesis and anterior hemi-epiphysiodesis to arrest growth on the convex side, instrumented stabilization (growing rods) and instrumented fusion.

Idiopathic scoliosis (Fig. 10.4)
Idiopathic scoliosis is the most common type of scoliosis in children.

Classification
- Infantile before age of 3yrs.
- Juvenile between 4 and 9yrs.
- Adolescent idiopathic scoliosis after 10yrs of age.

These age distinctions have prognostic significance.

Epidemiology

Prevalence of idiopathic scoliosis is 0.5%.

Aetiology

The aetiology is unknown and is probably multifactoral. Disorganized skeletal growth, hormonal factors (melatonin) and a neurological deficit (posterior column lesion) have been implicated in the development of idiopathic scoliosis.

Clinical

Most children present with a deformity of the trunk, different shoulder heights, asymmetrical chest or waist creases, or apparent limb length discrepancy. The history must include family history, birth history, developmental milestones (mental and physical) and neurological symptoms. On examination look for shoulder height asymmetry, protruding scapulae, hip asymmetry, frontal asymmetry, abnormal creases, hairy patches and café au lait spots. Palpate the curve. Drop plumb line to assess spinal balance. Bending confirms a postural or structural curve and establishes the degree of flexibility. In the most common curve pattern (right thoracic), the right shoulder is rotated forward and the medial border of scapula protrudes posteriorly. A complete neurological assessment is required. Hamstring tightness should be established. Measure leg lengths and if there is a discrepancy, correct using blocks to see if curve disappears (suggesting compensatory curve due to leg length discrepancy). Skeletal maturity must be assessed—Risser's sign used most often.

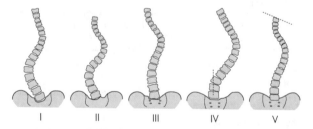

Fig. 10.4 King–Moe classification system for idiopathic scoliosis: type I, primary lumbar curve greater than the compensatory thoracic curve; type II, primary thoracic curve with compensatory lumbar curve; type III, short pure thoracic curve; type IV, long C-shaped thoracolumbar curve; type V, double thoracic curve with extension into cervical spine and compensatory lumbar curve.

Reproduced from Bulstrode et al., Oxford Textbook of Orthopaedics and Trauma, with permission from Oxford University Press.

Scoliosis in children 2

Infantile idiopathic scoliosis (under 3yrs of age)

Description
Association with congenital heart diseases, developmental dysplasia of the hip, breech, older mother, inguinal hernia and spinal cord anomalies. Some may resolve with time. Males tend to have left thoracic curves.

Investigation
Measurements of the curves are done by rib vertebral angle difference (RVAD) or Cobb angle. All need MRI scan to rule out spinal dysraphism.

Management
Serial body casting is the mainstay of treatment in infantile idiopathic scoliosis. Curves likely to deteriorate if they are >40° or if the rib vertebral angle difference is >20°.

Juvenile idiopathic scoliosis (3–10yrs of age)

Description
More common in females. Thoracic curve can be to the left or to the right. Lumbar curves are rare. About 70% of the juvenile idiopathic curves progress and will need some form of treatment. 50% will require surgery. There is high incidence of intraspinal pathology reported in this group.

Investigations MRI scan is essential.

Management
Curves of >40–45° will progress and will need surgery. Surgery varies depending on type of curve. Posterior fusion, anterior fusion or anterior + posterior fusion may be required. Crankshaft complication—anterior growth after posterior fusion alone may lead to rotation of the spine.

Adolescent idiopathic scoliosis

Description
The curve patterns in adolescent idiopathic scoliosis can be classified using the King classification system[1].

The likelihood of progression depends on the size of the curve, skeletal and physiological maturity—mature patients with small curves have a lower risk of progression.

Investigations
Plain radiographs—AP and lateral standing views, including pelvis, are used to characterize the deformity. Bending views are helpful in determining flexibility. Look for Risser's sign and measure Cobb angle.

MRI scan—used to exclude intraspinal pathology, if this is suggested by the clinical assessment.

Other tests—pulmonary function testing done in patients with moderate to large deformities.

Screening—the Adams forward bending test is simple and effective in identifying scoliosis.

Management

Non-operative treatment—observation or orthotic use. Observation includes interval X-rays or ISIS scans. Electrical muscle stimulation, physiotherapy, manipulation, and nutritional therapies are ineffective. Children with curves as small as 20° and who are a Risser 0 should be braced immediately. Bracing can be effective in reducing curve progression in older children with modest curves (20–39°). It is recommended that bracing should be for 23h/day. Problems include psychological stress, poor compliance, and pressure effects (local pain).

Operative options—the goals are safely to correct the deformity and achieve a solid bony fusion. One can use a posterior or anterior approach. An anterior release can be performed prior to posterior fusion. Modern instrumentation allows for adequate curve correction.

Intraoperative monitoring during scoliosis surgery can allow early recognition and treatment of spinal cord dysfunction. Somatosensory and motor evoked potentials are commonly used to monitor spinal cord function. Stagnara wake-up test may also still be employed if the surgeon desires. Complications include excessive bleeding, infections including delayed infections, usually caused by low-virulence organisms such as *Propionibacterium acnes*, and spinal cord or nerve root injury. Other complications include a pneumothorax, vascular or visceral injury, pseudarthrosis, persistent pain, progressive deformity or broken instrumentation. Clinical outcomes are strongly linked to curve magnitude. Regardless of treatment, scoliosis patients have a higher self-reported rate of arthritis and poorer perceptions of their overall health and body image, and more back pain.

Neuromuscular scoliosis

Description Typically long C-type curves that involve entire thoracic and lumbar spine—may extend from the neck to the sacrum.

Classification

- Neuropathic: CP, spinocerebellar degeneration (Friedreich's ataxia), myelomenigocele, syringomyelia, cord tumour or trauma, spinal muscular atrophy, LMN problems (poliomyelitis)
- Myopathic: arthrogryposis, muscular dystrophy, myotonia, NF, mesenchymal, Marfan disease, Ehler–Danlos, homocystinuria
- Miscellaneous: postlaminectomy, post-trauma.

Management

Non-operative treatment—bracing, wheelchair modification.

Operative options—spinal fusion with instrumentation. Aim for a balanced spine with head centred over pelvis.

Reference

1 King H, Moe J, Bradford D, et al. The selection of fusion levels in thoracic idiopathic scoliosis. J Bone Joint Surg Am 1983;**65A**:1302–13.

Kyphosis in children

Definition Kyphosis is an excessive curvature of the spine in the sagittal plane. Normal angles: wide variation, but 40° is the average thoracic curve, it increases with age and peaks at 14yrs.

Classification

Congenital kyphosis:
- Type I: failure of segmentation
- Type II: failure of formation
- Type III: mixed.

Acquired kyphosis:
- Scheuermann's disease
- Postural round back
- Inflammatory
- Metabolic
- Post-traumatic
- Iatrogenic
- Neoplastic.

Congenital kyphosis

Description

Congenital deformities in the sagittal plane similar to those in the coronal plane. Congenital deformities rarely seen in the sagittal plane alone; they are associated with other vertebral anomalies, nervous system anomalies or pathology related to other organ systems. May be breakdown of skin, abdominal viscera compression, pulmonary impairment (>100° thoracic region) and poor sitting posture. A severe angular deformity may develop with a gibbus at the apex. Congenital kyphosis often progresses rapidly if untreated and may lead to paralysis (type I).

Investigation

- Radiographs—AP and lateral erect and lateral hyperextension are used to characterize the deformity.
- CT scan—used to define bony anatomy, especially in planning surgery.
- MRI scan—to evaluate the spinal canal and neural elements.

Management

Non-operative treatment—almost no role for non-operative treatment, bracing is not effective. Traction contraindicated because of paralysis risk.

Operative options—posterior *in situ* fusion alone can be used to treat children <5yrs with curves <50° since some correction of kyphosis occurs with growth. Anterior fusion may be indicated for older children and those with modest curves. Anterior + posterior fusion is usually necessary for children >5yrs with curves >50°. Instrumentation may aid in the correction of the deformity. Children with secondary neurological deficits should have a decompression of neural elements.

Scheuermann's kyphosis

The most common cause of acquired kyphosis in children.

Description

AVN of the ring apophysis occurs as a result of excess mechanical stress. Herniation of disc material occurs through endplates (Schmorl's nodes).

Epidemiology

The incidence of kyphosis due to Scheuermann's disease is 0.4–0.8%. Male to female ratio appears to be equal. It does not occur in children <10yrs.

Aetiology

The aetiology of Scheuermann's disease remains unknown. It is a defect of endochondral ossification.

Clinical

Pain is a common complaint and is usually at the apex of the curve; it is often self-limiting. The cosmetic effects of the kyphosis often concern adolescents. Examination reveals an adolescent with poor posture, increased kyphosis and tight hamstrings. Backache or tenderness may be found. The deformity becomes more prominent with the Adams forward bending test. Neurological deficits are rare.

Investigations

Radiographs—erect AP and standing views, and a lateral hyperextension view are indicated. Criteria for diagnosis include irregular endplates, narrowing of the disc spaces, three vertebrae with wedging of >5° and kyphosis >45°. Associated radiographic findings include disc space narrowing, endplate irregularities, spondylolysis and scoliosis. Lumbar disease, which is less common, does not have wedging. There is an increased incidence of spondylolysis in Scheuermann's disease.

Management

Bracing or surgery can be used to correct the kyphosis.

Non-operative treatment—patients with curves <50° are treated with observation and physical therapies. In skeletally immature patients with significant kyphosis that is painful or deteriorating, bracing is used. It should be continued to skeletal maturity. Bracing is most effective where the apex of the kyphosis is below T7 or the curve is small.

Operative options—surgery is usually undertaken if the kyphosis is >75°. The most reliable surgery is an anterior release followed by posterior instrumented fusion.

Postural roundback deformity

A modest kyphosis of 40–60° is usually found. It is correctable and vertebral morphology is normal. If diagnosed after 13yrs Scheuermann's disease needs to be excluded. Rehabilitation includes postural and hyperextension exercises. Bracing may be required.

Spondylolysis and spondylolisthesis in children

Description

Spondylolysis is a fatigue fracture of the pars intra-articularis. The most common location is at L5. Bilateral superior articular processes are in continuity with the pedicles and vertebral body, but most of the lamina, spinous process and inferior articular processes are detached.

Spondylolisthesis is the anterior slippage of one vertebra on another.

Spondylolisthesis

Classification

Wiltse and Neman classification:

- Type I: congenital or dysplastic
- Type II: isthmic
  - IIa: spondylolysis
  - IIb: isthmic elongation
  - IIc: acute fracture
- Type III: degenerative
- Type IV: traumatic
- Type V: pathological.

Aetiology

Spondylolysis is associated with erect posture, sports involving hyperextension activities. Inherited form identified.

Spondylolisthesis only affects humans. 90% occurs in the lumbar spine at L5. Majority are isthmic, i.e. associated with a spondylolysis. Dysplastic spondylolisthesis is rare and occurs due to congenital changes in upper part of the sacrum. The disc below the listhesis usually pathological and the disc above may be degenerate. May be lumbar scoliosis due primarily to rotation with forward slippage of one vertebra on another.

Natural history

The vast majority settle as the slip stabilizes. Patients with some forms of isthmic spondylolisthesis develop back and leg pain symptoms. It is difficult to predict who will become symptomatic. Risk of progression is young age, females, type of slip, degree of the angle of slip and radiological evidence of instability.

Clinical

Most children with spondylolisthesis are asymptomatic. It is the most common cause of back pain in adolescents and is associated with sporting activities and occasionally trauma. Back pain usually begins with walking or standing. It is activity related. The pain can radiate to buttock, lateral aspect of the thigh or calf. When severe, it can cause gait disturbances, numbness or muscle weakness, and signs of cauda equina compression may develop. Claudication may signal lateral recess stenosis.

Examination

On examination there is flattening of the back (loss of lordosis) and a spinous process step-off may be palpable. Hamstrings are usually tight. The examination must include an assessment of distal neurology.

Investigations

Radiographs—plain X-rays are indicated and a lateral view will show the extent of slip. The film should be centred on the lumbosacral junction. The percentage slip is calculated by measuring the relative displacement of one vertebra to an adjacent vertebra. The slip is graded: grade I, <25%; grade II, 25–50%; grade III, 50–75%; grade IV, 75–100%; grade V, >100% (spondyloptosis) (Fig. 10.5). The slip angle can also be measured on a lateral radiograph: the actual defect is to the pars interarticularis and can be seen in 80% of lesions, ~15% of which are seen on oblique views (Scottie dog sign of La Chapelle).

- CT scan—can demonstrate lysis but lesion may be missed if tomogram is not in the same plane
- MRI scans—to assess compression of neural elements and state of the disc
- Bone scans—may be hot in the acute phase and if so suggests more likely to unite.

Management

Non-operative treatment—rest, analgesia and if symptoms do not settle lumbosacral orthosis may be helpful.

Operative options—indications for surgery include: slip >50% or progressing in adolescents. Persistent back and/or leg pain unresponsive to non-operative treatment. Significant neurological deficit.

Grade I and II: *in situ* fusion or repair of the pars defect using a lag screw or wires has been recommended. A decompression may be necessary if there is nerve root compression.

Grade III–V: extended *in situ* fusion and decompression. A posterior inter-transverse fusion without instrumentation.

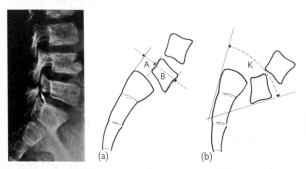

Fig. 10.5 Spondylolysis (arrow) of L5 on lateral radiograph. (a) Calculation of the amount of vertebral slip according to Laurent and Einola[1]: slip (%) = A/B×100. (b) Measurement of lumbosacral kyphosis as the angle between the posterior wall of S1 and the anterior (or posterior) wall of L5.

Reproduced from Bulstrode *et al.*, *Oxford Textbook of Orthopaedics and Trauma*, with permission form Oxford University Press.

Reference

1 Laurent L, Einola S. Spondylolisthesis in children and adolescents. *Acta Orthop Scand* 1961;**31**:45–64.

Back pain in children

Epidemiology

In older, school-aged children, back pain is more common, occurring in 10–30% of these children.

Aetiology

The causes of back pain in children include: slipped vertebral apophysis and spondylolisthesis, a herniated disc, osteomyelitis, TB, discitis, spinal cord tumours, eosinophic granuloma, metastatic disease (neuroblastoma).

All children under 12yrs of age with pain for >1 month, night pain, a rigid spine, painful scoliosis, abnormal neurology, weight loss, fever or a history of NF should be assessed and investigated as a matter of urgency.

Clinical

Children presenting with back pain require careful evaluation. The pain must be fully characterized. A full neurological history must be obtained. A history of trauma is important, in particular of any history of a traumatic event related to recreational or sporting activities. The signs may be difficult to elicit in young children. Look for swelling, deformity, skin lesions and examine gait carefully. Range of motion of the spine is important. Assess if there is any leg length discrepancy and examine joints. Neurological examination must include power, tone, reflexes—deep tendon and abdominal reflexes, sensation (light touch, pin-prick, vibration sense and proprioception) and nerve root tension signs.

Investigations

These are very important in evaluating a child with back pain, especially if there are constitutional symptoms. One should request:

Laboratory

FBC, ESR, CRP. Further studies may be necessary such as rheumatoid screen or HLA B27 status.

Radiology

Plain X-rays—should be obtained. Look for spondylolisthesis, fractures and erosions of endplates, and assess the overall shape of the spine.

MRI scan—used to look for discitis, disc degeneration, disc prolapse and pathology involving the spinal cord (syrinx) or nerve roots.

Herniated disc

Clinical

Herniated discs occur in children. They often present with back pain radiating into the lower limbs. On examination signs of radiculopathy may be elicited.

Investigations

The investigation of choice is MRI.

Management

Non-operative treatment—rest and pain control (analgesia and anti-inflammatory medication). Treated for up to 3 months this way.

Operative option—if pain persists or if there is deterioration in neurology, surgery needs to be considered and is usually discectomy without fusion. In children with a congenitally narrow canal, a decompression may be necessary.

Back pain in children: presentation and treatment of specific disorders

Slipped vertebral apophysis

Description
Occurs in lower lumbar spine when fusion between vertebral ring apophysis and central cartilage is incomplete. The ring apophysis with adjacent disc is displaced into vertebral canal. It is associated with heavy lifting and vigorous activities.

Clinical
Pain radiating into one or both limbs. The symptoms and signs are similar to those of an acute herniated disc.

Investigations
Radiology—X-ray may show a small bone fragment (edge of ring apophysis) within the spinal canal. It is rarely diagnosed on plain films.

MRI scan or CT (better at detecting bone fragment) are more likely to show the lesion.

Differential diagnosis
Disc herniation.

Management
Non-operative treatment—usually unsuccessful.

Operative options—most patients require surgery to excise the disc and ring apophysis. Simple disc excision is not adequate.

Discitis (see 📖 p. 510)

Spondylolisthesis (see 📖 p. 502)

Deformity
Idiopathic scoliosis rarely causes pain. If a deformity is painful ⚠—look for syringomyelia, infection or neoplasm.

Scheuermann's disease (see 📖 p. 501)

Traumatic back pain
Check for NAIs. Fractures are usually painful, and post-traumatic kyphosis can cause severe back pain, particularly if there is progressive vertebral collapse.

Spinal neoplasm

Type of tumours

They can be benign or malignant and intrarosseous or extraosseous. The most common benign tumours involving the spine are osteoid osteoma, osteoblastoma, aneurysmal bone cyst and eosinophilic granuloma. Malignant tumours include neuroblastoma, Ewing's sarcoma and osteosarcoma. Children with acute lymphocytic leukaemia sometimes present with back pain.

Clinical

Children with spinal tumours often present with back pain. There should be a suspicion that there is a tumour if the child is young, <10yrs, the pain is constant (with or without night pain) or if there is a neurological deficit.

Investigation

An MRI scan is the investigation of choice as some tumours causing back pain are extraosseous and are unlikely to be detected with a bone scan.

Management

Treatment depends on the type of tumour. The most common tumours osteoid osteoma and osteoblastoma are excised. A paediatric oncologist should be involved in the care of all children with spinal tumours.

For further reading, see Brown et al.[1]

Reference

1 Brown R, Hussain M, McHugh K, et al. Discitis in young children. *J Bone Joint Surg Br* 2001;**83**:106–11.

Spinal infections in children

Spinal infections in children are uncommon.

Pyogenic infections

Pathology

With colonization of the endplates by the causative organism, there is spread to the disc space and the infection develops. Untreated the infection spreads into the adjacent vertebral bodies destroying the bone and forming abscesses.

Clinical

Children present at any age. Symptoms include fever, reluctance to walk, back pain or abdominal pain. There are often reduced spinal movements, loss of lumbar lordosis and local tenderness. There may be a positive SLR. Neurological deficits are uncommon.

Investigations

Laboratory:

Require FBC, ESR and CRP. Results may be normal. Blood cultures may be positive.

Radiology:

Plain X-rays—are usually negative early in the disease, but may be useful in excluding other pathology. Later, disc changes and destruction of bone may be seen.

MRI scans—is the imaging modality of choice as it can demonstrate bony as well as soft tissue changes.

Differential diagnosis

It includes pyogenic tuberculous infections and neoplasms, especially osteoblastoma.

Management

Non-operative treatment—early management is IV antibiotics covering *S. aureus*, later oral agents can be used. Bed rest and bracing not indicated, unless there is vertebral collapse.

Operative options—surgical debridement is indicated in those patients with drainable collections or who respond poorly to antibiotic therapy.

Tuberculous osteomyelitis

Bone involvement, including that of vertebrae, relatively common in children. The anterior spine is usually involved and the most common region involved is the thoracolumbar junction.

Clinical

Back pain is the most common presenting symptom. These children often have flu-like symptoms. Gait abnormalities occur due to psoas involvement or neurological deficits. Children with longstanding disease may present with an obvious deformity of the spine. With involvement of the cervical spine, the child may have difficulty swallowing or breathing due to pressure on the adjacent structures by a paravertebral abscess. Children, unlike adults, are rarely paralysed by TB of the spine.

Investigations

Radiology:

X-rays—may show extent of vertebral involvement. A deformity, usually kyphosis, can be seen and monitored with serial X-rays.

MRI scans—demarcate soft tissue involvement, associated collections and effects of the infection on neural elements (compression of cord or nerve roots).

Management

Non-operative treatment—the disease is primarily treated with long-term chemotherapy.

Operative options—drainage, debridement or stabilization (anterior, posterior or both) may be required. Late deformity or development of neurological deficit may require reconstructive surgery.

Discitis in children

Definition

Benign, self-limiting infection or inflammation of the intervertebral disc or endplate.

Epidemiology

Discitis is uncommon in children. It usually affects children <10yrs old but is more common in toddlers (1–3yrs) than in older children. The lumbar spine is the most common location.

Aetiology

The aetiology is unclear. Most researchers believe the condition may represent a brisk host response to a low grade pathogen which does not produce a progressive vertebral osteomyelitis. Non-infective processes and trauma have been suggested.

Clinical

The clinical findings are non-specific and include refusal to walk, back pain, inability to flex the lower back and a loss of lumbar lordosis. There are usually no systemic symptoms and children are typically afebrile. They may present with hip or abdominal pain or they may have a limp or refuse to sit, stand or walk. On examination there is often tenderness over the spine and paravertebral muscle spasm, which results in loss of flexion and decreased lumbar lordosis. It is often difficult to make a diagnosis in children under 3.

Differential diagnosis

Includes osteomyelitis, tuberculous spondylitis and postoperative discitis.

Investigations

Laboratory

Laboratory tests can be unhelpful as WCC is often normal; ESR may be elevated. Most blood cultures are sterile, but when an organism is identified, it is usually *S. aureus*. Biopsy may be indicated for children who fail to respond to non-operative management, for older children and adolescents in whom a non-staphylococcal infection is suspected or in those thought to have TB or tumour.

Radiology

X-rays are normal early in the disease. Later, disc space narrowing and irregularities of adjacent vertebral endplates are seen. In adults, vertebrae usually fuse but in children the disc space is usually preserved. In only 20% of children with discitis is there fusion of the adjacent vertebrae.

Bone scan

Bone scan demonstrates increased uptake of isotope in infected disc space—may be useful in early diagnosis of discitis (within 1 week of symptoms developing).

MRI scan

In very early discitis an MRI scan is a more sensitive investigation than a bone scan. It can demonstrate a paravertebral inflammatory mass and epidural collections. It may prevent the need for biopsy. An MRI scan also helps guide treatment.

Management

Bed rest and if symptoms severe an orthosis should be considered. Empirical oral or IV antibiotics are prescribed. If no organism is cultured a cephalosporin is used. Most children have a mobile pain-free spine within 18–20 months of treatment being started.

Further reading

1 Brown R, Hussain M, McHugh K, *et al.* Discitis in young children. *J Bone Joint Surg Br* 2001;**83**:106–11.
2 Jansen BR, Hart W, Schreuder O. Discitis in childhood. 12–35-year follow-up of 35 patients. *Acta Orthop Scand* 1993;**64**:33–6.

Lower limb malformations—introduction

Congenital limb deficiencies affect ~1 in 2000 live births, with the slight majority involving the upper limb. Most in the lower limb are longitudinal (reduction/absence of bone(s)/soft tissue in long axis of the limb). A few are transverse (proximo-distal limb development normal to level of deficiency, which superficially resembles amputation). True intrauterine amputation is rare but can occur with amniotic bands.

Most lower limb reduction anomalies are sporadic; some, for example tibial hemimelia, may be part of generalized syndrome of limb abnormalities. Maternal smoking during pregnancy has been implicated as a factor. Much of our prosthetic knowledge is based on work subsequent to thalidomide; an antiemetic prescribed during late 1950/60s for morning sickness in pregnancy which caused severe limb reduction anomalies, many in physicians' children.

The lower limb bud appears at 4 (intrauterine) weeks, major development is complete by 6, with most anomalies occurring between these times. Modern recommendations for more descriptive nomenclature, e.g. 'longitudinal deficiency, fibula total, tarsus partial, rays 4 and 5 total', have not caught on in place of Latin-based terminology, in this case *fibula hemimelia* (half-limb).

Molecular biologists are increasingly identifying key molecules (morphogens) whose graded concentrations orchestrate embryological limb development e.g. SHH (sonic hedgehog) active in the ZPA (zone of polarizing activity, the signalling centre of the developing limb bud). These molecules may represent a target for future therapeutic interventions.

In the meantime, management must be multidisciplinary with careful counselling and reassurance for parental feelings of responsibility and guilt. Paediatricians and geneticists should be involved if a wider syndrome is suspected for skeletal survey and careful phenotyping. Surgery indicated in the minority, may be
• Reconstructive—limb lengthening, hip stabilization
• Growth modifying—timed epiphysiodesis for length equalization
• Ablative—amputation to facilitate prosthetic limb fitting.

Amputation should not be delayed if clearly indicated and done through joint to prevent long bone overgrowth relative to skin. Also maximizes end-bearing and proprioceptive stump properties and flare of condyles/malleoli aid prosthetic suspension/rotational control.

Proximal focal femoral deficiency

Characterized by a variably short femur, associated with apparent loss of continuity between the shaft and the neck (pseudarthrosis; some will ossify). More common than tibial dysplasia, but less so than fibular hemimelia.

Look also for signs of acetabular dysplasia and proximal femoral deformity which may include coxa vara (severe) hip abduction/flexion contracture and external rotation deformity (femoral retroversion). Also exaggerated anterolateral femoral bow, hypoplastic lateral femoral condyle, absent cruciate ligaments and frank knee instability. Associated with fibula hemimelia in about half of cases. Bilateral in 15%.

Clinical appearance is characteristic: very short, fleshy thigh which is flexed, abducted and externally rotated. Foot at level of mid tibia or normal knee in severe cases.

Various classifications (Aitken[1]—Table 10.4) focus on potential for ossification of the femoral shaft to the proximal segment and status of the hip. Gillespie's is simpler:
- Group I—femur 40–60% short but hip and knee can be made functional. Overall leg 20–30% short, foot at level of mid-tibia
- Group II— femur shorter, hip/knee cannot be made functional. Foot at level of knee.

Management

Should be multidisciplinary in specialist centre. Genetic counselling difficult as genotype–phenotype relationships not clearly delineated as yet. Prenatal counselling appropriate if identified on US scan.

Gillespie group I and Aitken type A/B can be treated with femoral lengthening (cross knee joint with fixator if joint unstable) after release of hip contractures, valgus proximal femoral osteotomy ± correction of pseudarthrosis and acetabular osteotomy.

Prosthetic management of more severe cases facilitated by:
- Judicious femoral lengthening to improve lever arm of retained limb segment
- Fusion of femur to pelvis if no hip joint, knee assumes function of hip
- If stable hip but very short femur, amputate foot through ankle (Syme's amputation) and fuse knee (function similar to above-knee amputation)
- Van Nes rotationplasty; creates a knee joint by attaching ankle backward to distal femur (function similar to below-knee amputation).

Dror Paley (Baltimore, USA) has extended the indications for reconstruction with his 'superhip' and 'superknee' operations, but these are highly complex and extensive procedures which are yet to permeate the mainstream.

Reference

1 Aitken GT. Proximal femoral focal deficiency—definition, classification, and management. In: Aitken GT, ed. *Proximal Femoral Focal Deficiency. A Congenital Anomaly.* Washington, DC: National Academy of Sciences;1969.

Table 10.4 Aitken Classification

Aitken type	Appearance	Morphology
A		Femoral head present and ossifies to shaft coxa vara and short femur
B		Head present but segment does not ossify to shaft, dysplastic acetabulum
C		No femoral head (or ossicle only), acetabulum poorly defined
D		Femur extremely short or absent

Developmental dysplasia of the hip

Due mostly to abnormal intrauterine development of the acetabulum with 2° femoral changes. Vast majority of cases detectable at birth[1].

Dysplasia—a hip that can be provoked to dislocate or is subluxed/dislocated but relocatable ((+)ve Ortolani sign: see opposite).

Dislocation—irreducibly dislocated hip ((−)ve Ortolani sign), with 2° changes: shortening (Galeazzi sign), restricted abduction, asymmetric gluteal folds.

Teratological dislocation—a separate entity occurring in association with neurological disorders, arthrogryposis and certain syndromes.

Screening

The principle is simple; treatment for DDH diagnosed within first 3 months of life is 80–95% effective. Late presenting DDH requires more invasive treatment with a less predictable outcome.

Literature on the subject is vast and confusing[2]. Screening based on risk factors (opposite), clinical examination and US screening or a combination. Universal US screening (Austria, parts of Scandinavia) associated with lowest rates of late presentation, but expensive. Spontaneous resolution rate of early-diagnosed neonatal hip instability/dysplasia is high, and direct evidence of improved functional outcome from intervention secondary to screening is lacking. Most UK/North American centres reserve US for neonates with risk factors or abnormal clinical findings; selective US screening cheaper, but majority of 'true DDH' (those hips which actually go on to require treatment) have no or few risk factors. Clinical examination is a heavily operator-dependent test.

Investigations

Ultrasound

- Pioneered by R. Graf in Austria and T. Harcke in the USA in the 1980s
- Visualizes femoral head before ossification (usually age 3–6 months, but often delayed in DDH) allows x-ray imaging
- Graf described alpha angle (osseous acetabular development) and beta (cartilage) on static views
- Harcke used stress coronal and transverse views (real-time or dynamic ultrasonography).

Radiograph

- Can draw Perkin's and Hilgenreiner's lines (through triradiate cartilages and vertically down from acetabular edge, respectively) to infer position of unossified head by relative position of the ossified metaphysis
- Acetabular index a measure of ongoing acetabular dysplasia
- Shenton's line; restoration a key endpoint in reduction of dislocation or subluxation.

Ortolani and Barlow clinical tests

Useful up to 6 weeks of age:
- Ortolani test: abduction and gentle elevation of dislocated femoral head→'clunk' of reduction
- Barlow's 'provocation' test: gentle depression of adducted hip→palpable subluxation or dislocation of unstable hip.

Consistent epidemiological risk factors for DDH

- Positive family history
- Female gender (but too broad for use in screening)
- Breech position.

Additional risk factors may include:

- Maternal primiparity
- High birth weight
- Oligohydramnios
- Congenital anomalies.

Treatment

Aim: to achieve a stable, concentric femoral head reduction with full range of hip motion for normal acetabular growth and development. Protocols based on age of presentation:

0–3 months High rate of spontaneous resolution of transient instability in first 6 weeks of life so can monitor with US. Persisting abnormality and dislocation treated with splintage: Pavlik harness loosely applied and regularly checked (to minimize rate of AVN or femoral nerve palsy). Reserve rigid splints, e.g. Von Rosen, for those with ligamentous laxity that fail to stabilize in harness.

For Ortolani-negative hip dislocation, must check for reduction at 1–2 weeks and abandon splintage if no improvement.

Should all be followed to skeletal maturity in case of non-resolving acetabular dysplasia; normal radiograph at 6 months associated with very low risk of this.

3–12 months 'Delayed' presentation or failed splintage likely to require surgical intervention with arthrogram, closed reduction and spica casting in Salter's 'human position': 90–100° flexion and 50–70° abduction. If reduction poor quality then management controversial: some wait until appearance of ossific nucleus before performing open reduction (theoretical reduced risk of AVN as ossified head less vulnerable to compression), others proceed direct to open reduction via medial approach—the 'open-assisted closed reduction'[2] (which puts the medial circumflex arterial branch to the femoral head at risk).

12 months to 2yrs Closed reduction now unlikely to succeed even after adductor tenotomy/psoas release. Formal open reduction now required via an anterior approach that gives best access to displaced femoral head and capsule for reefing. Can combine with procedure, e.g. Salter osteotomy[3], to redirect the acetabulum as persistent dysplasia now incresingly likely even if good quality reduction achieved.

≥2yrs Open reduction now inevitable. Preoperative traction to facilitate reduction now largely abandoned in favour of femoral shortening osteotomy. Beware treating older child with bilateral dislocations and >7–9yrs.

Untreated dislocation produces abnormal gait, risk of ipsilateral knee symptoms and hip pain from the 3rd decade. Studies of treatment for late presenting dislocation (>1.5yrs) are few but expect ~50% rate of hip replacement by age 50yrs in this group.

References

1 Weinstein SL, Mubarak SJ, Wenger DR. Developmental hip dysplasia and dislocation Part 1. *Instr Course Lect* 2004;**53**:523–30.

2 Shipman SA, Helfand M, Moyer VA, *et al.* Screening for developmental dysplasia of the hip: a systematic literature review for the US preventive services task force. *Pediatrics* 2006;**117**: e557–76.

3 Salter RB, Dubos JP. The first fifteen years personal experience with innominate osteotomy in the treatment of congenital dislocation and subluxation of the hip. *Clin Orthop Rel Res* 1974;**98**:72–103.

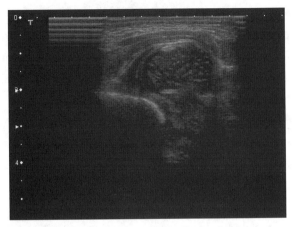

Fig. 10.6 Neonatal ultrasound of dislocated femoral head.

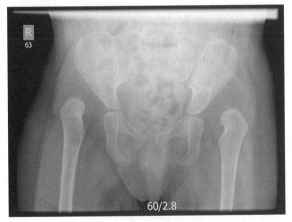

Fig. 10.7 Late presenting bilateral DDH in 18 month female.

Perthes disease—aetiology and presentation

Temporary interruption of blood supply to bony nucleus of proximal femoral epiphysis (aetiology unknown) causes increased bone density and impaired epiphyseal growth. Dense bone then resorbed and replaced (revascularization) but altered mechanical properties of the head cause flattening and enlargement. Incidence 1 in 1200, ~10% bilateral.

Aetiology

Theories:
- Disrupted *blood flow*: compromised arterial inflow, venous congestion, thrombophilia (silent coagulopathy)
- Underlying *systemic disorder* or skeletal dysplasia—delayed skeletal maturation common, hormonal abnormalities in some children
- *Environmental influences*—poor nutrition, parental smoking
- *Trauma*—associated with attention deficit disorder.

Typical child is male (4–5:1 M:F ratio), aged 4–8yrs with short stature, delayed skeletal maturation and hyperactivity. Painless limp a common presentation; symptoms, if present, may radiate from groin. to anterior thigh or knee

Examination reveals antalgic or Trendelenburg gait, limited hip motion especially in abduction and internal rotation, hip flexion contracture ± mild femoral shortening.

Radiographic stages

- Initial (osteonecrosis)—smaller ossific nucleus in femoral head which is lateralized and shows increased density. Subchondral fracture and metaphyseal lucencies appear
- Fragmentation—segments demarcate within femoral head, increased density lost
- Reossification—new woven bone appears to replace lucencies between fragments
- Residual—femoral head reossified, remodels up to skeletal maturity
- Stages 2 and 3 characterized by '*creeping substitution*'; revitalization of the femoral head of dead bone by invading vascular connective tissue carrying osteoclasts (bone resorption) and osteoblasts (replace with immature bone).

Four patterns of resultant deformity are seen:

- Coxa magna: ossification of hypertrophied articular cartilage, which is still nourished by synovial fluid
- Premature physeal arrest: central arrest causes coxa breva with trochanteric overgrowth; lateral coxa valga with oval epiphysis
- Irregular head formation: collapse of epiphyseal trabeculae 2° to resorptive repair processes and abnormal stresses, also iatrogenic from attempts at 'containment'
- Osteochrondritis dissecans.

History

Known as Legg– (Harvard, 1874–1939), Calve– (Paris 1875–1954), Perthes (Rhineland 1896–1927) disease, but pictures in Kohler's atlas (1905) and a description by Fragenheim (1909) predated all their work. Nonetheless, these individuals are credited with popularizing the condition.

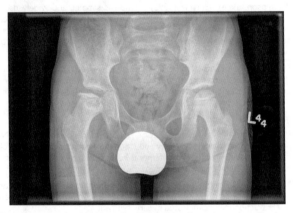

Fig. 10.8 7 yrs male with Herring C collapse, subluxation and metaphyseal cystic change.

Perthes disease—classification and treatment

Can be based on extent of head involvement and 'at risk' signs (Catterall, 1971) and extent of subchondral fracture, present in ~50% of cases (Salter/ Thompson, 1984). Herring (1992) method is simpler and widely used, divides epiphysis into 3 pillars: if lateral 15–30% pillar height is normal then group A, maintained >50% group B, <50% group C. A B/C group was later added with a thin or poorly ossified lateral pillar or exactly 50% loss of height.

Clinical course of untreated Perthes disease is inferred rather than known; disease severity varies greatly but correlates directly with extent of radiographic involvement, duration of disease and age of child (early onset <6yrs mild symptoms, 6–9yrs moderate, and >9yrs have worst outcome).

Treatment

Mostly based on 'Containment theory'[1]; in a pig model of (induced) AVN, holding hips within acetabulum by abduction during revascularization produced modelling into rounded femoral heads. Despite lack of scientific proof from clinical trials, containment the goal for a range of procedures:

Non-operative: motion therapy to maintain abduction, cast (Petrie) or brace (Atlanta Scottish Rite) in abduction (± adductor tenotomy). Bed rest ± traction may be indicated in early synovitic stage.

Operative: femoral varus osteotomy, acetabular redirectional (innominate) osteotomy, acetabular augmentation by a 'shelf' (Staheli) or medial displacement osteotomy (Chiari).

The best available evidence at present is Herring's propective study[2] (compromised by a retrospective change in classification—the B/C group) which found:
• Group A children fare well regardless of age at onset of disease
• Patients aged 8yrs chronological or 6yrs skeletal at time of onset with hip in B or B/C group do better with surgical treatment (varus femoral osteotomy or innominate osteotomy) than non-operative (no treatment, motion therapy or bracing)
• Group B hips <8yrs old have favourable outcomes unrelated to treatment type
• Group C hips frequently have poor outcomes unrelated to treatment.

Prognosis

Most important predictors of long-term outcome are shape of healed femoral head (compared with Moses spherical template) and congruency with acetabulum which constitutes the Stulberg class:

- I/II: spherical, congruent femoral heads, do not develop arthritis
- III/IV: degrees of femoral head flattening but acetabular changes maintain 'aspherical congruency', develop mild/moderate arthritis in late adult life
- V: loss of head shape but acetabulum unchanged so 'aspherical incongruency', develop severe arthritis by age 50yrs.

Future directions

May be pharmacological, aimed at tipping the balance during revascularization from osteoclast resorption towards osteoblast new bone formation; bisphosphonate improved femoral head sphericity in rat and piglet model of the disease, RANKL (essential for osteoclast formation) inhibition with osteoprotegrin (shorter acting than bisphosphonates) preserved femoral head structure in a piglet model.

References

1 Salter RB, Bell M. The pathogenesis of deformity in Legg–Perthes disease; an experimental investigation. *J Bone Joint Surg Br* 1968;**50**:436.
2 Herring JA, Kim HT, Browne R. Legg–Calve–Perthes disease. Part II: prospective multicenter study on the effect of treatment on outcome. *J Bone Joint Surg Am* 2004;**86**:2121–34.

Slipped capital femoral epiphysis

Incidence is ~1 in 100 000; so commonly seen by paediatric orthopaedic surgeons but rarely so by GPs and physiotherapists to whom they initially present. This and typical complaint of knee rather than hip pain cause problems; early diagnosis is critical.

SCFE describes posterior and inferior rotation of femoral head epiphysis on neck through (hypertrophic zone of) relatively weak physeal cartilage. Actually epiphysis stays within acetabulum and femoral neck rotates away anteriorly and externally.

Aetiology unknown, but typical child is male, obese, adolescent and in accelerated pubertal phase of growth. Endocrine disturbance (thyroid imbalance, hypogonadism, panhypopituitarism) also associated, particularly in younger children (typical age range 10–16yrs boys; 9–15yrs girls). More common in Afro-Caribbeans, Polynesians and Down syndrome.

Presentation

Hip, thigh or knee pain, antalgic gait and progressive loss of internal hip rotation, particularly in hip flexion, as slip progresses.

Most common is chronic presentation (>3 weeks symptoms) for which average time to diagnosis is >6 months. Critical classification is Loder's into stable/unstable[1], as defined by ability or not to weight bear ± crutches. AVN of femoral head occurs in upto half of latter, almost none of former.

Severity is measured by slip angle (Figs 10.9 and 10.10); between a line along the femoral neck on lateral view and another line perpendicular to the epiphysis. <30° mild; >30 to <60° moderate and >60° severe.

Contralateral slip (within 6 months) rate up to 60%, but much less if triradiate cartilage has closed on plain film (occurs half way through pubertal growth spurt).

Plain AP and lateral hip radiographs confirm SCFE. Klein's line drawn up upper side of femoral neck on both views should pass through edge of epiphysis but will miss with SCFE. In chronic slips, 'frog leg' lateral with hips flexed, abducted and externally rotated gives best view but should be avoided in unstable slips (may worsen the slip; request cross table lateral).

Management

Pin *in situ* for the majority.

This arrests incremental progression and secondary deformity. A single screw in centre of epiphysis usually suffices (Fig. 10.11); starting point must be anterior on femoral neck as epiphysis has slipped posteriorly. Best is reverse-cutting 7.3mm cannulated screw. Slip progression after fixation unlikely with ≥5 screw threads across into the epiphysis; achieving this without joint penetration is difficult (need exact centering of screw in epiphysis and careful screening with image intensifier). 3.5 threads the minimum required to pass.

Acute unstable slips which are moderate or severe are very controversial. Reasonable to place on traction table under general anaesthetic if within 24h of presentation as may spontaneously reduce. If not, can open hip joint and reduce taking an anterior wedge of femoral neck to avoid tension on critical posterolateral vessels to femoral head. If presentation >24h, can do same but prolonged bed rest a while to allow secondary inflammatory changes to subside is advisable.

Complications

- *AVN*—almost exclusively in unstable slips and usually after treatment. Untreatable at present and potentially devastating.
- *Chondrolysis*—aetiology unknown, seen in particular but not exclusively with joint penetration of screw fixation.
- *Secondary OA*—in proportion to severity of slip.

Controversies

Where to start? Contralateral prophylactic pinning not routine, but probably should be in younger child. Even with diligence to spot the symptoms early, contralateral slip probably no more benign than first side[2].

Whether, which, when and by what means to open and reduce epiphysis. In general; further the correction from the epiphysis, the less the risk of subsequent AVN. Correct unstable slips through physis acutely but consider intertrochentric osteostomy to correct secondary deformity in chronic severe slips.

References

1 Loder RT, Richards BS, Shapiro PS, et al. Acute slipped capital femoral epiphysis: the importance of physeal stability. *J Bone Joint Surg Am* 1993;**75**:1134–40.
2 Yildirim Y, Bautista S, Davidson RS. Chondrolysis, osteonecrosis and slip severity in patients with subsequent contralateral SCFE. *J Bone Joint Surg Am* 2008;**90**:485–92.

Slipped capital femoral epiphysis: images

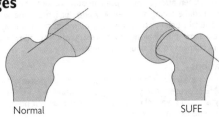

Fig. 10.9 Trethowan or Klein's line reveals how a slip alters the relationship of the femoral neck to the epiphysis: SUFE = slipped upper femoral epiphysis.

Reproduced from Bulstrode et al., *Oxford Textbook of Orthopaedics and Trauma*, with permission from Oxford University Press.

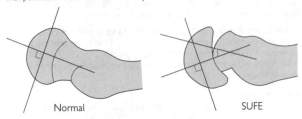

Fig. 10.10 The extent of epiphyseal displacement is expressed in degrees or as a proportion of femoral head displacement on the neck: SUFE = slipped upper femoral epiphysis.

Reproduced from Bulstrode et al., *Oxford Textbook of Orthopaedics and Trauma*, with permission from Oxford University Press.

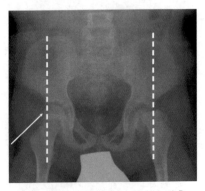

Fig. 10.11 Severe, acute unstable SCFE in a 13yr-old-child with Down syndrome. Klein's line misses the epiphysis altogether.

Fibular hemimelia

Most common of the lower limb reduction anomalies: occurs in 1:25 000 live births. Longitudinal deficiency of lateral portion of lower limb, in which part or all of fibula is missing and varying degrees of tibial shortening. A range of associated deficiencies, from the ground up:

- Lateral ray deficiencies. <3 rays unlikely to provide a functional foot so indication for amputation
- Hindfoot coalitions ± 'ball and socket' ankle joint
- Equinovalgus ankle with apex anterior tibial bow and a skin dimple
- Lateral femoral condylar hypoplasia ± cruciate ligament deficiency/ absence
- Femoral shortening ± PFFD commonly.

Treatment

Depends on severity, mild forms managed with shoe raise ± orthotics and subsequent contralateral epiphysiodesis. For more severe forms, debate ranges between amputation with prosthetic fitting vs limb reconstruction, with rapid developments in both fields.

<3 ray foot and anticipated shortening >30% indications for amputation.

Children with non-functional upper extremities will need feet for daily activities so amputation not an option.

Reconstruction involves

- Correction of tibial bow and ankle deformity with resection of fibular anlage (posteromedial deforming tether)
- Staged lengthening(s) with circular frame.

Tibial hemimelia

- Partial or total absence of the tibia
- Rare (1 in a million)
- Often AD inheritance, should see geneticist
- Typical appearance of absent distal tibia with overlong fibula that curves round so lateral malleolus prominent and foot equinovarus
- May be associated central ray deficiencies ('Lobster claw').

Treatment

- Commonly to centralize fibula
- If absent knee joint, brown procedure was to fuse fibula into intercondylar notch. Results poor cf. below-knee amputation.

Choice of amputation

Syme is through ankle; stump does not subsequently enlarge in the young child so excellent cosmesis.

Boyd retains the os calcis (fused to distal tibia) to stabilize the heel fat pad (for end-bearing stump) but has a problematic rate of non-union.

Blount's disease

Growth disorder of the medial aspect of the proximal tibial physis causing tibia vara, internal torsion of the proximal tibia ± distal femoral deformity.

W.P. Blount (Milwaukee, Wisconsin) first fully described the condition in 1937. Affected children are otherwise healthy; majority are bilateral.

Risk factors

- Obesity (>95th centile for age)
- Female gender
- Afro-American, West Indies or Finland origin
- Early walking age.

Differential causes of tibia vara

- Physiological bow legs ('U' coronal profile rather than 'V' of Blount's)
- Metabolic, e.g. rickets
- Skeletal dysplasia, e.g. metaphyseal chondrodysplasia, Ollier's disease, focal fibrocartilaginous
- Dysplasia.

Diagnosis

Tibia vara is physiological up to the age of 2yrs[1] and so the diagnosis of infantile Blount's is difficult and should not be made before then. Typical features are a sharp angular deformity in an obese toddler that has walked early, with a fragmented medial metaphyseal beak on radiographs (taken with patella facing forwards, as internal torsion may lead to an 'obliquogram').

The metaphyseal–diaphyseal[2] angle can be helpful: <9° likely to be normal, >15° abnormal but in between is a grey area.

An adolescent form is generally milder, with a subgroup which is not obese.

Management

Early treatment is essential in an attempt to prevent premature bone bridge fusion of the medial physis.

Observe up to age 2–3yrs, bracing probably not effective.

Simple corrective osteotomy for early cases may suffice.

For more advanced cases, need to consider any of the following in addition:
- Physeal bar resection (epiphysiolysis), or completion lateral hemiepiphysiodesis
- Medial hemiplateau elevation
- Corrective osteotomy distal femur for (commonly varus, but can be valgus) deformity
- Gradual correction of tibia with frame restoring alignment, length, and rotation.

References

1 Salenius P, Vankka E. The development of the tibiofemoral angle in children. *J Bone Joint Surg Am* 1975;**57**:259–61.
2 Levine AM, Drennan JC. Physiological bowing and tibia vara. *J Bone Joint Surg Am* 1982;**64**:1158–63.

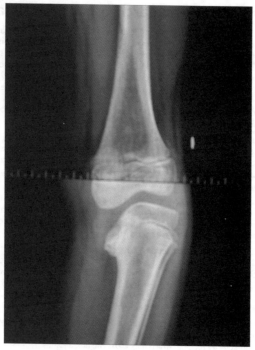

Fig. 10.12 Radiograph of left knee Blount's disease in 8 yrs female.

Congenital pseudarthrosis of the tibia

This is perhaps the most difficult condition of all in Children's Orthopaedics to manage. Fortunately it is rare (1 in 140 000 live births). The deformity consists of a short limb with characteristic apex antero-lateral tibial bow above the ankle joint[1]. Fracture through the abnormal bone underlying the bow is inevitable, usually before 2nd birthday, and does not easily unite (Fig. 10.13). The foot is initially inverted and medially displaced secondary to the bow, but later the ankle may go into valgus, especially if there is associated fibula pseudarthrosis, necessitating corrective surgery here too.

Aetiology is unknown. Over half are associated with **NF** and 6% of patients with NF type 1 develop CPT. Any association with **fibrous dysplasia** is less clear; both this and NF can have café au lait spots but these may not appear until the child is older so early prefracture diagnosis (which is important) is not straightforward.

Histopathologically the lesions consist of highly cellular fibrovascular tissue with thickened periosteum, but whether this is primary or secondary to fracture is not known. The tibia is the bone most commonly affected, but forearm bones may also have pseudarthroses.

There are various classifications, but really the only important factor in deciding management is whether the tibia has fractured. Up to this point, the child should be treated in a tibial (clam shell-type) orthosis for weight bearing with the ankle free to maintain motion. The aim is to delay fracture, and therefore surgery, for as long as possible because the results of fixation are almost certainly better in older children.

The number of reported interventions reflects the peculiar difficulty with obtaining lasting union in this condition:
- *Intramedullary rodding*, which may cross the ankle joint.
- *Ilizarov or spatial frame*: commonly after resection and compression. Either side of the abnormal tissue with a more proximal corticotomy for distraction to restore length.
- Resection and filling of void with *free vascularized fibular* autogenous bone graft.
- More recently, early reports suggest the adjuvant application of bone morphogenetic protein (*BMP-2*) around the pseudarthrosis with intramedullary stabilization gives dramatically improved union rates.

Typically multiple procedures are required with no guarantee of successful union. Amputation is rarely considered early in the management[2] but should be included in discussions in case the CPT later fails to heal (see 📖 p. 531).

Indications for amputation and prosthetic fitting:

- Failure of union after 3 surgical attempts
- Significant predicted limb length discrepancy (lengthening potentially hazardous as corticotomy may not unite)
- Permanently deformed foot with resultant poor function
- Functional loss resulting from prolonged medical care and hospitalization.

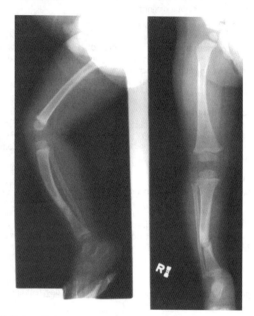

Fig. 10.13 2-yr-old child presenting with fracture through CPT.

References

1 Vander Have KL, Hensinger RN, Caird M, et al. Congenital pseudarthrosis of the tibia. *J Am Acad Orthop Surg* 2008;**16**:228–36.
2 McCarthy R. Amputation for CPT: indications and techniques. *Clin Orthop Rel Res* 1982;**166**:58–61.

Knee disorders: idiopathic anterior knee pain

Description AKP is common in adolescents. It can result from a number of musculoskeletal conditions and the diagnosis may be difficult. In the absence of definable pathology the condition is usually referred to as idiopathic AKP. The term chondromalacia patella has been used interchangeably with AKP; this should not be done—chondromalacia patella is a surgical finding and not a diagnosis.

Aetiology In most children with AKP there is no true mechanical derangement of the knee. The aetiology is unclear but is probably multifactorial. It is thought that the combination of genetic or developmental factors (dysplasia of patellofemoral joint or joint laxity) and acquired problems (repetitive loading or direct trauma) result in the knee becoming unbalanced or unstable and that the changes which occur in patellar tracking eventually lead to the onset of pain.

Differential diagnosis

The differential diagnosis includes Osgood–Schlatter disease, Sinding–Larsen–Johansson disease, OCD, bipartite patella, patellar stress fracture, plicae, complex regional pain syndrome, foreign body, neuroma or tumour. There are also non-organic causes of AKP.

Clinical

Patients complain of AKP with an insidious onset. The pain is poorly localized and usually made worse by physical activity (running, jumping, squatting) or prolonged sitting with the knee flexed. Patients sometimes report giving way, and this is usually due to quadriceps inhibition. The history should include limitations in activity, previous treatment and symptoms related to the other knee. Assess gait, the alignment of the lower limbs and patellar tracking (Q angle, lateral tilt, lateral tracking), stability and range of movement of both knees. In idiopathic AKP there is usually a full range of movement. There may be maltracking of the patella, crepitus or wasting of the quadriceps. The lumbar spine, hips, ankles, feet and lower limb neurology must also be assessed.

Investigations

Radiology: X-rays of the knee should include AP, lateral, tunnel and skyline views. An MRI scan may be helpful in excluding chondral and ligamentous lesions.

Management

Non-operative: idiopathic AKP is managed by modifying activities to reduce stress on the knee, with exercises to improve flexibility and strength, and analgesia. Some patients benefit from using a knee or foot orthosis, especially if there is malalignment or instability. Operative options: soft tissue or bone (post skeletal maturity) realignment procedures, trochleaplasty.

Knee disorders: osteochondritis dissecans

Description

OCD is an idiopathic lesion of bone and cartilage resulting in loss of continuity with subchondral bone. There may be separation of overlying articular cartilage. The most common site in the knee is the lateral aspect of the medial femoral condyle.

Epidemiology Usually seen in adolescents. Male to female ratio is 2:1. Lesions are bilateral in 20% of patients.

Aetiology

The cause of OCD is unknown. Significant direct trauma, repetitive microtrauma, vascular insufficiency and abnormal ossification within the epiphysis have been implicated in this disorder.

Clinical

Adolescents present with activity-related pain, swelling, catching, locking and giving way. On examination there may be a limp and the knee may be tender and swollen (effusion). Extension may be blocked by a loose body. With medial femoral condyle lesions pain may be reproduced by flexing the knee to 90° and rotating the tibia medially while extending the knee. If positive, pain will occur at ~30° of knee flexion (Wilson's sign).

Investigations

Radiology: AP, lateral, tunnel, and skyline are views. Tunnel view shows the intercondylar notch.

MRI scan: demonstrates size and extent of the lesion contrast (IV gacolinium) may indicate whether or not lesion is likely to be stable.

Arthroscopy: can be both diagnostic and therapeutic.

Management

Treatment depends on the lesion stage (subchondral stability, integrity of overlying cartilage) and skeletal age of the patient. There is considerable debate as to the best treatment. Early lesions in skeletally immature patients have the best prognosis.

Non-operative treatment: activity modification with or without use of crutches, immobilization and anti-inflammatory drugs.

Operative options: surgery is indicated in skeletally mature patients with a locked knee or symptomatic loose body. The loose body can be removed or reattached but will have swollen if detached > 6 weeks. Unstable lesions can be fixed or debrided and the subchondral bone drilled (improves vascularity). With larger defects chondral grafting may be considered.

Other knee disorders in children

Congenital absence of anterior cruciate ligament

Rare and usually co-exists with other dysplastic conditions of the lower limb. Often well tolerated but may become a problem if corrective treatment, such as leg lengthening, is undertaken.

Discoid meniscus

Description

A discoid lateral meniscus is one that is round rather than crescent shaped. Approximately 90% occur on the lateral side of the knee.

Epidemiology

Discoid menisci are present in 5% of population and are often bilateral.

Clinical

Pain is the most common complaint, but clicking, swelling or locking are other presenting symptoms. The findings on examination include joint line tenderness, clicking, an effusion, loss of flexion or extension, a positive grinding test (Apley) or thigh muscle wasting.

Investigations

Radiology: plain X-rays may, but rarely, show widening of the lateral joint space, flattening of the lateral femoral condyle, tilt of the lateral tibial condyle, hypoplasia of the lateral tibial spine and a more proximal position of the fibular head. An MRI scan is the most appropriate investigation to diagnose and characterize a discoid meniscus.

Management

Asymptomatic discoid menisci do not require treatment. If it becomes symptomatic, due to a tear or meniscal instability, a partial or total meniscectomy may be necessary.

Meniscal injuries

These injuries are rare in childhood but may occur in contact sports. They may occur with ruptures of the ACL. In general, meniscal injuries should be managed non-operatively. In children with episodes of locking, arthroscopy is recommended. Peripheral tears should be repaired. Partial meniscectomy should only be carried out for lesions that cannot be repaired.

Congenital talipes equinovarus (clubfoot)

Description

Common birth defect affecting 1 in 1000 live births, 3:1 males.

Majority idiopathic, but may be associated with additional malformations (risk ~50% in males with bilateral involvement), chromosomal abnormalities or genetic syndromes, e.g. arthrogryposis.

Characteristic appearance (Fig. 10.14) of hindfoot equinus and varus, midfoot varus and cavus.

Severity before and after treatment is graded according to appearance of lateral foot border (straight or curved), extent of equinus ('empty heel pad sign'), extent of (un)covering of lateral talar head.

Affected foot and calf always smaller; extent proportionate to severity.

Diagnosis is a clinical one; radiographs are not useful in early management.

History

In the 1950s an orthopaedic surgeon in Iowa, Ignatio V. Ponseti, began reporting good results with a staged technique of serial stretch and casting for idiopathic clubfoot. The central tenets of the technique are shown in Table 10.5. He was largely ignored by the wider orthopaedic community who dismissed his cases as mild variants; the results of non-operative treatment were considered poor and extensive release was preferred. In the mid 1990s the long-term results of the Ponseti technique were confirmed to be excellent[1], far better than for operative release and almost comparable for function to unaffected feet. By the turn of the century it began to be embraced worldwide by a range of practitioners, some in the most basic of settings since no specialist equipment is required. Good results are now being reported in non-idiopathic deformities such as arthrogryposis[2].

Recurrence

For idiopathic clubfoot the success rate of Ponseti's technique, in Iowa at least, approaches 100%, but there is a strong tendency to relapse. Corrected feet are placed in abduction 'boots and bars' to be continued at night up until the age of 4yrs ideally. Tolerance becomes difficult after ~2yrs of age, when relapses should still respond to repeat manipulation and casting. After age 2.5yrs transfer of the tibialis anterior tendon, a strong forefoot supinator if there is residual medial displacement of the navicular on the talus, to the lateral cuneiform is effective for preventing recurrence. It is an option for the non-brace-tolerant and also older child with relapse in whom the foot remains supple.

In reality, the technique is a fluid and progressive elevation and abduction of the first ray about the talus, unlocking the midfoot and hindfoot as the first ray swings around. Critical is to correct each sequential deformity before moving on to the next, otherwise correction will stall.

Once correction complete, final cast stays on for 3 weeks before application of abduction brace (boots and bars) full time for 3 months or until walking, then at night and naptime only.

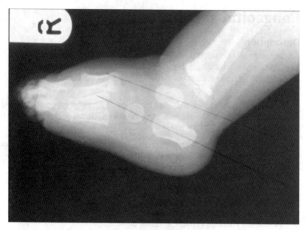

Fig. 10.14 Radiograph of a child with congenital talipes equinovarus.
Reproduced from Bulstrode *et al.*, *Oxford Textbook of Orthopaedics and Trauma*,
with permission from Oxford University Press.

Table 10.5 Ponseti technique (mnemonic CAVE)

Deformity	Manipulation and position of cast	Pitfalls
Cavus	Elevate (supinate) first ray	Dorsiflexion is all that is required—first cast to correct cavus only
Adduction (midfoot)	Abduct first ray using counterthumb pressure against the uncovered lateral talar head	Avoid cuboid as a fulcrum (Kite's error) which will lock the hindfoot in varus Foot remains supinated, do not attempt to force into pronation
Varus (hindfoot)	Correction follows with further abduction of first ray, allowing the os calcis to abduct under the talus	If the midfoot cavus has not been corrected the correction will stall at this point.
Equinus (hindfoot)	Talar head now covered, hindfoot varus corrected (os calcis abducts into valgus under talus) and foot elevated with forepart in maximal abduction	15° ankle dorsiflexion must be achieved; otherwise percutaneous release of heelcord is indicated (in ~70–80% of cases)

References

1 Cooper D, Dietz F. Treatment of idiopathic clubfoot. *J Bone Joint Surg Am* 1995;**77**:1477–89.
2 Boehm S, Limpaphayom N, Alaee F, et al. Early results of the Ponseti method for clubfoot in distal arthrogryposis. *J Bone Joint Surg Am* 2008;**90**:1501–7.

Congenital vertical talus

Description

An uncommon condition of fixed dorsal (and lateral) dislocation of the navicular on the talus. Produces a 'rocker bottom' sole appearance which is characteristic and made up of a hindfoot fixed in equinus and a midfoot which is dorsally dislocated.

The majority have associated abnormalities, e.g. arthrogryposis, spinal dysraphism, myopathy. Idiopathic congenital vertical talus is therefore a diagnosis of exclusion.

Diagnosis, usually made in the neonate, is confirmed by lateral radiographs taken in maximum dorsi and plantar flexion. The navicular ossifies between 3 and 5yrs of age so the line of the first ray is extrapolated to infer its long axis. Even in plantar flexion, the navicular remains dorsally dislocated; if it appears partially to reduce the milder diagnosis of 'oblique' talus is made. The blob of ossification seen in front of the talus is the cuboid, which will be confirmed by an AP view. The dorsiflexion view shows that the os calcis remains fixed in equinus.

Treatment for this fixed deformity is classically surgical[1], with an extensive release of the talonavicular joint and posterolateral tethers, through separate posterior and medial incisions or a single 'Cincinatti' incision as used in posteromedial club foot release.

More recently, a new '**reverse Ponseti**' technique[2] is reported and gaining popularity; 4–6 weekly manipulations followed by casting in plantar flexion and adduction progressively to relocate the talonavicular joint, followed by a more limited open reduction and pinning of the talonavicular joint, and percutaneous tendo-achilles release.

References

1 Laaveg SJ, Ponseti IV. Long-term results of treatment of congenital club foot. *J Bone Joint Surg Am* 1980;**62**:23–31.
2 Dobbs MB, Purcell DB, Nunley R, *et al*. Early results of a new method of treatment for idiopathic congenital vertical talus. *J Bone Joint Surg Am* 2006;**88**:1192–200.

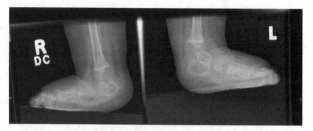

Fig. 10.15 Lateral radiographs of right congenital vertical talus in maximum dorsi flexion.

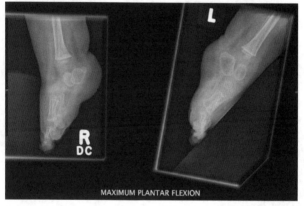

MAXIMUM PLANTAR FLEXION

Fig. 10.16 Lateral radiographs of right congenital vertical talus in maximum plantar flexion.

Tarsal coalition

Description

AD condition affecting 1% of population. Failure of mesenchymal segmentation and differentiation produces abnormal bridge between tarsal bones. Most common coalitions occur between calcaneum/navicular (CNC) and talus/calcaneum (TCC). Undergo metaplasia from fibrous syndesmosis to cartilaginous synchondrosis to bony synostosis during childhood and adolescence; affected joints usually become symptomatic at 8–12yrs for CNC and 12–16yrs for TCC if motion causes pain (75% are asymptomatic).

Coalition is the most common cause of a rigid flat foot[1]. Pain felt in medial hindfoot by sustentaculum tali (felt as a prominence just below and in front of medial malleolus) for TCC and in sinus tarsi (depression in front of distal fibula) for CNC; both may produce lateral heel pain from fibular impingement if marked hindfoot valgus (old name 'peroneal spastic flat foot').

Imaging

Standing AP ankle radiograph to exclude valgus in tibio-talar joint

- AP foot weight-bearing radiograph—increased angle between long axes of talus and calcaneum (planovalgus), may see CNC on this or more likely with an *oblique view* of foot
- Lateral foot weight-bearing radiograph will show flattened/inverted angle between talus and first metatarsal long axes (planovalgus), may also see 'ant-eaters sign' (dorsal beaking of talus in CNC)
- Harris–Beath view (taken from behind in the plane of the subtalar joint with foot plantarflexed) may show a TCC of the middle facet
- CNC usually seen on plain films, TCC harder. *CT* visualizes middle facet of subtalar joint to identify and map extent of TCC, order also for CNC if surgery planned as high rate of co-existent TCC
- MRI may be indicated for diagnosis of fibrous coalition or synovitis without definite bone bridge.

Treatment

Below-knee walking cast (for 4–6 weeks) should relieve pain; otherwise consider possibility that coalition is incidental to another diagnosis. Follow with moulded orthotic insole.

Surgery indicated if symptoms recur: resection of coalition and interposition of bone wax, fat or other material. Caution required if extensive TCC (hindfoot may collapse further into valgus) and/or severe flat foot deformity; consider lateral column lengthening osteotomy (especially if calcaneo-cuboid joint significantly proximal to talonavicular on AP radiograph) or hindfoot fusion.

For 'flat feet' see Pes planovalgus (see 🕮 p. 544).

Reference

1 Mosca VS. Flexible flatfoot and tarsal coalition. In: Richards BS, ed. *Orthopaedic Knowledge Update: Paediatrics 2*. American Academy of Orthopaedic Surgeons, 2002:215–22.

Pes cavus

A high arched foot secondary to fixed plantar flexion of the first ray.

Unlike flexible pes planovalgus (PPV), pes cavus deformity is fixed, progressive and commonly (60–70%) associated with underlying neurological abnormality. The first ray points to the cause of the deformity: down (towards the foot) in PPV where the cause is intrinsic laxity or tight heel cord commonly (tarsal coalition or congenital vertical talus for fixed deformity), up in pes cavus (towards the spinal cord and brain).

50% of those with neurological abnormality have HMSN (hereditary motor and sensory neuropathy), also common with CP (classically hemiplegia), myelomeningocele. Types I–III HMSN commonly present to orthopaedics; the hypertrophic (I) and Dejerine–Sottas (III) forms are demyelinating with reduced or absent reflexes and delayed nerve conduction on studies, but the axonal type (II) is normal for these tests. Look for first dorsal interosseous wasting, a common sign, and also ask about family history as most forms are inherited.

The plantar flexed first ray is associated with tight plantar fascia and a pronated forefoot. The hindfoot goes into secondary supination or varus, which becomes fixed with time. The Coleman block tests for mobility of the subtalar joint; if the first ray plantarflexion is accommodated by a block under the heel and lateral border, the hindfoot varus will correct to neutral or physiological valgus unless this secondary deformity has become fixed. This is critical to operative planning.

Management

- Establish or exclude underlying abnormality
- Appropriate orthotics; generally accommodative for fixed deformity to spread load and relieve pressure areas
- Surgery may be inevitable, follow these principles[1]:
  - *Correct fixed bony and soft tissue deformities while preserving joint motion*, e.g. first ray dorsiflexion osteotomy and plantar fascia release ± hindfoot lateral displacement osteotomy depending on results of Coleman block test
  - *Balance the muscle forces*, e.g. tibialis posterior transfer to dorsum of foot
  - *Leave open options for the future* Pes cavus is a progressive deformity so recurrence highly likely. Avoid early resort to arthrodesis.

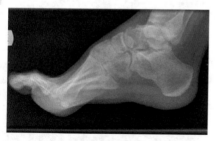

Fig. 10.17 Pes cavus.

Reference

1 Mosca V. The cavus foot (Editorial). *J Paediatr Orthop* 2001;**21**:423–4.

Pes planovalgus (flat foot)

Loss of medial longitudinal arch with midfoot sag, valgus hindfoot and abduction and supination of the forefoot in relation to the hindfoot (*plano-abductio-valgus*) (Fig 10.18).

Flexible flat foot

Characterized by mobility of subtalar joint; ask child to stand on tip-toe and the hindfoot is seen to invert when looking from behind.

Associated with benign hypermobility; also with syndromal cause (Ehlers–Danlos, Marfan syndrome, osteogenesis imperfecta, Down syndrome).

Rigid flat foot

Hindfoot maintained in valgus; stiffness often symptomatic on rough ground (loss of subtalar accommodation) or a cause of recurrent ankle sprains or stress fracture in foot.

Differential diagnosis includes tarsal coalition and congenital vertical talus ('Persian slipper' appearance to foot with os calcis in equinus and navicular dorsally dislocated on the talus), also accessory navicular and neuromuscular disease.

Management

Most flexible flat feet in children require reassurance only and will resolve into adulthood; a few are symptomatic in the area under the uncovered head of talus and will respond to a moulded foot orthosis.

No indication for treatment of flexible flat foot if asymptomatic; orthotics will not change the shape of the foot in the longer term.

Examine for tightness of tendo-achilles with knee extended. Failure to address this may lead to a 'midfoot break' (secondary midfoot abduction); treat with stretching, serial casting or botulinum toxin injection to calf.

Occasionally require surgical release ± corrective hindfoot or lateral column osteotomy.

Rigid flat foot requires correction of underlying cause; usually surgical[1].

Calcaneovalgus foot

Classic 'packaging defect' secondary to cramped intrauterine environment. Neonatal presentation with dorsum of foot applied to anterior surface of tibia (opposite deformity to clubfoot) and apex anterolateral bow of tibia.

Management

Parental reassurance that bow will correct spontaneously in first years of life and foot position will improve ± simple stretching/splintage. Risk of fracture very low (cf. congenital pseudarthrosis of tibia).

Warn, however, that residual limb length discrepancy is common, usually small but not always so and needs follow-up to skeletal maturity in case of requirement for limb equalization procedure.

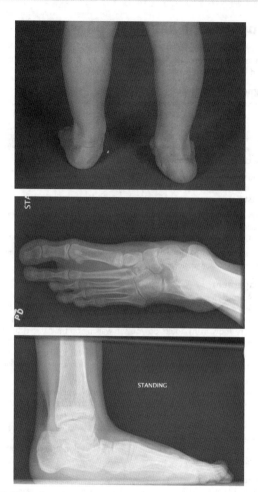

Fig. 10.18 Pes planovalgus.

Reference

1 Mosca VS. Flexible flatfoot and tarsal coalition. In: Richards BS, ed. *Orthopaedic Knowledge Update: Paediatrics 2.* American Academy of Orthopaedic Surgeons, 2002:215–22.

Idiopathic or habitual toe walking

Tip-toe walking is relatively common in toddlers up to the age of 4–5yrs. Habitual toe walkers will have done so since their earliest steps; this should be sought in the history. It also runs in the family in ~50%.

Diagnosis of exclusion

The same diagnosis for persistent or new-onset toe walking beyond this age is one of exclusion, primarily of an underlying neurological disorder. Top of the list comes CP (spastic diplegia), typically associated with a flexed knee during gait, followed by muscular dystrophy in boys, of which Duchenne's (X linked) is the most common. Gower's sign is a useful test in the clinic; ask also about delayed motor milestones.

Consider also HMSN (Charcot–Marie–Tooth disease) especially if later onset ~6yrs of age after previously normal walking. Examine for cavovarus feet, 1st dorsal interosseous wasting and ask about family history.

Always examine the spine in case of underlying spine/cord anomaly. A midline pit, hairy tuft, lipoma or other abnormality should prompt MRI evaluation for underlying tethered cord, syrinx or diastematomyelia.

Toe walking may also be associated with learning disorders and autism. Also with calf haemangioma.

Management[1]

For confirmed idiopathic toe walking, management can be tricky, with high recurrence rates and often considerable parental pressure to intervene. Reassurance is helped by the fact that persistence beyond skeletal maturity is rare (how many adults do you see walking on their toes?) but there are theoretical concerns about development of a secondary midfoot break and PPV for untreated calf contracture. This may be a particular issue with joint laxity; stabilize the midfoot when testing for ankle dorsiflexion to avoid spurious motion through this region.

Dynamic tightness may respond to physiotherapy and night splints. There is also recent interest in the use of botulinum toxin calf injections. Fixed contracture ('congenital short tendo-achilles') may require serial casting or surgery (percutaneous heelcord release or lengthening of the gastrocnemius aponeurosis). Again there is a high recurrence rate (30–60%) and a risk of over-correction, which is a disaster (weak push-off and no good surgical rescue option).

Reference

1 Eastwood DM, Menelaus MB, Dickens DR, et al. Idiopathic toe-walking: does treatment alter the natural history? *J Paediatr Orthop B* 2000;**9**:47–9.

Metatarsus adductus

Medial deviation of the forefoot (through the midtarsal joints) in isolation is a common (~1:1000 live birth) neonatal foot deformity.

It should be differentiated from *clubfoot*, in which there is hindfoot equinus and varus with midfoot cavus, and *skew foot*, a less common congenital deformity of metatarsus adductus combined with midfoot abduction and hindfoot valgus.

As a cause of in-toeing (and tripping) in the toddler metatarsus adductus should be differentiated from persistent femoral neck anteversion and internal tibial torsion. Progressive deformities ± cavus presenting in older age groups should prompt investigation for a more proximal spinal abnormality.

Most forms are a '*packaging*' rather than a '*manufacturing*' defect reflecting a tight intrauterine environment. Examine also for other packaging problems such as torticollis, plagiocephaly and hip dysplasia.

Management

The majority (>85%) are flexible and resolve without treatment[1]. Radiographs are not usually helpful. The heel should be stabilized in one hand while the other is used to abduct the forefoot. Those forefeet which correct to the midline can be managed expectantly ± a reverse counter shoe. Those which do not should undergo serial stretch and casting in the first year of life. The heel bisector line[2], which should pass through the 2nd/3rd web but goes laterally in metatarsus adductus, is a useful guide to severity, flexibility and response to treatment.

Surgery is very rarely required for resistant feet. Options include:
• Tarso-metatarsal osteotomies—largely abandoned because of stiffness and recurrence
• Multiple basal metatarsal osteotomies
• 'Cut and shut' tarsal osteotomies— a closing wedge cuboid and opening wedge cuneiform osteotomy, transferring the bone wedge across the foot.

References

1 Ponseti IV, Becker JR. Congenital metatarsus adductus. *J Bone Joint Surg Am* 1966;**48**:702–11.
2 Bleck EE. Metatarsus adductus: classification and relationship of outcomes to treatment. *J Pediatr Orthop* 1983;**3**:2–9.

Paediatric trauma

Growing bones

'Children should not simply be considered little adults'

Mercer Rang

Unique properties of the immature skeleton include:
- Presence of growth plates (physis, epiphyseal plate)
- Great capacity to remodel which is inversely proportional to age
- Different biomechanics from those of adult musculoskeletal system.

Bone growth: occurs by two mechanisms

Intramembranous ossification Increases diameter of bones and completely forms cranial and facial bones as well as part of clavicle. Mesenchyme-derived cells develop sites of ossification without cartilage precursor.

Endochondral ossification All other skeletal growth. Primary ossification centres develop in long bones (all present by 12 weeks of gestation) with secondary centres appearing at extremities at variable times after birth (exception in distal femur; secondary centre present at birth).

The physis

Between the secondary (epiphyseal) ossification centre and the meta-physics and responsible for longitudinal bone growth. Has several zones (from epiphysis to metaphysis).
- Reserve (or germinal)
- Proliferative (zone of growth)
- Hypertrophic (zone of transformation and calcification).

Physeal chondrocytes proliferate and then increase in volume, principally by fluid swelling, preparing around them a matrix scaffold on which osteoblasts build as the chondrocytes undergo a form of apoptosis, or 'chondroptosis', in the zone of calcification. Vascular loops from the metaphysis then invade and osteogenesis (with remodelling) begins[1].

Biomechanics and response to injury are determined by: strength and attachment of local ligaments, the perichondral ring and the shape of the physis. The smooth capital femoral physis is less resistant to shear or torsion than the 'W'-shaped distal femoral one, but injury to latter indicates greater disruption (a Salter–Harris II injury here is less likely to have a benign outcome despite adequate reduction). Likewise, proximal tibial physis is relatively protected by collateral ligaments which bridge it but take origin from the distal femoral epiphysis (the more commonly injured physis). The perichondral ring is uniquely vulnerable to injury and predisposes to eccentric physeal arrest and the rapid accumulation of secondary angular deformity.

Remodelling

A poorly understood process but various observations in clinical practice and fracture management are salient:

Wolff's Law (1892) Bones respond to their physical environment ('form follows function'); BMD (formation) is directly proportional to load.

Volkman's Law (1862) The physis responds to load but if deformity induces excessive forces across it growth may be inhibited (e.g. Blount's disease).

Angular remodelling Influenced by age (<8yrs do better), location of deformity (close to physis good), orientation (in plane of movement of adjacent joint good).

Rotational correction Very limited.

Translational correction Side to side displacement remodels very well, especially in prepubertal bone where 100% displacement may be entirely remodelled in 1–2yrs (so 'bayonet apposition' acceptable if alignment and rotation corrected).

Length correction Postfracture overgrowth occurs—physeal stimulation by a variety of factors but probably mainly vascular. Peaks at 3 months and complete by 18 months. Effects minimal in upper limb but produces 0.5–2cm length in lower limb, most noticeable in femur.

Biomechanics

The immature skeleton has:
- More bone per unit area
- Enhanced vascularity
- Thicker periosteum.

The implications are:
- Different fracture patterns and propagation, e.g. greenstick, torus, buckle
- Greatly reduced healing times and much lower rates of non-union
- Intact periosteum can aid reduction and healing, but if torn and incarcerated in fracture will have opposite effect and require open procedure
- Relatively more energy transfer to fracture the bone (thus greater local tissue damage than is seen in adult, e.g. rib fractures = lung contusion in a child)
- Special fracture types, e.g. triplane ankle fracture reflects course of physeal closure around adolescence, tibial spine avulsion the immature version of ACL rupture when chondroepiphysis fails before ligament (see also dislocations and fractures pp. 394 and 396).

Reference

1 Bush P, Hall A, Macnicol M. New insights into function of the growth plate. *J Bone Joint Surg Br* 2008;**12**:1542–7.

Physeal injuries

Physeal fracture is the commonest cause of growth arrest, but other causes exist.

Salter and Harris[1] in Canada established and popularized the principles of physeal fracture with their 1963 classification (see opposite and Fig. 11.1) on which current management of physeal fractures is based:

- Fractures which do not disrupt the continuity of the germinal layer of the physis (types I, II) should not lead to growth arrest
- Injuries which segment the growth plate and epiphysis (types III, IV) risk physeal arrest if not accurately reduced
- Growth arrest after physeal injury presumed due to bony bar forming across the gap of an unreduced fracture.

Their work coincided with that of Langenskiold (1975) identifying such a 'bony bridge'.

However, there is no guarantee of uneventful healing even with type I, II fracture patterns; the cell biology and healing responses of the physis are not well understood[2].

Physeal stress injury patterns also seen; commonly in gymnasts' wrists as *epiphysiolysis*.

Growth arrest lines described by Harris (radiodense lines parallel to physis moving away with time) represent self-limiting injury in a variety of forms from which the growth plate recovers.

Growth arrest

If a discrete bony bar is identified on CT or MRI scan which can be resected, usually via a metaphyseal window, this may be worthwhile if there is significant growth remaining. Various materials, including fat and bone cement, interposed to prevent reformation.

Remember that longitudinal shortening alone is easier to correct (at skeletal maturity) than angular deformity. Thus, for peripheral physeal bar causing eccentric growth arrest and angular deformity, consider completing the epiphysiodesis if bar resection not feasible. For paired bones, e.g. forearm, lower leg, may need to arrest other bone to prevent secondary joint deformity.

Non-traumatic physeal injury

- Chemotherapy (side) effects
- Infection, especially meningococcal septicaemia
- Neurological disease
- Burns
- JIA
- Uraemia
- Endocrine disease
- Malnutrition
- Thalassaemia.

Salter–Harris classification of physeal injury

- Type I: through the physis
- Type II: through the physis with metaphyseal fracture
- Type III: epiphyseal fracture
- Type IV: epiphyseal fracture extending across the physis to the metaphysic
- Type V: crush
- Type VI: perichondral ring inury.

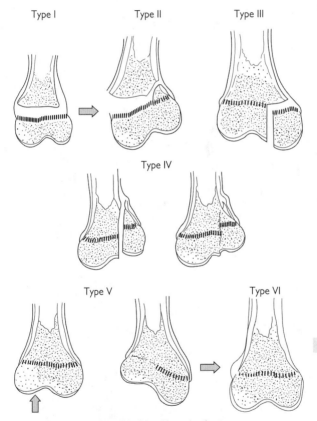

Fig. 11.1 Rangs modification of the Salter–Harris classification.

Reproduced from Bulstrode *et al.*, *Oxford Textbook of Orthopaedics and Trauma*, with permission from Oxford University Press.

References

1 Salter TB, Harris WR. Injuries involving the epiphyseal plate. *J Bone Joint Surg Am* 1963;**45**:587–622.
2 Bush PG, Hall AC, Macnicol MF. New insights into function of the growth plate—review article. *J Bone Joint Surg Br* 2008;**90**:1541–7.

Birth trauma

Injuries occurring during delivery are less common now with improved obstetric care. Nonetheless, obstetric brachial plexus palsy (OBPP) can be a cause of substantial subsequent morbidity with severe secondary shoulder dysplasia.

Birth injuries associated with

- Breech presentation
- Shoulder dystocia
- Excessive birth weight >4kg (maternal diabetes)
- Premature or very small neonates
- Osteogenesis imperfecta.

Clavicle fracture

Most common injury (~40%), usually middle third. Causes pseudoparalysis of limb but beware 5% associated brachial plexus injury. Treat expectantly and with reassurance.

Brachial plexus injuries (OBPP)

Uncommon (0.6–2.6 per 1000 live births) distraction injury primarily to upper roots typically when shoulders become stuck after head delivered. For patterns of injury see opposite. Majority recover spontaneously but those without biceps function at 3 months have a poor prognosis. Microsurgical plexus reconstruction in this group is controversial because of mixed results, must be performed early (within 6 months). Internal rotation contracture of affected shoulder the common *sequela* causing glenoid dysplasia and posterior dislocation. Options for the orthopaedic surgeon:

- Early splintage in external rotation and abduction ± botulinum toxin injections to internal rotators of shoulder
- Open or arthroscopic anterior release of shoulder capsule, subscapularis and rotator interval
- Transfer of tendons of latissimus dorsi and teres minor into rotator cuff external rotators
- Salvage derotation osteomy of proximal humerus; brings forearm away from body but does not address the prominent humeral head dislocated posteriorly.

Humeral fracture

- Usually transverse midshaft
- Shortening or angulation will usually correct spontaneously
- Transphyseal separation at elbow and proximal humerous also possible.

Femoral fracture

- Mostly midshaft and transverse
- Treat in gallows traction, hip spica or strapping of thigh to chest.

Cervical injuries

- Cord injury may occur during breech delivery
- May be a differential diagnosis for neuromuscular disorder in a 'floppy baby'.

Gilbert and Tassin classification of OBPP

- C5/6: full recovery in 90%
- C5/6 + partial C7 injury: full recovery in 50–75%
- C5/6/7 + partial C8/T1 injury: full recovery in 33%
- C5/6/7/8/T1: full recovery not possible.

Non-accidental injury

'Victoria had the most beautiful smile that lit up the room. The purpose of this Inquiry (is) to find out why this once happy, enthusiastic little girl, brought to this country to enjoy a better life, ended her days the victim of almost unimaginable cruelty.' *Laming report on the death by physical abuse of Victoria Climbie.*

Physical abuse is defined as any form of physical injury not consistent with the account of its occurrence or where there is knowledge or reasonable suspicion that the injury was inflicted, or knowingly not prevented, by a person in charge of a child. 7% of children suffer serious physical abuse by parents or carers, 6% are neglected at home because of parental absence or drug and alcohol problems[1]. In 2007 a United Nations report placed the UK bottom of 21 economically advanced countries for the well-being of its children and adolescents.

Any orthopaedic practitioner dealing with children **must** know the signs of NAI to ensure prompt recognition and protection of the child from further injury. Particular suspicion should be aroused by long bone injuries in children of prewalking age. Where doubt exists, admit the child for protection pending further investigations. Failure to recognize NAI carries a 20% risk of further injury and a 5% risk of permanent neurological damage or death.

Features in history
80% of cases in children <2yrs old.
- Delayed presentation
- Implausible or changing story of injury mechanism
- Unwitnessed injury
- Domestic disharmony or step-parental, drug, and alcohol abuse.

Examination
Be suspicious of the silent, watchful, abnormally still child
- Injuries of various ages
- Bite marks, cigarette burns, scalds, finger tip bruises
- Bruises on arm, leg or face from gripping
- Subconjuctival haemorrhage ('shaken baby').

Radiology
Skeletal survey indicated if reasonable suspicion at this stage, looking for fractures at various stages of healing and injuries highly specific for NAI:
- Posterior rib fractures
- 'Corner' and 'bucket handle' metaphyseal fractures
- Complex or wide skull fracture
- Digital injury
- Lateral clavicle fracture
- Bilateral or multiple diaphyseal fractures.

Differential diagnosis
- Osteogenesis imperfecta
- Juvenile OP
- Caffey's disease—cortical hyperostosis resembling fracture with no history of injury
- Haematological disorders—haemophilia, leukaemia.

Management
Admit for protection of child from further injury and refer to paediatric team for further evaluation and referral to appropriate services.

Manage the injury(s) as appropriate.

Reference
1 Royal College of General Practitioners. *The Role of Primary Care in the Protection of Children from Abuse and Neglect*. October 2002.

Paediatric hand injuries

The hand is the most common site of injury in children. It is central to function and seemingly trivial injuries may have serious consequences.

Soft tissue injuries

- Crush injuries often as a result of finger trapped in a door
- Finger tip or pulp amputations should be thoroughly irrigated and the amputated part applied as a 'biological dressing' if clean
- If amputation occurs proximal to the nail fold referral for replantation or reconstruction is indicated
- Nail bed avulsion or lacerations should be repaired carefully under general anaesthetic; associated distal phalanx fracture is an open injury.

Tendon and nerve injuries

- Flexor tendon injuries should be repaired and protected postoperatively; stiffness is rarely a problem
- Extensor tendon injuries are rare, but a mallet finger (which is a Salter–Harris III fracture of the distal phalanx extensor tendon insertion) should be splinted in hyperextension for 4–6 weeks
- Nerve injuries should be referred for consideration of repair.

Fractures by anatomical location

- Metacarpal and phalangeal fractures common after relatively minor trauma. Usually physeal but heal quickly and rarely cause growth disturbance.
- Distal phalanx fracture mallet finger as above; variant in older adolescents is the *Seymour* fracture, a Salter–Harris II injury of distal phalanx (physis is proximal into which extensor tendon inserts) commonly with disruption of dorsal skin. Needs washout and repair of nail fold; always suspect open injury, especially if blood is seen
- Proximal phalangeal fractures usually Salter–Harris II of base of proximal phalanx. In little finger, abduction deformity may give 'extra octave' sign. Reduce displaced fractures under block with MCPJ flexed (tightens collaterals to manipulate against), then buddy strap as for undisplaced
- Boxers' fracture (5th metacarpal) seen in adolescents; manage as for adults
- Fracture of thumb metacarpal is uncommon, may be: (i) metaphyseal and impacted (reduce closed and splint); (ii) Salter–Harris type II with medial or lateral angulation (closed reduction and cast or percutaneous pinning as required); (iii) type IV which is the paediatric equivalent of a Bennett's intra-articular fracture dislocation of the thumb base (requires anatomical reduction and stable fixation).

Paediatric wrist injuries

Distal radial fractures

The distal radius is a common site for injury but has enormous remodelling potential due to proximity of the physis. Depending on energy transfer and fracture stability, up to 25° angulation in the sagittal plane can be accepted under age 12; then up to 15° over this age and less (10°) in radial deviation.

Manage complete fractures with closed reduction if angulation unacceptable; high rate of loss of position in cast prompts consideration of K-wiring although this in itself has the potential for complications (infection, extensor tendon irritation, injury to superficial radial nerve).

Can attempt remanipulation if position lost and soft tissue outline on radiograph suggests significant deformity, but beware excessive force in vicinity of the physis.

Physeal injuries

- Most commonly Salter–Harris II fractures
- Reduce by gentle traction (finger-traps helpful) and then gentle pressure in distal and volar direction to minimize shear force across physis (reduces risk of injury and growth arrest)
- Never attempt manipulation after 5–7 days; high risk of physeal injury. Most will remodel, or do later corrective osteotomy
- Look critically for associated ulnar styloid fracture or ulnar physeal injury (high rate of ulnar physeal arrest).

Torus (buckle) fractures managed symptomatically in a plaster or splint for short period (2–3 weeks).

Greenstick fractures

- The periosteum remains intact so they reduce easily but require careful 3-point moulding in cast to prevent redisplacement.

Fractures and dislocations of the carpus

- Rare injuries in children
- The most commonly injured carpal bone is the scaphoid.
  - Scaphoid fractures are very rare before the age of 10
  - The most common site is the distal pole and this may result in AVN of the scaphoid
  - Diagnosis and treatment are as for adult scaphoid fractures.

Paediatric forearm injuries

The forearm is made up of the radius and ulna bound together by the interosseous membrane. It is possible to break either of the bones in isolation but most commonly both bones break. If only one bone appears broken, check carefully for dislocation of the other one.

Isolated fracture of the ulna

- Rare in children, results from a direct blow to ulna
- Managed non-operatively in cast.

Fracture of both bones of forearm

- Can be plastic deformation, greenstick or complete (see opposite)
- Reduce by 3-point pressure centred on apex of deformity and cast likewise above elbow to control rotation
- Residual ulna angulation influences forearm appearance; radial angulation reduces forearm rotation
- Can probably accept up to 20° angulation under age 8, no more than 10° at >10yrs
- Unstable fractures require fixation; intramedullary wires effective but may require limited open reduction to pass fracture site
- For children within 1yr of skeletal maturity, open anatomical reduction and plate fixation is preferred as remodelling potential is very limited
- No definitive evidence for or against plate removal, but risk of nerve injury higher when removing plates. Wires generally removed
- Complications include refracture (higher with diaphyseal fracture and residual angulation) so avoid immediate return to impact sport, compartment syndrome (recognize early and decompress) and nerve injury (usually neurapraxia).

Fracture–dislocations

- A **Monteggia** fracture is one of the ulna associated with radiocapitellar dislocation.
  - Results from fall on outstretched arm in forced pronation
  - Key to diagnosis is detecting the radial head dislocation (often missed). A line along the axis of the radius should bisect the capitellum (or its ossification centre) in any x-ray view
  - Beware mistaking this injury for congenital radial head dislocation (radial head small and convex and capitellum hypoplastic)
  - Check neurology, particularly posterior interosseous nerve
  - Accurate reduction of ulna key to relocate radial head. Incomplete fracture or plastic deformation managed closed; operate for complete fractures to stabilize with intramedullary wire or plate
  - Complications include redislocation of the radial head (so careful x-ray follow-up is essential until union) and compartment syndrome

- A **Galeazzi** fracture is a fracture of the distal 1/3 of the radius with a dislocation of the distal radioulnar joint. Clue to diagnosis is tenderness over lower end of the ulna
  - Mechanism probably axial load with forced rotation
  - Reverse deformity and hold in cast
  - If radius short consider plating
  - Variant with distal ulnar physeal injury easily missed and high rate of subsequent physeal arrest. Needs reduction ± wiring.

Fracture types

Plastic—forces exceed elastic limit of bone causing plastic deformation but fall short of the ultimate strength of the bone. Require prolonged 3-point pressure force to correct otherwise high rate of recurrent deformity.

Greenstick—convex cortex fails completely but concave side deforms plastically. This facilitates reduction, and rotational deformity is unlikely.

Elbow injuries in children 1

- Account for ~10% of paediatric fractures, i.e. common; supracondylar fractures especially so
- Clinical examination difficult with swollen elbow and uncooperative child; try to establish whether tender medially, laterally or both
- X-ray interpretation made difficult in young child as much of elbow is cartilaginous (anlage). Look for displacement or absence of ossification centres; requires knowledge of sequence and rough timing of appearance.

Ossification centres appear as follows: mnemonic 'CRMTOL' is helpful
- Capitellum 6 months–2yrs
- Radial head 2–4yrs
- Medial epicondyle 6–8yrs
- Trochlea 8yrs
- Olecranon 8–10yrs
- Lateral epicondyle 8–12yrs.

NB: centres appear later in boys.

Classic situation of an elbow dislocation postreduction in which the humero-ulnar joint is less than congruent, the humeral trochlear ± olecranon centres are present but the medial epicondylar centre is absent. Diagnosis is medial epicondylar avulsion with incarceration in the joint after reduction; requires open reduction and fixation.

Supracondylar fractures

- Usually a fall onto an outstretched hand
- Peak incidence in 5–8yr olds. In younger child, **transphyseal separation** can occur (consider NAI in such cases) and is harder to identify radiographically
- Check for associated forearm fracture (up to 10%); high risk of compartment syndrome with double level injury
- Neurovascular exam imperative
  - Risk of injury to brachial artery
  - Risk of nerve damage to radial nerve (especially in posteromedially displaced fractures), median nerve (anterior interosseous branch, test for by 'O' sign which requires thumb FPL flexion), ulnar nerve (vulnerable with medial placement of K wires for fixation)
- Tenderness and swelling is both medial and lateral
- A 'pucker sign' suggests the proximal fragment has pierced brachialis. This can be milked inferiorly at time of reduction or may require an open procedure. Ecchymosis at the fracture is associated with development of compartment syndrome
- Vast majority are extension injuries (98%), remainder flexion or unstable in both directions. Former implies intact posterior periosteal hinge against which to reduce. See Gartland classification on p. 565.

- Reduce by aligning fragments in coronal plane with correction of rotation and then flexing up with gentle traction. Fracture occurs through thin bone surfaces like 2 knife edges; if rotation not corrected, the blades will tilt (usually into cubitus varus: 'gunstock' deformity)
- Other feared complication is compartment syndrome as discussed; requires early diagnosis and emergent forearm fasciotomy
- Check for radial pulse at end of reduction; if lost and fails to return with elbow extension consider exploration via anterior approach with vascular or plastic surgeon.

Gartland classification of supracondylar fractures

- Type 1: undisplaced fractures—treat in above-elbow plaster or collar and cuff.
- Type 2: displaced with intact periosteal hinge—require MUA ± K wire. A line along anterior humeral cortex should pass through the capitellum for satisfactory reduction on lateral view.
- Type 3: complete displacement ('off-ended')—requires MUA + K wire or ORIF. Use a 2/3 lateral wire configuration if possible to avoid injury to/entrapment of ulnar nerve.

Lateral condylar mass fracture

- Tenderness and swelling lateral only
- Radiographs deceptive in younger child—cartilage fragment of lateral condyle separates with small sliver of metaphyseal bone. Oblique views helpful
- Fracture is intra-articular so only minimal displacement acceptable. Consider arthrogram to assess whether articular surface intact
- Displaced fractures require open reduction with visualization of joint surface, anatomical reduction and pinning or screw fixation
- Non-union rate fairly high, especially in unstable pattern (Milch classification) so watch carefully during healing for displacement.

Milch classification of lateral condylar mass fractures

- Type 1: fracture line runs lateral to trochlear groove, i.e. does not go into humero-ulnar joint.
- Type 2: fracture line medial to trochlear groove; essentially a fracture dislocation of the elbow and unstable.

Elbow injuries in children 2

Medial condylar fractures
- Rare pattern fracture
- Diagnosis and treatment similar to lateral condylar fractures.

Medial epicondylar fracture
- 3rd most common fracture around elbow in children
- Peak age 11–12yrs old; more common in boys than girls
- 50% associated elbow dislocation
- Medial epicondyle traction apophysis for medial collateral ligament (does not contribute to humeral growth)
- Generally managed non-operatively; significant displacement or associated elbow dislocation are relative indications for fixation with surgery (mandatory if incarcerated in joint postreduction).

Radial head and neck fractures
- Most involve neck of radius
- Pain on supination and pronation forearm
- If <30° angulation manage non-operatively
- If >30° require MUA ± direct K wire ('joystick') or intramedullary wire (Metazieau technique) to flip back into place
- Avoid open reduction whenever possible; stiffness inevitable. Sometimes required when radial head/neck buttonholes out through capsule.

Olecranon fractures
- Rare in children, but seen with osteogenesis imperfecta
- Check for radial head dislocation (variant of Monteggia fracture)
- Open and fix if significant displacement.

Elbow dislocation
- 90% posterior dislocations, fall onto outstretched hand
- Most will reduce closed with sedation. Then brief immobilization (2–3 weeks) and early motion
- If there is an incarcerated bony fragment (usually medial epicondyle) or unstable fracture–dislocation, then open and fix
- Complications include neurovascular injury, elbow stiffness, compartment syndrome, recurrent instability, myositis ossificans.

Pulled elbow
- Injury results from traction to arm with hand in pronation and elbow extended; often when child lifted or swung by arm
- Radial head subluxes under annular ligament
- X-rays unremarkable; diagnosis clinical
- Reduce closed by supinating forearm with thumb over radial head, followed by elbow flexion.

Paediatric shoulder and arm injuries

Humeral shaft fractures

May occur as birth injuries or in older children secondary to trauma. Obstetric humeral and elbow fractures associated with pseudoparalysis which may mimic brachial plexus palsy. A spiral fracture of the humeral shaft should always alert clinician to possibility of NAI. Transverse fractures suggest direct blow to the humerus.

The wide, multidirectional range of glenohumeral motion and the circumferential muscle coverage of the humerus allow a good deal of angular and rotational deformity to be accepted without functional or cosmetic deficit. Consequently most injuries can be managed non-operatively in a sling, a U-plaster or functional brace.

Proximal humeral fractures

- Peak incidence of physeal injury in adolescence (sports injuries) and newborns (obstetric injury and NAI)
- Displacement usually anterolateral (muscle pull against intact posteromedial periosteum)
- Metaphyseal fractures common in 5–12yr age group
- 80% of humeral growth from proximal physis so remodelling potential is excellent
- Most injuries managed by closed reduction as necessary and a sling
- In young children up to 70° of angulation may be acceptable due to huge remodelling potential; in adolescents less deformity is acceptable and open reduction occasionally indicated
- Rare complications include humerus varus, axillary nerve injury and osteonecrosis.

Clavicle fractures

- Most common fracture in children
- Clavicle is the first bone to ossify (intramembranous ossification)
- Mechanism of injury is a fall onto an outstretched hand
- 80% occur in the shaft, 15% are lateral fractures
- The lateral fragment is pulled down by the weight of the arm whilst the medial fragment is pulled up by the sternomastoid muscle
- Neurovascular and respiratory examination to exclude injury to brachial plexus, or a pneumothorax
- Normally managed in a sling until pain free (2–4 weeks)
- Open fractures (rare) may require ORIF.

Acromioclavicular joint injury

- Rare in children as CC ligaments remain intact
- Treatment as for adults.

Scapular fractures

- Rare in children
- If present usually indicate a significant injury—look for associated injury and consider NAI
- Managed non-operatively as surrounding musculature splints fragments.

Anterior shoulder dislocation

- Rare in children, becoming more common in adolescents with increasingly vigorous sports participation
- Mechanism of injury is a fall with the arm in abduction, extension and external rotation
- Examination reveals squaring of shoulder and the humeral head is palpable anteriorly
- X-ray axillary or scapular-Y view confirms anterior dislocation
- Neurovascular examination for axillary nerve injury (sensation over regimental patch and deltoid contraction postreduction)
- Treatment is closed reduction under sedation, rest in broad arm sling and then physiotherapy
- Anterior dislocations in young athletes have a high risk of recurrence; increasing interest in early (or even acute) arthroscopic anterior repair of detached glenoid labrum and bone (Bankart repair).

Posterior dislocation

- Much less common than anterior
- Mechanism of injury is a fall with shoulder adducted, flexed and internally rotated or following an epileptic seizure
- Examination reveals restricted external rotation
- On AP X-ray the humeral head may be the shape of a light bulb with head central on shaft rather than offset medially (drumstick or lollipop sign)
- Posterior dislocation is easily missed; key to diagnosis is limited external rotation of the shoulder and careful review of the X-ray. Axillary view is diagnostic and a modified view should always be possible
- Reduced with traction applied to the shoulder in 90° of abduction, followed by external rotation.

Paediatric spinal injuries

Anatomy

In children:
- Vertebral column is mobile
- Facet joints are shallow and oriented horizontally
- Spinal ligaments and joint capsules can withstand significant stretching
- Nuchal muscles are weak—increased translation during flexion and extension
- Large head to body ratio in children <8yrs shifts axis of rotation to the upper cervical spine (greatest movement is at C2/3 compared with C5/6 in adults).

Prevalence

Spinal injuries are rare in children, <1% of all fractures in children involve the spine. RTAs are the most common mechanism of injury.

Clinical

Presenting symptoms are variable, but a spinal injury must be suspected when a child has:
- Lost consciousness
- Pain related to neck or back, guarding, rigidity, torticollis, numbness, weakness or radicular symptoms
- Autonomic disturbances can occur (bladder or bowel dysfunction)
- A neurological deficit (radicular or myelopathic) or unresolved pain within 1 or 2 weeks of an injury.

The injuries sustained include fractures, dislocations and soft tissue injuries without significant bony or articular injury. The most common injury to the spine is a fracture. Facet dislocations are uncommon in children but when they occur they are usually associated with neurological sequelae. Partial spinal cord injuries are often incomplete and may improve, but children with complete spinal cord injuries normally do not recover. Progressive neurological deficits can develop if instability is not recognized. Children with spinal cord injuries are at risk of developing scoliosis.

It is important clinically to establish which patients are at risk of having a significant spinal injury, and the results of the NEXUS study are helpful.

NEXUS study

Low-risk patients must meet all five criteria:
- Absence of midline cervical tenderness
- No evidence of intoxication
- Normal level of alertness
- No focal neurological deficit and
- No painful distracting injuries.

If a patient fulfils all five of the NEXUS criteria, plain radiographs are of marginal value. In this study 1% of patients who did not meet the NEXUS criteria had a cervical spine injury. Therefore, serial assessment is important in managing children with cervical injuries.

Investigations

Differences in radiographs of children and adults
Synchondroses occur in all cervical vertebrae: there are three synchondroses at C2 that close between the ages of 3 and 7yrs. That at the dens-arch is most prominent, and is most frequently mistaken for a fracture. The distinguishing feature of the dens-arch synchondrosis from a fracture is that the synchondrosis is visible on an oblique but not on a straight lateral X-ray film. Subaxial vertebrae in young children have synchondroses between the posterior and anterior elements, and these can also be mistaken for fractures. Prominent vascular channels in the ossification centres have a similar appearance to fractures.

Pseudosubluxation: in the upper cervical spine of children is considered a normal finding. In 40% of children under 8yrs, >3mm of anterior displacement is present at C2/3 and in 14% at C3/4.

Plain radiographs
AP, lateral and odontoid views are often requested when a cervical injury is suspected. The value of an odontoid view in young children is of questionable value. Instability of the cervical spine is assessed using flexion and extension views, but should only be obtained if the child has no neurological deficit. If there is a neurological deficit an MRI scan is indicated.

CT scans
These are of limited value in children under 10yrs as most injuries in this age group are ligamentous. In children older than 10yrs, 20% of cervical injuries are ligamentous and no fracture is identified. A CT scan may be useful in planning surgery.

MRI
An MRI scan can be used to clear the cervical spine. If a child has neurological symptoms or signs and normal findings on X-ray films and a CT scan, an MRI scan may show a ligamentous or disc injury that would otherwise be missed.

Evaluating cervical stability
In a normal study there should be <3.5mm displacement of one vertebral body relative to an adjacent vertebral body and angular displacement between vertebral bodies should not exceed 11°. In children flexion and extension views are not as reliable as in adults.

Spinal cord injury without radiographic abnormality (SCIWORA)
SCIWORA is found primarily in children. A child with this injury usually has signs of a myelopathy but with no evidence of a fracture or instability on plain X-ray films or tomograms. The factors that predispose children to SCIWORA are a more tenuous spinal cord blood supply and greater elasticity in the vertebral column in relation to that of the spinal cord. Flexion or extension injuries are the most common mechanism. An MRI scan is best for evaluating patients with SCIWORA as it will show ligamentous or disc injuries, spinal cord compression, spinal cord signal changes and soft tissue or spinal cord haemorrhage.

Treatment

Most spinal injuries in children can be managed with immobilization of the injury (cervical collar, halo jacket or thoracolumbar orthosis). With advances in surgical techniques and instrumentation, internal fixation surgery has become more common. Surgical management is aimed at ensuring early stability of the vertebral column and protection of the spinal cord, facilitating early mobilization and return to normal activities. Indications for surgery include highly unstable injuries, significant deformities, progressive deformities and compression of neural element (decompression and fixation).

For further reading, see Cirak et al.[1] and Hoffman et al.[2]

References

1 Cirak B, Ziegfeld S, Knight VM, et al. Spinal injuries in children. *J Pediatr Surg* 2004;**39**:607–12.
2 Hoffman JR, Schriger DL, Mower W, et al. Low-risk criteria for cervical spine radiography in blunt trauma: a prospective study. *Ann Emerg Med* 1992;**21**:1454–60.

Paediatric pelvic injuries

Paediatric pelvic fractures are uncommon. In young children, the pelvis is predominantly cartilage whose elasticity implies greater trauma if fracture has occurred. Look first, therefore, for other serious and potentially life-threatening injuries (head, chest, abdomen and genitourinary; see opposite). In fact the majority of pelvic fractures will be managed non-operatively with a good prognosis; in the acute setting it is the associated injuries which are more important.

Other differences to adults are that children are more likely to injure intra-abdominal organs, single breaks in the pelvic ring can occur and avulsion injuries (of vulnerable apophyseal cartilage plates) are common.

Fracture types

- **Avulsion:** of attached powerful muscle insertions: ischium (hamstring origin), ASIS (sartorius and iliotibial band), AIIS (rectus femoris), iliac crest (hip abductors). Common in sporting adolescents. Treat with rest and crutches only
- **Iliac wing or blade:** common pedestrian vs car injury. Adult problem of non-union not seen in children, fixation not required
- **Pubis or ischium:** if pelvic ring not involved then stable and heal with bedrest and mobilization as comfortable, but infers high energy transfer so again look first for and manage other serious injuries
- **Sacrum:** may be associated with anterior pelvic fractures. SIJ injuries are rare in isolation
- **Pubic symphysis:** separation has differing normal limits according to age; stress views in lateral compression may be helpful
- **Double breaks**
  - **Straddle** (vertical pubic rami fractures): worst prognosis due to associated injuries
  - **Malgaigne** (anterior and posterior pelvic ring injuries) may require fixation for severe displacement or external stabilization in older children with haemorrhage
  - **Multiple crushing** injuries to pelvis (usually fatal).

Further imaging

- CT
  - If doubt about diagnosis on plain X-ray
  - If operative intervention is planned
- MRI
  - Better delineation of soft tissue injuries
  - Absence of ionizing radiation.

Complications

- Injury of triradiate cartilage leading to premature closure and risk of subsequent acetabular dysplasia
- Heterotopic bone formation, especially where open reduction required
- Osteonecrosis if associated femoral head/neck fracture
- Sciatic nerve palsy
- Leg length discrepancy.

Signs of pelvic fracture
Described by Milch
- Destot sign
  - Superficial haematoma beneath inguinal ligament or in the scrotum
- Roux sign
  - Decreased distance from the greater trochanter to the pubic spine on the affected side in lateral compression fractures
- Earle sign
  - Bony prominence or large haematoma and tenderness on rectal examination.

Associated injuries
- Skull, cervical, facial and long bone fractures
- Diaphragmatic rupture
- Blunt chest trauma
- Splenic/liver laceration
- Damage to major blood vessels
- Retroperitoneal bleeding
- Rectal tears
- Rupture or laceration of urethra/bladder.

For further reading, see Holden et al.[1] and Beaty and Kaiser[2].

References
1 Holden C, Holman J, Herman MJ. Paediatric pelvic fractures. *J Am Acad Orthop Surg* 2007;**15**:172–7.
2 Beaty JH, Kaisser JR. *Rockwood & Wilkins' Fractures in Children*, 6th edn. Baltimore, MD: Lippincott Williams & Wilkins, 2006.

Hip fractures in children

Uncommon, but almost always associated with high energy trauma (or pathological fracture through bone cyst).

Tenuous blood supply predisposes to AVN, rate determined by type and degree of initial displacement. Physis contributes 0.3–0.4cm length per year.

The classification of Delbet is useful:
- Type I: fracture–separation of the epiphysis
- Type II: transcervical fracture of femoral neck (most common)
- Type III: basal (cervico-trochanteric) fracture
- Type IV: intertrochanteric fracture.

Type I has a strong association with hip dislocation, Type II is the most common. pattern. Type IV has the best prognosis. Hip dislocation associated also with temporal head frature, classified by pipkin.

History
Ask about mechanism of injury, speed of impact if RTA, and other injuries. Antecedent hip symptoms if pathological fracture suspected.

Examination
Examine affected limb for deformity, pain on movement.

Look for associated injuries and assess neurovascular status of limb.

Investigations
Plain films will usually make the diagnosis; USS or MRI may be indicated for occult fracture.

Treatment
- Emergent if displaced or associated dislocation
- Closed reduction and pinning or hip screw/plate if anatomic, otherwise require open reduction. Operating table set-up must allow conversion to an open procedure if necessary. The capital femoral physis may need to be crossed to achieve stable fixation
- For dislocation, if gentle attempt at closed reduction unsuccessful then open from direction of dislocation
- Children <2yrs of age, reasonable to treat with closed reduction and hip spica.

Complications
- AVN of femoral head (20–50%, displaced type I and II common)—may take 2–3yrs to develop after fracture
- Coxa vara—observe initially as many correct
- Non-union—can treat this and coxa vara with subtrochanteric valgus osteotomy
- Physeal arrest causing limb length discrepancy.

Femoral injuries in children

Shaft fractures

- Common injuries, beware NAI in children below walking age. In older children, associated with high energy transfer and likely additional injuries
- Treatment depends on age and socioeconomic factors—prolonged periods in a hip spica in older child will be poorly tolerated, not least by a working parent(s).

Birth–1yr

Immediate hip spica or Pavlik harness. Gallows traction (skin traction to overhead beam) can be used up to 2yrs—but is falling out of favour as definitive treatment.

Up to age 5–6yrs

Immediate reduction and hip spica application under general anaesthetic. Beware applying traction through the leg portion of the cast (so-called 90°–90° method); associated with skin breakdown in popliteal fossa and compartment syndrome. Better to achieve reduction with appropriate moulding in one-leg above-knee spica and then complete to 1 1/2 spica. Position hip/knee in 45° flexion so child can sit.

Acceptable results have been reported in this age group with flexible nailing, but usually unnecessary (may be indicated in rare situation of poly-trauma).

6yrs to skeletal maturity

Flexible IM nails inserted retrograde and advanced to the fracture site prior to reduction the mainstay of treatment. May require supplementary support in older children in whom complication rate is higher. Some prefer trochanteric entry rigid locked nails in older children, but there remains a risk of femoral head AVN from arterial damage in the piriformis fossa prior to closure of the proximal femoral physes. Risk is very low, but the complication is essentially untreatable—delayed or malunion on the other hand is treatable.

Very proximal or distal fractures, long spiral or severely fragmented—reduction harder to obtain and hold with flexible nails. Options are an external fixator, with disadvantages of long time in frame, knee stiffness and risk of refracture (stress shielding in frame, pin holes), or plating; associated with extensive exposures and blood loss, but can ameliorate using a long plate/indirect reduction technique with fewer screws in a 'near–far' percutaneous construct[1]. This is also an option for older, heavier children.

Complications

- Leg length discrepancy; often overgrowth. Poorly understood, may be increased vascularity at physis, but need to follow for this. Between 1 and 10yrs expect 0.9cm overgrowth (range 0.4–2.5); can allow fracture to shorten this amount in closed treatment

- Angular deformity and rotational malunion: various guidelines for acceptable limits. Can accept up to 30–40° varus/valgus or pro/recurvatum and the same rotation up to 2yrs with expectation of remodelling, but becomes less effective with increasing age. 2–10yrs allow up to 15 and 30° angulation and rotation, respectively.

Distal femoral physeal injuries

The distal femoral physis undulates, so traumatic separation associated with significant energy transfer (cartwheel injury the historical name; may resemble knee dislocation on presentation). The body's largest and fastest growing physis so even Salter–Harris I/II injuries not benign (angular deformity common after type II); magnitude of displacement predicts risk of growth disturbance.

Require careful neurovascular examination. Oblique views may be helpful if minimally displaced.

Treat type I/II with closed reduction and pins or screws. Type III/IV requires anatomical restoration of articular surface and physis (may necessitate open reduction).

Follow for angular deformity or limb length discrepancy 2° to partial or complete physeal arrest.

Reference

1 Rozbruch S, Muller U, Gautier G, et al. The evolution of femoral shaft plating technique. *Clin Orthop Rel Res* 1998;**354**:195–208.

Knee injuries in children[1]

Fracture of the tibial intercondylar eminence

- Adolescent version of a cruciate ligament tear, most common age group 8–13yrs
- Can follow hyperextension injury, fall from bike or direct blow
- Child typically has pain and large effusion with inability to weight-bear
- X-ray will show fragment in centre of knee, CT aids assessment of displacement
- If undisplaced or fragment reduces in extension, treat in long leg cast in 10–15° flexion for 4–6 weeks
- Irreducible fragments may have flipped over a meniscal edge; need reduction and fixation at arthrotomy or with arthroscopic-assisted technique. Can use countersunk minifragment or headless cannulated screws or a tension band suture technique. Avoid multiple passes through the physis, or all together if possible.

Tibial tubercle fractures

The tibial tubercle is part of the proximal tibial physis (a traction apophysis). Osgood–Schlatter disease is recurrent superficial microfractures of this region.

Injuries common in adolescents: jumping or rapid quadriceps contraction with a flexed knee. Cause local pain, swelling and difficulty with active knee extension.

Injury may be through the apophyseal secondary centre of ossification (type I), between this and the metaphysis (II) or intra-articular (III) according to Ogden classification. Fix displaced type I and type II/III after closed or open reduction with screws and washers.

There is a risk of genu recurvatum if anterior growth arrest follows.

Patella injuries

- Fracture uncommon as high ratio of cartilage to bone in children
- Beware *sleeve fracture*; radiograph shows a small distal bony fragment only, which carries with it a large portion of the cartilaginous articular surface
- Reduce and fix if >3mm separation of fragments; suture ± drill holes, tension band wiring are options
- Dislocation common, especially in girls with increased Q angle (ASIS to centre patella, thence to tibial tubercle). Most spontaneously reduce but up to 60% will recur. Present with tense effusion and diffusely painful patella. Get plain films in search of associated osteochondral fragment; if large and displaced will require reduction and fixation (cannulated minifragment or headless screw) at arthrotomy. MRI may be indicated to demonstrate true size of fragment.

Knee soft tissue injuries

Meniscal injuries rare prepuberty, except with discoid lateral meniscus (3–5% of population).

Ligamentous injuries may be increasing in children; treatment controversial but ACL reconstruction probably best deferred until close to maturity as modern intra-articular techniques may cause premature physeal arrest.

Proximal tibial epiphyseal fractures

Uncommon injuries but beware associated risk of popliteal artery damage (vessel closely apposed in the popliteal fossa and tethered by the anterior tibial branch passing anteriorly above the interosseous membrane). Salter–Harris I/II injuries can usually be reduced closed and treated in cast; III/IV require closed reduction and fixation with pins or screws, but open exploration required if vascular compromise.

Reference

1 Flynn JM, Scaggs D, Sponseller PD, *et al.* The operative management of pediatric fractures of the lower extremity. *J Bone Joint Surg Am* 2002;**84**:2288–300.

Leg injuries in children[1]

Tibial shaft fracture

- Among the most common lower extremity injuries in children
- Mostly treated closed with casting
- Can accept up to 10° deformity in coronal and sagittal planes but no malrotation
- Tendency of distal fractures to recurvatum can be treated by casting with ankle in equinus for 4 weeks—persistent stiffness unusual in children unless associated soft tissue injury.

Indications for surgical treatment

- Soft tissue injury: open fracture, compartment syndrome
- Polytrauma (including head injury)
- Floating knee
- Failure to maintain adequate closed reduction.

Options

- IM flexible nailing—antegrade balanced nails, entry point posterior to apophysis to prevent recurvatum 2° to anterior epiphysiodesis. Technically harder than for femur and requires supplementary cast or brace
- External fixator—severe or open soft tissue injury the main indication. Application is simple and quick, problem of long time (in frame) to union with stress shielding and risk of refracture after frame removal
- Plating.

Proximal tibial metaphyseal fracture

- Commonly occurs aged 2–8yrs
- May require open reduction if soft tissue interposition
- May heal in valgus which can remodel (cosen's fracture)—if not consider corrective osteotomy or timed proximal hemiepiphysiodesis.

Reference

1 Flynn JM, Scaggs D, Sponseller PD, et al. The operative management of pediatric fractures of the lower extremity. J Bone Joint Surg Am 2002;**84**:2288–300.

Ankle injuries in children

The Salter–Harris classification is the most widely used descriptive system for these injuries. The adult Lauge–Hansen classification modified for children is based on mechanism of injury but, like its adult counterpart, is difficult to commit to memory.

Beware the juvenile Tillaux and triplane fracture variants of adolescence; anatomical reduction of the physis is generally less important at the age at which these fractures occur, but the joint surface must be reduced to within 2mm (axial or 'step') displacement. Modern digital imaging software can be used to assess this on CT scans.

Implanted subchondral metalwork should be removed after fracture healing to prevent increased local stress on the overlying cartilage, which may predispose to OA.

Distal tibial fractures

- Salter–Harris I and II: closed reduction and casting if displaced, allow weight bearing after 3–4 weeks. Occasionally need reduction and pinning if unstable
- Salter–Harris III and IV: truly undisplaced fractures can be treated as above, but require weekly follow-up with radiographs to check for displacement. Displaced fractures require closed reduction and cannulated screw fixation, occasionally may need to reduce open.

Eccentric physeal injuries should be followed for partial growth arrest causing angular deformity.

Juvenile Tillaux and triplane injuries

The distal tibial physis closes around a central 'bump', beginning in an anteromedial direction. The posterior and lateral portions of the physis are the last to fuse. As adolescents approach skeletal maturity, physeal injuries occur around this 'bump', separating off an anterolateral fragment (of Tillaux) and sometimes a posterior (coronal) spike. The combination of the two is called triplane because the fracture plane is sagittal in the epiphysis, axial in the physis and coronal in the metaphysis. There are many variants of the triplane fracture pattern and so CT is indicated to assess displacement and plan (cannulated) screw fixation. Key is to visualize and reduce the joint surface (Tillaux fragment), but the posterior spike will need to be adequately reduced to facilitate this (may require a small posterior incision to facilitate).

Distal fibular fractures

The usual injury is a Salter–Harris I fracture; a diagnosis of suspicion unless there is a small metaphyseal fragment indicating a type II injury. Treatment in a walking cast until symptoms subside is reasonable.

Foot injuries in children

Serious foot injuries are fairly uncommon in children, with the exception of mechanical lawnmower injuries which can mandate amputation.

Fractures of the talus

Undisplaced require only a non-weight-bearing cast until union (usually 6–8 weeks). Displaced neck fractures should be treated surgically; reduced closed if possible, stabilized with percutaneous screws. AVN is the most common complication of these fractures, usually present within 6 months. Fractures of talar body and head are very rare.

Fractures of the os calcis

Usually from a fall. Non-displaced and extra-articular fractures treated in cast. Occasionally ORIF or percutaneous pin fixation required for significant displacement.

Tarso-metatarsal injuries

Excessive foot swelling, ecchymosis and inability to bear weight are clues to the diagnosis of an injured Lisfranc (tarso-metatarsal joint). Order AP, lateral and oblique (medial border of 4th metatarsal should line up with that of cuboid) weight-bearing plain radiographs, but may need CT to diagnose. A fracture of the cuboid may be associated. Critical for displaced injuries is to reduce the 2nd metatarsal base into its recessed position relative to those either side (usually held there by Lisfranc's ligament to medial cuneiform) and fix there to maintain the coronal arch of the foot. There is negligible movement here but arch restoration is critical for foot shape.

Metatarsal fractures

Relatively common injuries. Mostly treated with a walking cast, even moderate displacement remodels well. 5th metatarsal base fractures can be difficult to diagnose because of the apophysis and sesamoids present at this level.

Phalangeal fractures

Treated by neighbour strapping; likewise dislocations of MTPJs and IPJs after closed reduction.

Puncture wounds

Puncture wounds from, for example, treading on nails should be irrigated well and, if cellulitic, treated with antibiotics. *Pseudomonas* ('trainer sole' contaminant) should be covered. Consider surgical exploration only for puncture wounds that do not settle after 2–3 days.

Lawnmower injuries

Typically occur when a child is playing too close to a lawnmower on a wet, sloping surface. Usually severe soft tissue and bone destruction, or even traumatic amputation, with highly contaminated wounds. Require cephalosporin and aminoglycoside antibiotic cover ± penicillin for agricultural dirt. Multiple debridements (vacuum dressings useful in between) and plastics coverage usually required, may need to counsel parents and child for amputation.

Rehabilitation

Chapter 12

Rehabilitation

Physical therapy

Physiotherapy is a healthcare profession concerned with human function and movement. It uses physical approaches to promote, maintain and restore function and maximize an individual's potential[1].

Modern physical therapy uses a wide range of diagnostic and treatment modalities:

- Active exercises to mobilize joints, strengthen muscles and improve motion
- Hydrotherapy allows either assistance (buoyancy reduces effect of gravity) or resistance to motion. Indications include joint stiffness, musculoskeletal strains, arthritis and strengthening in neuromuscular conditions
- Passive joint movement to maintain movement otherwise inhibited by pain or paralysis and prevent contracture
- Neuromuscular electrical stimulation (NEMS) may be useful while a patient is recovering after nerve injury to maintain muscle power or increase contractile strength in certain neuromuscular conditions (muscle re-education)
- US therapy; heats deep tissues by high frequency sound waves; may provide beneficial effects through other mechanical or chemical means
- Interferential stimulation (IFC). Used for pain relief, increased circulation and muscle stimulation (applies two medium frequency currents simultaneously; waveforms superimposed which causes an interference 'beat')
- Acupuncture may be practised by physiotherapists
- TENS used for pain control and promotion of healing: sensory TENS (high rate) for acute phase or postoperative pain, motor TENS (low rate) for subacute pain or trigger points
- Cryotherapy used to reduce pain and swelling by superficial vasoconstriction. Cold also decreases nerve conduction velocity.

Specialist roles

Hand therapy: an integral part of any hand service to coordinate and direct rehabilitation and splinting after injury or operation.

Back pain rehabilitation (non-operative): a proven effective form of management for certain types of chronic back pain. Specialist physiotherapists directing these programmes may also have a role as independent practitioners triaging spine outpatient referrals.

Specialty trained physiotherapists: may offer non-operative treatment modalities such as intra-articular injection, manipulation in appropriate clinics, e.g. shoulder. Also extended roles in management of children's conditions, e.g. DDH (Pavlik harness application and supervision), club-foot (serial casting according to the method of Ponseti).

Reference

1 Atkinson K, Coutts F, Hassenkamp A-M. *Physiotherapy in Orthopaedics*, 2nd edn. London: Elsevier Churchill Livingstone, 2005.

Orthotics and prosthetics

Orthosis

An externally applied device used to control the motion of a body segment to:
- compensate for muscle weakness
- control an unstable joint
- reduce a dynamic deformity to its fixed component.

Named with respect to anatomy, e.g. ankle–foot orthosis (AFO), knee–ankle–foot orthosis (KAFO), or to function, e.g. hip abduction spinal orthosis (HASO). Less commonly named after people or places. e.g. Boston brace, a thoracolumbar spinal orthosis.

Leaf spring AFO—allows dorsiflexion in stance, prevents foot drop in swing.

Hinged AFO—as leaf spring but better ankle varus/valgus control.

Ground reaction AFO (GRAFO)—used for 'crouch gait' (weak plantar-flexors); block excess ankle dorsiflexion in stance so ground reaction force moves in front of knee and passively extends it.

Prosthesis

A device that replaces a missing limb or body segment.

A prosthetist, as part of your multidisciplinary team, will assess:
- Premorbid function (vocational and recreational)
- Cognitive state
- Expected function postoperatively.

Preferred levels of amputation for prosthetic fitting (always discuss with prosthetist where possible) are 1 inch per foot of height below the knee joint (below-knee amputation) and 15cm above the medial joint line (above-knee). Following amputation, a preparatory prosthesis may be fitted; the definitive one requires a well-healed, stable stump.

Prosthetic elements

- Socket with a means of suspension
- Shank (body) ± an articulation
- Terminal device, e.g. SACH (solid ankle cushioned heel), dynamic response (better force absorption)

Indications for amputation and prosthesis (PATTIN)

- **P**eripheral vascular disease
- **A**nomaly (congenital)
- **T**rauma
- **T**umour
- **I**nfection
- **N**erve injury.

For further reading, see Colbum and Ibbotson[1] and Bodeau[2].

References

1 Colbum J, Ibbotson V. Amputation. In: Turner A, Foster M, Johnson S, eds. *Occupational Therapy and Physical Dysfunction: Principles, Skills & Practice*, 4th edn. London: Churchill-Livingstone, 1997.
2 Bodeau VS. Lower limb prosthetics. eMedicine article (2002), www.emedicine.com.

Walking aids

Provide an extension of the upper extremities to help transmit body weight and provide support for a patient. Patients need upper limb strength, coordination and proper hand function. Indications are to:
- Improve balance
- Redistribute forces across or unload a weight-bearing limb
- Provide tactile feedback in patients lacking proprioception.

Canes

- Consists of handle, shaft, end piece and ferrule (rubber bit on the end)
- Can be wood or aluminium: latter lighter and height-adjustable
- Types include:
  - Single point or C-cane: basic cane with single point at base
  - Functional grip cane: better grip and more comfortable than C-cane to hold
  - Quad cane: has 4 legs at base. Provides additional support but may slow patient down
- Size cane from tip to level of greater trochanter with patient upright. (elbow should be flexed ~20°)
- Hold on the **opposite** side to the affected hip (reduces joint reaction force in contralateral hip) and same side for affected knee.

Crutches

Better stability than cane as there are two points of contact with body.

With crutch placed 3 inches lateral to the foot, the hand piece height should produce 30° elbow flexion with wrist in maximal extension and fingers in a fist.
- Often used bilaterally
- Made of aluminium, height adjustable
- Transfer 40–50% of patient's body weight (non-axillary; axillary crutches transfer more but can cause nerve palsies due to pressure)
- Hands are free to perform tasks.

Crutch gaits
- *Four-point*
  - Left crutch, right foot, right crutch, left foot
  - Always 3 points of contact with ground
  - Used for ataxic gaits
- *Three-point* (non-weight bearing)
  - Both crutches down with weaker limb, followed by stronger, unaffected limb
  - Used for lower limb fractures/amputations
- *Two-point*
  - Left crutch and right foot, then right crutch and left foot
  - Faster than four-point gait
  - Reduced weight bearing in both legs
  - Used for bilateral weakness or ataxia
- *Swing-through gait*—for patients with good upper limb and abdominal muscle strength.

Frames and walkers
- Provide maximum support
- Slower for patient
- May encourage bad posture
- Limited use outside home.

Standard pick-up walker
Requires upper extremity strength to pick up walker and place forward.

Rolling walker (wheeled)
For patients with poor coordination and upper body strength, e.g. Kaye walker for CP child.

Others: forearm support walkers (for patients with forearm deformities) and stair-climbing walkers.

Aids to daily living

Many patients require additional help on discharge from hospital with activities of daily living: mobility, self-care, communication and ability to use environmental hardware. Assessment is undertaken by occupational therapists and physiotherapists, who may prescribe a number of assistive devices.

Problems and solutions

Mobility—see preceding section.

Self-care: dressing, feeding, toileting, bathing and grooming

Problems faced by orthopaedic patients include:

- Limited hand movement and loss of fine motor control
  - Eating: built-up utensils, universal cuff with utensil hold
  - Dressing: button hook, zipper hook, velcro closure, sock aid, long shoe horn, elastic shoelaces
  - Bathing: long handled sponges, wash mitts
  - Grooming: built-up combs and brushes, electric toothbrush, electric razors with customized handles
- Loss of function in one hand
  - Plate guards and rocker knife to aid eating
- Impaired coordination and tremor
  - Weighted utensils to provide accuracy of movements
- Impaired range of motion of shoulder/proximal weakness
  - Reachers to open cupboards and pick up objects
- Impaired mobility for toileting
  - Raises for toilet seat, bars around toilet, commodes
- Impaired mobility for bathing
  - Tub transfer benches, hand-held showers, grab rails on bath/shower, shower chairs.

Communication

- Difficulty holding pens: built-up pens
- Difficulty typing: typing stick
- Impaired vision to read: large print book/magnifying glasses, talking clocks/watches
- Difficulty using telephone: push-button dialling, voice-activated/speaker phones
- Difficulty calling for help: buzzers requiring minimal pressure, community alarm connected to local emergency services.

Environmental hardware

Keys, light switches, doors and windows can also be modified for ease of use.

Occupational therapy referral necessary

- Dressing aids
- Toileting/bathing aids
- Home adaptations (grab rails, ramp access, stair rail, etc.); require a home assessment by an occupational therapist, should be discussed with them
- Feeding aids
- Wheelchairs.

Physiotherapy referral necessary

- Walking aids (sticks, crutches, walking frames); physiotherapist assessment required to prescribe appropriate equipment. Proper instruction important; not uncommon for various items to be used incorrectly and therefore inefficiently.

Specialist services required

- Prosthetic limbs—specialist field, needs suitable assessment and multidisciplinary approach to prescribe and train in the most appropriate prosthesis. Regional services exist and should be consulted early; when amputation being considered, advice from rehabilitation consultant is essential from the outset.
- Orthotics—referrals can be made for specially adapted footwear (e.g. shoe raises in leg length discrepancy and custom-made shoes). Seek advice from the orthotist in each situation if necessary.
- For further reading, see Foti et al.[1]

Reference

1 Foti D, Williams Pedretti L, Lihle SM. Activities of daily living. In Williams Pedretti L, Early MB, eds. *Occupational Therapy: Practice Skills for Physical Dysfunction*, 4th edn. St Louis, MO: Mosby Year Book, 1996:463–506.

Long-term management of head injury

Head injury has a major impact on the patient, their family and society as a whole. Careful assessment, setting achievable goals and the involvement of a multidisciplinary team will aid the ultimate goal of community reintegration, but this may take many years. The goals of neurorehabilitation are to prevent and minimize complications and to maximize recovery and function.

Issues in neurorehabilitation and some solutions

Medical problems

- Nutrition
  - Build up to full oral intake once gag reflex and swallowing has been assessed to be present and safe
  - Involve dieticians to ensure adequate calorific intake
  - Patient's ability for oral intake may be compromised and/or unsafe. Enteral feeding via nasogastric tube or percutaneous gastrostomy/jejunostomy may be preferable
- Neuroendocrine complications
  - Reduced antidiuretic hormone (ADH) secretion (from posterior pituitary) causing diabetes insipidus; severe water loss and hypernatraemia. May require synthetic vasopressin (DDAVP)
  - Conversely, may be increased secretion of ADH; syndrome of inappropriate ADH secretion (SIADH) causing hyponatraemia
  - Cerebral salt wasting syndrome; loss of both sodium and water in the urine, with loss of circulating volume and hyponatraemia
  - Sodium imbalances may affect conscious level and may precipitate seizures
- Seizures secondary to underlying brain injury
  - Treated with long-term carbamazepine or sodium valproate. Benzodiazepines and phenytoin are reserved for acute treatment of seizures or status epilepticus
- Pulmonary complications
  - Increased risk of pneumonia secondary to immobility, inability to clear secretions and aspiration due to impaired gag reflex
  - Chest physiotherapy invaluable in rehabilitation
  - Tracheostomies for long-term ventilation prior to rehabilitation; consult intensive care/outreach team before any decision to wean
- Bowel and bladder function
  - Depending on severity of brain injury, may be loss of voluntary control which should be assessed by continence nurse and appropriate specialists
- Musculoskeletal injuries
  - Fix long bone fractures early where possible to facilitate care and rehabilitation. Consider prophylaxis for heterotopic ossification (oral indomethacin). Regular and early physiotherapy to prevent joint contracture. Antispasmodics such as baclofen may be required for spasticity.

Cognitive and behavioural problems
- Cognitive state may be assessed using tools such as the Wechsler Adult Intelligence Scales, incorporates: memory and learning, attention, verbal and perceptual abilities, reasoning and organizational ability
- Mood
  - Patients and families prone to depression
- Behavioural problems
  - Personality changes, aggressive behaviour and anxiety
  - Family distress: address this to optimize rehabilitation following discharge of patient into community
- Deterioration in sexual relationships
  - Should be discussed and referred as appropriate.

Social problems
Occupational therapists will assess level of function and needs of patient:
- Assessment of level of disability using scales such as the Barthel Index or Disability Rating Scale
- Assessment of ability to perform ADL and provide aids if required
- Prevocational assessment and training
- Gentle reintroduction into household activities
- Supported work programmes
- Community reintegration: there may be a need for transitional living arrangements prior to reintegration.

For further reading, see Rose and Johnson[1].

Reference
1 Rose FD, Johnson DA, eds. *Brain Injury and After: Towards Improved Outcome*. Chichester: John Wiley & Sons, 1996.

Community services

Intermediate care

Recommended for patients requiring further therapeutic intervention out of the acute setting. Facilitates short-term focused rehabilitation therapy in medically stable patients with appropriate healthcare professionals: occupational therapy, physiotherapy, speech and language therapy. Decision to refer based on multidisciplinary assessment:

• Domiciliary (home-based)—patient safe to return home but needs further therapy
• Inpatient—usually based in nursing or residential homes according to a goal-focused rehabilitation programme
• Community hospital; referrals generated by ward team while in acute hospital or by GP in primary care. Patient remains under care of own GP who has local 'admission rights'. Places cannot be provisionally booked, a postoperative assessment is required.

Social services care packages

Local social worker or care manager organizes appropriate package of care based on multidisciplinary assessment ± individual case conference to address particular needs, e.g. washing, dressing, feeding (healthcare assistant).

Other community services

Red Cross

• Medical equipment loans not covered by NHS, e.g. wheelchairs for outdoor use.

Age concern

• Arrange delivery of shopping
• Carer support
• Telephone support for isolated or vulnerable individuals.

Home from hospital schemes

• Support visits after discharge from hospital.

Disability services

The Disability Discrimination Act defines a disabled person as someone with 'a physical or mental impairment which has a substantial and long-term adverse effect on his ability to carry out normal day-to-day activities'. Handicap is a disadvantage, resulting from an impairment or disability, that interferes with a person's efforts to fulfil a role that is normal for that person. In essence, handicap is a social concept representing the environmental consequences of impairment or disability.

Provision of services to maximize independent function of those with disabilities is central to the modern welfare system, but many services are still provided by non-governmental or charitable agencies. There are also commercially run 'Resource Centres' in most major towns and cities.

Identifying services

- For most doctors the most useful first point of contact is the occupational therapy service in the locality
- The internet is also very helpful
  - www.direct.gov.uk/disabledpeople gives excellent general information and provides the option to search for local providers of services
  - The local government website should yield the telephone number, and possibly name, of the disability services department/officer and links to services
  - Support groups are also very helpful, e.g. MS Society, STEPS for children with congenital clubfoot and other conditions.

Disabled access

Access to services, employment and recreation is enshrined in law. The Disability Discrimination Act of 1995 protects disabled people in education, employment, property matters, access (to goods, facilities and services) and lays out minimum standards for public transport. It has been implemented in stages over 10yrs.

Common services include provision of mobility aids, dial-a-ride, shopmobility, care at home, meals on wheels, etc.

Appendices

Drugs used to treat arthritis

Inflammatory joint disease is a complex disease to treat. Aggressive suppression of the immune system aimed at treating the cause exposes the patient to side effects, opportunistic infection and potential oncogenesis. Simply relieving the symptoms with analgesia and anti-inflammatory drugs is not disease modifying, and therefore results in joint damage and disability. A balance in risk must be struck, taking into account the potential destructiveness of the disease (natural history), patient's age, functionality and the toxicity of the drugs. Knowing the natural history of the disease and using biomarkers such as anti-CCP antibody and CRP, combination therapies may be deemed the most effective therapeutic option. The early use of DMARDs, including the biologic agents, gives the best chance for complete disease control.

Below is a table classifying the various treatment options available.

A1. Drugs which control symptoms

Class of drug	Examples
Analgesics	Paracetamol
	Paracetamol/codeine combinations, e.g. co-codamol
	Dihydrocodeine
	Opiates, e.g. tramadol, buprenorphine, nefopam and morphine
NSAIDs	Aspirin
	Diclofenac
	Ibuprofen
	Piroxicam
	Naproxen
COX-2-specific NSAIDs ('coxibs')	Celecoxib
	Etoricoxib

A2. Disease-modifying drugs (DMARDs)

Type of arthritis	Drugs	
Rheumatoid arthritis	Biologics	Gold
Psoriatic arthritis	Anti-TNF drugs	Hydroxychloroquine
Spondyloarthropathy	Adalimumab	Leflunomide
Connective tissue diseases	Etanercept	Methotrexate
	Infliximab	Azathioprine
	Anti-IL-6	Ciclosporin
	Tocilizumab	Sulfasalazine
	B-cell therapy	
	Rituximab	
	Anti-IL-1	
	Anakinra	
Acute crystal arthritis (treatment for acute attack of gout and pseudogout)	Colchicine	
	Corticosteroids	
Gout (prevention of further attacks)	NSAIDs	
	Reduce uric acid production	
	Allopurinol	
	Febuxostat	
	Uricosuric	
	Sulfinpyrazone	
	Benzbromarone	

Symptom-controlling drugs

NSAIDs

NSAIDs relieve pain and stiffness by reducing inflammation; however, they do not influence the progression of inflammatory joint disease. Cyclo-oxygenase-2 (COX-2)-specific NSAIDs ('coxibs') have a similar mechanism of action, but their specificity results in fewer gastric side effects. NSAIDs are flexible regarding their administration. 'Slow-release' NSAIDs can be taken once a day. NSAIDs can be applied topically to the joint as a cream or gel for local pain relief. There is debate regarding the efficacy of this route of administration.

Disease-modifying drugs

Gold

Although its mechanism of action remains unknown, intramuscular injections of gold (sodium aurothiomalate) have been proven to be effective in reducing inflammation, pain, swelling and stiffness. Trials have shown a 30% decrease in swollen joints compared with treatment with a placebo. Gold is, however, no longer used as first-line therapy as it has a 50% chance of side effects within the first 2yrs of prescription. Anecdotal evidence suggests that it works best in RhF-positive disease or palindromic-onset rheumatoid disease.

Hydroxychloroquine

This antimalarial treatment has been exploited in the treatment of RA due to its capacity to interfere with antigen processing. Antigens are not displayed in the major histocompatibility complex (MHC) to the same degree, and antigenic recognition by CD4+ T cells cannot occur. This leads to fewer autoantibodies, damping down the destructive effects of arthritis on the joints. This drug is a weak antirheumatoid drug when used alone; however, in combination, it is considered safe and effective. Patients are generally started on a higher dose (e.g. 400mg/day) which is gradually reduced so patients with well controlled disease may take 200mg 2–3 times a week. It is thought to be effective in the connective tissue diseases for controlling rash, especially photosensitivity and non-erosive joint disease.

Leflunomide

The proposed mechanism of action for this designer immunomodulatory agent involves it inactivating rUMP (ribonucleotide uridine monophosphate), a pyrimidine which is integral in cell cycle progression. Therefore, autoimmune lymphocytes cannot mature. Leflunomide is taken daily as a tablet, as 10 or 20mg dose. The onset of action is slightly delayed; patients may wait 4–6 weeks before they feel the effects. The main side effect is diarrhoea which occurs in 17% of cases. Hypertension may also occur in 8–9%. Leflunomide is often used in combination with hydroxychloroquine and/or methotrexate. It has been shown to be useful as a DMARD in spondyloarthropathy and psoriatic arthritis.

Methotrexate

Methotrexate is currently the first-line disease-modifying treatment for RA and it is the most commonly used DMARD in the western world. It is involved in apoptosis and may also promote Th2 (T-helper 2) dominance through the expression of certain cytokines which lead to the immune imbalance. However, its main function is disrupting the activation of folate which thereby prevents DNA replication. It inhibits the enzyme dihydofolate reductase. Its effects on the immune system act to reduce inflammation. It is administered once a week as an injection or in tablet or syrup form. The main side effects include mild liver dysfunction, minor GI upset, a 3–5% incidence of idiosyncratic allergic alveolitis and bone marrow suppression. The side effects are, however, far less frequent than those of older DMARDs such as gold and penicillamine.

Azathioprine

Azathioprine is a pro-drug which when metabolized, is converted to active agents which inhibit purine synthesis. Therefore, leukocyte proliferation is halted. This suppression of the bone marrow increases the patient's susceptibility to infection. Azathioprine is taken once or twice a day and patients are usually started on a low dose of 25–50mg which is raised as necessary. The TPMT (thiopurine methyltransferase) enzyme is involved in its metabolism and there are known polmorphisms of this enzyme which are associated with the haematological or marrow side effects. Gene testing of the enzyme polymorphism is often performed and the index of suspicion for side effects is lowered if the gene is of the wild type.

Ciclosporin

Ciclosporin inhibits calcium-dependent signalling pathways in T cells which lead to inhibition of the release of lymphokines. This acts as an immuno-suppressant. Ciclosporin is taken as a capsule twice a day, and grapefruit should not be consumed within an hour of taking the drug. There can be renal side effects and an increase in BP and gum hyperplasia. Ciclosporin is not usually used as a single agent.

Sulfasalazine

Sulfasalazine is a pro-drug, the main metabolite of which is 5-aminosali-cylic acid (5-ASA). 5-ASA inhibits cyclooxygenase and lipoxygenase, thereby reducing prostaglandin formation and therefore inflammation. Sulfasalazine impedes the progress of the disease. This is also often used in combination with other agents and seems to be more effective in the spondyloarthropathy group of disease (HLA B27 positive).

Biologics

Anti-TNF agents

Adalimumab is a fully humanized soluble anti-TNF monoclonal agent used to combat the raised levels of TNF in the blood and synovial fluid which acts to promote inflammation and joint destruction. The normal dose for treating RA is 40mg injected every other week by subcutaneous injection.

Etanercept is an antibody to the soluble receptor for TNF. Etanercept is administered by subcutaneous injection once or twice a week.

The incidence of opportunistic infections associated with its use, such as TB, is thought to be less for the receptor antibody, etanercept than for the soluble TNF molecule antibodies.

Infliximab, a chimeric human–mouse antibody, inhibits TNF but also reduces the genomic expression of interleukin-1 (IL-1) and IL-6. These inflammatory cytokines play a role in promoting osteoclast action and therefore bone loss. It is administered by IV infusion.

B-cell therapy

Rituximab is an anti-B cell therapy (blocking CD20 on B cells) used to prevent the production of autoantibodies, primarily RhF. Therefore, ritux-imab is less likely to be prescribed if the patient's arthritis is seronegative. It is usually prescribed if methothrexate and the anti-TNF therapies are not effective. Like infliximab, it is administered via IV infusion, given twice with a 2 week interval. The CD19 level is used as a surrogate marker of efficacy.

Anti-IL-1 (Anakinra) is used for periodic fever syndromes, and Tocilizumab (anti-IL-6) is in the final stages of study. Data suggest that it is extremely effective for systemic onset juvenile arthritis and RA.

There are a number of other new agents in phase III studies, and a number of new small molecule agents (e.g. Imatinib) that are currently undergoing further research.

Conclusion

Patients with RA are usually offered both symptom-relieving medication and DMARDs to manage their disease effectively. Research is currently being channelled into discovering new drugs as the understanding of the disease is increasing. Therefore, drugs can be targeted at factors involved in the pathophysiology. Combining drugs with different mechanisms of action can be complementary and therefore achieve an improved outcome.

Further reading

Bentin J. Mechanism of action of cyclosporin in rheumatoid arthritis. *Clin Rheumatol* 1995;**14**:22–5.

Clark P, Tugwell P, Bennett KJ, et al. Injectable gold for rheumatoid arthritis. *Cochrane Database Syst Rev* 1997;(**2**)CD000520.

Integrative Medical Arts Group, Inc. Methotrexate [Online]. Available from: http://home.caregroup.org/clinical/altmed/interactions/Drugs/Methotrexate.htm (Accessed 9 July 2009).

MedicineNet.com. Sulfasalazine [Online]. Available from: http://www.medicinenet.com/sulfasalazine/article.htm (Accessed 9 July 2009).

AO classification of fractures

Reproduced from the Müller AO *Classification of Fractures*, with permission from Springer Verlag.

1 Humerus

11 proximal; 3 types according to topography and extent of bony lesion

| 11-A1 | 11-A2 | 11-A3 | 11-B1 | 11-B2 | 11-B3 | 11-C1 | 11-C2 | 11-C3 |

11-A extra-articular unifocal fracture

11-A1 tuberosity
11-A2 impacted metaphyseal
11-A3 nonimpacted metaphyseal

11-B extra-articular bifocal fracture

11-B1 with metaphyseal impaction
11-B2 without metaphyseal impaction
11-B3 with glenohumeral dislocation

11-C articular fracture

11-C1 with slight displacement
11-C2 impacted with marked displacement
11-C3 dislocated

12 diaphysis

| 12-A1 | 12-A2 | 12-A3 | 12-B1 | 12-B2 | 12-B3 | 12-C1 | 12-C2 | 12-C3 |

12-A simple fracture

12-A1 spiral
12-A2 oblique (≥ 30°)
12-A3 transverse (< 30°)

12-B wedge fracture

12-B1 spiral wedge
12-B2 bending wedge
12-B3 fragmented wedge

12-C complex fracture

12-C1 spiral
12-C2 segmental
12-C3 irregular

13 distal

| 13-A1 | 13-A2 | 13-A3 | 13-B1 | 13-B2 | 13-B3 | 13-C1 | 13-C2 | 13-C3 |

13-A extra-articular fracture

13-A1 apophyseal avulsion
13-A2 metaphyseal simple
13-A3 metaphyseal multifragmentary

13-B partial articular fracture

13-B1 sagittal lateral condyle
13-B2 sagittal medial condyle
13-B3 frontal

13-C complete articular fracture

13-C1 articular simple, metaphyseal simple
13-C2 articular simple, metaphyseal multifragmentary
13-C3 articular multifragmentary

2 Radius/Ulna

21 proximal

| 21-A1 | 21-A2 | 21-A3 | 21-B1 | 21-B2 | 21-B3 | 21-C1 | 21-C2 | 21-C3 |

21-A extra-articular fracture

21-A1 ulna, radius intact
21-A2 radius, ulna intact
21-A3 both bones

21-B articular fracture

21-B1 ulna, radius intact
21-B2 radius, ulna intact
21-B3 one bone, other extra-articular

21-C articular fracture of both bones

21-C1 simple
21-C2 one artic. simple, other artic. multifragmentary
21-C3 multifragmentary

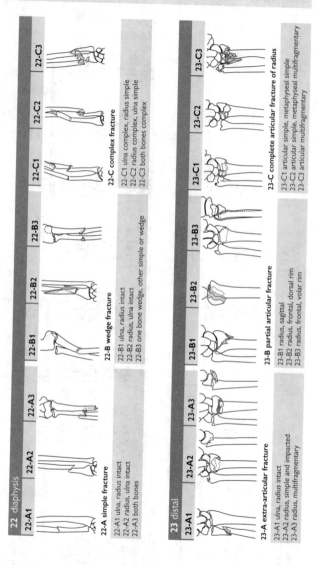

22 diaphysis

| 22-A1 | 22-A2 | 22-A3 | 22-B1 | 22-B2 | 22-B3 | 22-C1 | 22-C2 | 22-C3 |

22-A simple fracture

22-A1 ulna, radius intact
22-A2 radius, ulna intact
22-A3 both bones

22-B wedge fracture

22-B1 ulna, radius intact
22-B2 radius, ulna intact
22-B3 one bone wedge, other simple or wedge

22-C complex fracture

22-C1 ulna complex, radius simple
22-C2 radius complex, ulna simple
22-C3 both bones complex

23 distal

| 23-A1 | 23-A2 | 23-A3 | 23-B1 | 23-B2 | 23-B3 | 23-C1 | 23-C2 | 23-C3 |

23-A extra-articular fracture

23-A1 ulna, radius intact
23-A2 radius, simple and impacted
23-A3 radius, multifragmentary

23-B partial articular fracture

23-B1 radius, sagittal
23-B2 radius, frontal, dorsal rim
23-B3 radius, frontal, volar rim

23-C complete articular fracture of radius

23-C1 articular simple, metaphyseal simple
23-C2 articular simple, metaphyseal multifragmentary
23-C3 articular multifragmentary

3 Femur

31 proximal: defined by a line passing transversely through the lower end of the lesser trochanter

31-A1	31-A2	31-A3	31-B1	31-B2	31-B3	31-C1	31-C2	31-C3

31-A extra-articular fracture, trochanteric area

31-A1 pertrochanteric simple
31-A2 pertrochanteric multifragmentary
31-A3 intertrochanteric

31-B extra-articular fracture, neck

31-B1 subcapital, with slight displacement
31-B2 transcervical
31-B3 subcapital, displaced, nonimpacted

31-C articular fracture, head

31-C1 split (Pipkin)
31-C2 with depression
31-C3 with neck fracture

32 diaphysis

32-A1	32-A2	32-A3	32-B1	32-B2	32-B3	32-C1	32-C2	32-C3

32-A simple fracture

32-A1 spiral
32-A2 oblique (≥ 30°)
32-A3 transverse (< 30°)
32-A(1–3).1 = subtrochanteric zone

32-B wedge fracture

32-B1 spiral wedge
32-B2 bending wedge
32-B3 fragmented wedge
32-B(1–3).1 = subtrochanteric zone

32-C complex fracture

32-C1 spiral
32-C2 segmental
32-C3 irregular

33 distal

| 33-A1 | 33-A2 | 33-A3 | 33-B1 | 33-B2 | 33-B3 | 33-C1 | 33-C2 | 33-C3 |

33-A extra-articular fracture

33-A1 simple
33-A2 metaphyseal wedge and/or fragmented wedge
33-A3 metaphyseal complex

33-B partial articular fracture

33-B1 lateral condyle, sagittal
33-B2 medial condyle, sagittal
33-B3 frontal

33-C complete articular fracture

33-C1 articular simple, metaphyseal simple
33-C2 artic. simple, metaphyseal multifragmentary
33-C3 articular multifragmentary

4 Tibia/Fibula

41 proximal

| 41-A1 | 41-A2 | 41-A3 | 41-B1 | 41-B2 | 41-B3 | 41-C1 | 41-C2 | 41-C3 |

41-A extra-articular fracture

41-A1 avulsion
41-A2 metaphyseal simple
41-A3 metaphyseal multifragmentary

41-B partial articular fracture

41-B1 pure split
41-B2 pure depression
41-B3 split-depression

41-C complete articular fracture

41-C1 articular simple, metaphyseal simple
41-C2 artic. simple, metaphyseal multifragmentary
41-C3 articular multifragmentary

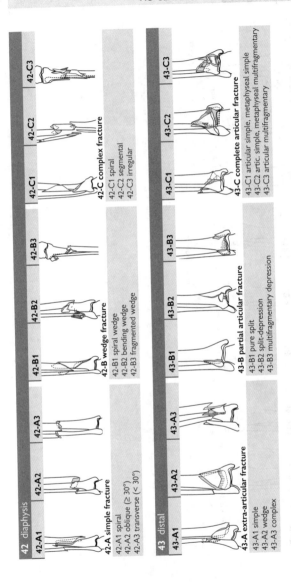

42 diaphysis

42-A1 | 42-A2 | 42-A3 | 42-B1 | 42-B2 | 42-B3 | 42-C1 | 42-C2 | 42-C3

42-A simple fracture
42-A1 spiral
42-A2 oblique (≥ 30°)
42-A3 transverse (< 30°)

42-B wedge fracture
42-B1 spiral wedge
42-B2 bending wedge
42-B3 fragmented wedge

42-C complex fracture
42-C1 spiral
42-C2 segmental
42-C3 irregular

43 distal

43-A1 | 43-A2 | 43-A3 | 43-B1 | 43-B2 | 43-B3 | 43-C1 | 43-C2 | 43-C3

43-A extra-articular fracture
43-A1 simple
43-A2 wedge
43-A3 complex

43-B partial articular fracture
43-B1 pure split
43-B2 split-depression
43-B3 multifragmentary depression

43-C complete articular fracture
43-C1 articular simple, metaphyseal simple
43-C2 artic. simple, metaphyseal multifragmentary
43-C3 articular multifragmentary

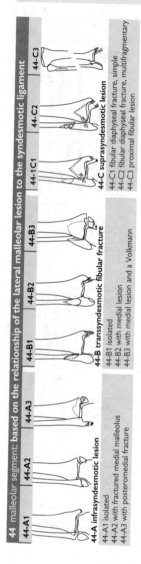

44 malleolar segment; based on the relationship of the lateral malleolar lesion to the syndesmotic ligament

| 44-A1 | 44-A2 | 44-A3 | 44-B1 | 44-B2 | 44-B3 | 44-1C1 | 44-C2 | 44-C3 |

44-A infrasyndesmotic lesion

44-A1 isolated
44-A2 with fractured medial malleolus
44-A3 with posteromedial fracture

44-B transsyndesmotic fibular fracture

44-B1 isolated
44-B2 with medial lesion
44-B3 with medial lesion and a Volkmann

44-C suprasyndesmotic lesion

44-C1 fibular diaphyseal fracture, simple
44-C2 fibular diaphyseal fracture, multifragmentary
44-C3 proximal fibular lesion

Index